METHODS IN MOLECULAR BIOLOGY™

Series Editor
John M. Walker
School of Life Sciences
University of Hertfordshire
Hatfield, Hertfordshire, AL10 9AB, UK

For further volumes:
http://www.springer.com/series/7651

Antibody-Drug Conjugates

Edited by

Laurent Ducry

Lonza Ltd, Visp, Switzerland

Humana Press

Editor
Laurent Ducry
Lonza Ltd
Visp, Switzerland

ISSN 1064-3745 ISSN 1940-6029 (electronic)
ISBN 978-1-4939-6026-2 ISBN 978-1-62703-541-5 (eBook)
DOI 10.1007/978-1-62703-541-5
Springer New York Heidelberg Dordrecht London

Softcover reprint of the hardcover 1st edition 2013

Printed on acid-free paper

Humana Press is a brand of Springer
Springer is part of Springer Science+Business Media (www.springer.com)

Preface

Antibody–drug conjugates (ADCs) represent a promising therapeutic approach for cancer patients by combining the antigen-targeting specificity of monoclonal antibodies (mAbs) with the cytotoxic potency of chemotherapeutic drugs. The FDA approval of Adcetris® (brentuximab vedotin) in 2011 and Kadcyla® (trastuzumab emtansine or T-DM1) in 2013 has validated the idea of making "armed" antibodies, attracting a lot of attention into this field. ADC technology has been an active area of research in recent years, resulting in a number of ADCs in development for various tumor types. The number of immunoconjugates or ADCs undergoing clinical trial will thus further increase, possibly replacing some of the existing naked monoclonal antibodies, and becoming the next generation of anticancer biotherapeutics.

Although the ADC concept is quite simple, successfully designing and developing such a "smart bomb" is a complex task. Despite a tremendous increase in our understanding in recent years, a lot of work is necessary in order to identify a suitable target; properly design the mAb, the linker, and the payload; as well as conjugate them in a reproducible and scalable fashion.

The success of the current conjugation technologies has been achieved thanks to the development of new methodologies. The aim of this book is to provide detailed protocols for many of the key ADC techniques necessary for working in the field. Each method is described by an author who has regularly used the technique in his or her laboratory. In addition, several review chapters are included to summarize the current knowledge and results in the ADC area. These should make this book useful to readers with no previous ADC experience as well as those already working in the field. It is my hope that this publication will further drive ADC development and thus help towards improving cancer treatments of the future.

Visp, Switzerland *Laurent Ducry*

Contents

Contributors

PIERRE-YVES ABECASSIS • *DSAR (Disposition, Safety & Animal Research), Sanofi, Vitry-sur-Seine, France*
CÉLINE AMARA • *DSAR (Disposition, Safety & Animal Research), Sanofi, Vitry-sur-Seine, France*
JAN ANDERL • *Heidelberg Pharma GmbH, Ladenburg, Germany*
NEIL H. BANDER • *Weill-Cornell Medical College, Cornell University, New York, NY, USA*
LOUISETTE BASA • *Protein Analytical Chemistry, Genentech Inc., South San Francisco, CA, USA*
SUNIL BHAKTA • *Genentech Inc., South San Francisco, CA, USA*
VÉRONIQUE BLANC • *Sanofi Oncology, Vitry-sur-Seine, France*
MARIE-PRISCILLE BRUN • *Natural Product and Protein Chemistry, Sanofi, Vitry-sur-Seine, France*
MICHELLE BUSCH • *Transitional Research, Genzyme, a Sanofi Company, Framingham, MA, USA*
YAN CHEN • *Protein Analytical Chemistry, Genentech Inc., South San Francisco, CA, USA*
PATRICK DENNLER • *Center for Radiopharmaceutical Sciences, Paul Scherrer Institute, Villigen, Switzerland*
WEIBING DING • *SLS Global Technical Support, Pall Corporation, Port Washington, NY, USA*
HEINZ FAULSTICH • *Heidelberg Pharma GmbH, Ladenburg, Germany*
ELIANE FISCHER • *Center for Radiopharmaceutical Sciences, Paul Scherrer Institute, Villigen, Switzerland*
WILLIAM J. GALUSH • *Early Stage Pharmaceutical Development, Genentech Inc., South San Francisco, CA, USA*
LAURENCE GAUZY-LAZO • *Natural Product and Protein Chemistry, Sanofi, Vitry-sur-Seine, France*
DIEGO A. GIANOLIO • *Drugs and Biomaterials R&D, Genzyme, a Sanofi Company, Cambridge, MA, USA*
JAY HARPER • *Oncology Research, MedImmune Inc., Gaithersburg, MD, USA*
TORSTEN HECHLER • *Heidelberg Pharma GmbH, Ladenburg, Germany*
MIRIAM I. HENSGEN • *Bioconjugates R&D, Lonza Ltd, Visp, Switzerland*
LIHUI HOU • *Transitional Research, Genzyme, a Sanofi Company, Framingham, MA, USA*
JAGATH R. JUNUTULA • *Genentech Inc., South San Francisco, CA, USA*
ADEELA KAMAL • *Oncology Research, MedImmune Inc., Gaithersburg, MD, USA*
MICHAEL KULKE • *Heidelberg Pharma GmbH, Ladenburg, Germany*
BENEDICT LAW • *Department of Pharmaceutical Sciences, College of Pharmacy, Nursing and Allied Sciences, North Dakota State University, Fargo, ND, USA*
ALEXANDRU C. LAZAR • *Analytical & Pharmaceutical Sciences, ImmunoGen, Inc., Waltham, MA, USA*

Joyce Lin • *Analytical & Pharmaceutical Sciences, ImmunoGen, Inc., Waltham, MA, USA*
Kedan Lin • *Early Development Pharmacokinetics and Pharmacodynamics, Genentech Inc., South San Francisco, CA, USA*
Shenlan Mao • *Oncology Research, MedImmune Inc., Gaithersburg, MD, USA*
Birte Nolting • *Biotherapeutics Research and Development, Pfizer, Pearl River, NY, USA*
Jun Ouyang • *Pharma Technical Regulatory, Genentech Inc., South San Francisco, CA, USA*
Anna Park • *Transitional Research, Genzyme, a Sanofi Company, Framingham, MA, USA*
Helga Raab • *Genentech Inc., South San Francisco, CA, USA*
Ingrid Sassoon • *Sanofi Oncology, Vitry-sur-Seine, France*
Roger Schibli • *Center for Radiopharmaceutical Sciences, Paul Scherrer Institute, Villigen, Switzerland*
Ben-Quan Shen • *Early Development Pharmacokinetics and Pharmacodynamics, Genentech Inc., South San Francisco, CA, USA*
James E. Stefano • *Transitional Research, Genzyme, a Sanofi Company, Framingham, MA, USA*
Jessica Steinmann • *Bioconjugates R&D, Lonza Ltd, Visp, Switzerland*
Patrick Strout • *Oncology Research, MedImmune Inc., Gaithersburg, MD, USA*
Bernhard Stump • *Bioconjugates R&D, Lonza Ltd, Visp, Switzerland*
Jay Tibbitts • *Drug Metabolism and Pharmacokinetics, UCB Celltech Slough, Berkshire, UK*
Anil Wagh • *Department of Pharmaceutical Sciences, College of Pharmacy, Nursing and Allied Sciences, North Dakota State University, Fargo, ND, USA*
Aditya A. Wakankar • *Late Stage Pharmaceutical Development, Genentech Inc., South San Francisco, CA, USA*

Chapter 1

Antibody–Drug Conjugate (ADC) Clinical Pipeline: A Review

Ingrid Sassoon and Véronique Blanc

Abstract

Biological therapies play an increasing role in cancer treatment, although the number of naked antibodies showing clinical efficacy as single agent remains limited. One way to enhance therapeutic potential of antibodies is to conjugate them to small molecule drugs. This combination is expected to bring together the benefits of highly potent drugs on the one hand and selective binders of specific tumor antigens on the other hand. However, designing an ADC is more complex than a simple meccano game, requiring thoughtful combination of antibody, linker, and drugs in the context of a target and a defined cancer indication. Lessons learned from the first-generation antibody–drug conjugate (ADC) and improvement of the technology guided the design of improved compounds which are now in clinical trials. Brentuximab vedotin (Adcetris®), an anti-CD30 antibody conjugated to a potent microtubule inhibitor for the treatment of Hodgkin's lymphoma and anaplastic large cell lymphomas, is the only marketed ADC today. A total of 27 ADC are currently undergoing clinical trials in both hematological malignancies and solid tumor indications. Among them, T-DM1 (trastuzumab emtansine), an ADC comprised of trastuzumab conjugated to DM1, via a non-cleavable linker, is showing very promising results in phase III for the treatment of HER2-positive refractory/relapsed metastatic breast cancer. Other compounds, such as CMC-544, SAR3419, CDX-011, PSMA-ADC, BT-062, and IMGN901 currently in clinical trials, targeting varied antigens and bearing different linker and drugs, contribute to the learning curve of ADC, as do the discontinued ADC. Current challenges include improvement of the therapeutic index, linked to a careful selection of the targets, a better understanding of ADC mechanism of action, the management and understanding of ADC off-target toxicities, as well as the selection of appropriate clinical settings (patient selection, dosing regimen) where these molecules can bring highest clinical benefit.

Key words Antibody–drug conjugate, Cancer, Cytotoxic, Linker, Antibody, Maytansine, Auristatin, Calicheamicin, T-DM1, SGN-35, CMC-544

1 Introduction

Decades of intensive research in oncology have been devoted to find drugs able to fight cancer and improve patient's life. Nowadays, cancer biologics (antibodies, peptides, and proteins) play an increasing role in the arsenal of therapeutic molecules, usually in combination with radiotherapy or chemotherapy. Despite clear

Laurent Ducry (ed.), *Antibody-Drug Conjugates*, Methods in Molecular Biology, vol. 1045,
DOI 10.1007/978-1-62703-541-5_1, © Springer Science+Business Media, LLC 2013

advantages of antibodies compared to small molecules in terms of (a) exquisite selectivity towards antigen-positive cells, leading to decreased off-target toxicity and (b) long half-life, only 13 therapeutic antibodies are marketed today for the treatment of cancer [1], highlighting the difficulty to identify targets whose modulation will impact tumor growth as well as the difficulty to identify antibodies with clinical efficacy as single agent. Arming antibodies or antibody fragments with toxins, cytotoxic drugs, and radionuclides can be viewed as a means of enhancing tumor-cell killing while sparing normal cells. Several of such armed molecules are marketed, namely, denileukin diftitox (Ontak®), an engineered protein combining interleukin-2 (which binds to IL2R) and Diphteria toxin, for the treatment of persistent or recurrent cutaneous T cell lymphoma, ibritumomab tiuxetan (Zevalin®), and ^{131}I-tositumomab (Bexxar®), two murine anti-CD20 antibodies conjugated to ^{90}Y and ^{131}I, respectively, for the treatment of relapsed/refractory follicular lymphoma, as well as the antibody–drug conjugate (ADC) brentuximab vedotin (Adcetris®), an anti-CD30 antibody conjugated to a potent microtubule inhibitor for the treatment of Hodgkin's lymphoma and anaplastic large cell lymphomas.

The concept of arming antibodies is not recent, as the use of ADC in animal models was already described in the literature in the 1970s, and clinical trials with murine IgG-based ADC were conducted in the 1980s, although with limited success. This is only in 2000 that the first ADC, gemtuzumab ozogamicin (Mylotarg®), an anti-CD33 antibody conjugated to calicheamicin (a very potent DNA binding drug), was approved in the USA for the treatment of acute myelocytic leukemia (AML), based on clear evidence of blast decrease in patient bone marrows [2, 3]. In 2010, the product was withdrawn from the market by the developer, Pfizer, following interim results from post-approval study (SWOG S0106), because of serious concerns about product's safety and failure to demonstrate clinical benefit [4].

This review will focus on ADC which are undergoing clinical trials (cf. Table 1). Lessons learned from first-generation ADC and improvement of the technology, both described in the first section, guided the design of improved compounds which are currently at different stages of clinical development. Adcetris® and the most advanced ADC in clinical trials will be described in a second section. The third section covers explored areas of improvement based on a thorough understanding of key parameters for ADC safety and efficacy retrieved from preclinical and clinical trials. The growing number of ADC in the clinic reflects the interest and confidence of clinicians and pharmaceutical companies that this approach can bring high benefit to cancer patients.

Table 1
ADC in clinical trials and launched

Drug names	Company	MAb mode	Target	Drug	Linker	Highest phase[a]	Indications
Adcetris® Brentuximab vedotin SGN-35	Seattle Genetics/ Takeda (Millenium)	Chimeric	CD30	Auristatin (MMAE)	vc	Launched 8.2011	Hodgkin's lymphoma ALCL
Inotuzumab ozogamicin CMC-544	UCB (Celltech) Pfizer	Humanized	CD22	Calicheamicin	Hydrazone AcBut	Phase 3 04.2011	ALL NHL (DLBCL)
T-DM1 Trastuzumab emtansine	Roche (Genentech) ImmunoGen	Humanized	Her-2	Maytansine (DM1)	SMCC	Phase 3 3.2009	Her2+ breast Gastric
Glembatumumab-vedotin CDX-011 CR-011-vcMMAE	Celldex (Curagen) Amgen (Abgenix)	Fully human	GPNMB (osteoactivin)	Auristatin (MMAE)	vc	Phase 2 4.2008	Breast Melanoma
IMGN-901 Lorvotuzumab mertansine	ImmunoGen	Humanized	CD56	Maytansine (DM1)	SPP	Phase 2 3.2012 SCLC	MCC, SCLC
SAR3419 HuB4-DM4	ImmunoGen/Sanofi	Humanized	CD19	Maytansine (DM4)	SPDB	Phase 2 9.2011	NHL, ALL
BT-062	Biotest	Chimerized	CD138 (Syndecan1)	Maytansine (DM4)	SPDB	Phase 1/2 8.2010	MM Solid tumors
IMMU-110 Milatuzumab-doxorubicin	Immunomedics	Humanized	CD74	Doxorubicin	Hydrazone	Phase 1/2 6.2010	Multiple myeloma
AGS-16M8F AGS-6MF	Astellas (Agensys)	Fully human	ENPP3	Auristatin (MMAF)	mc	Phase 1 8.2010	RCC

(continued)

Table 1
(continued)

Drug names	Company	MAb mode	Target	Drug	Linker	Highest phase[a]	Indications
AGS-22M6E ASG-22ME	Astellas (Agensys)	Fully human	Nectin-4	Auristatin (MMAE)	vc	Phase 1 5.2011	Solid tumors
AMG-172	Amgen	nd	nd	nd	nd	Phase 1 12.2011	Renal cancer
AMG-595	Amgen	Fully human	EGFRvIII	Maytansinoid	Non-cleavable	Phase 1 3.2012	Glioma
ASG-5ME AGS-5M2E	Astellas (Agensys)	Fully human	SLC44A4	Auristatin (MMAE)	vc	Phase 1 7.2010	Pancreas Prostate
BAY 94-9343	Bayer MorphoSys	Fully human	mesothelin	Maytansine (DM4)	SPDB	Phase 1 9.2011	Solid tumors
DEDN-6526A Anti-ETBR-vc-E	Roche (Genentech)	Humanized	ET8R (endothelin B)	Auristatin (MMAE)	vc	Phase 1 3.2012	Melanoma
IMGN 529 K7153A-SMCC-DM1	ImmunoGen	Humanized	CD37	Maytansine DM1	SMCC	Phase 1 2.2012	NHL
IMMU-130 hMN14-SN38	Immunomedics	Humanized	CEACAM5	SN-38	CL2	Phase 1 8.2011	Breast, colorectal, lung
MDX-1203	BMS (Medarex)	Fully human	CD70	MGBA	vc	Phase 1 7.2009	B-NHL ccRCC
PSMA-ADC PSMA-ADC-1301	Progenics	Fully human	PSMA	Auristatin (MMAE)	vc	Phase 1 9.2008	Prostate

RG-7450 DSTP-3086S	Roche (Genentech)	nd	nd	Auristatin	nd	Phase 1 3.2011	Prostate (CRPC)
RG-7458	Roche (Genentech)	nd	MUC16 (CA125)	Auristatin	nd	Phase 1 4.2011	Ovary
RG-7593 DCDT-2980S	Roche (Genentech)	Humanized	CD22	Auristatin (MMAE)	vc	Phase 1 10.2010	NHL
RG-7596 DCDS-4501A	Roche (Genentech)	nd	CD79b	Auristatin	nd	Phase 1 3.2011	CLL, NHL
RG-7598	Roche (Genentech)	nd	nd	Auristatin	nd	Phase 1 9.2011	MM
RG-7599	Roche (Genentech)	nd	MUC16 (CA125)	Auristatin	nd	Phase 1 7.2011	Ovary Lung (NSCLC)
RG-7600	Roche (Genentech)	nd	nd	Auristatin	nd	Phase 1 12.2011	Ovary Pancreas
SAR-566658 huDS6-DM4	ImmunoGen Sanofi	Humanized	Muc1 (CA6)	Maytansine (DM4)	SPDB	Phase 1 9.2010	Solid tumors
SGN-75 h1F6-vcMMAF	Seattle Genetics	Humanized	CD70	Auristatin (MMAF)	vc	Phase 1 11.2009	NHL RCC

[a]Current highest phase for cancer/first date/first indication
nd not disclosed

2 ADC Building Blocks

2.1 Definition of an ADC

An ADC can be defined as a prodrug. The antibody connected to the cytotoxic warhead (drug) via a linker serves as targeted delivery system to the tumor expressing the antigen/target recognized by the antibody. Ideally, in blood, after systemic administration, this prodrug is nontoxic. Upon binding of the antibody to the targeted tumor antigen and internalization of the complex into the cancer cell, the drug is then released in its active form and in sufficient quantity to kill the cell.

Designing an ideal ADC is more complex than a simple meccano game. On top of the careful choice of a target/antigen expressed in specific tumor indication, it requires finding the best combination between the antibody, the linker, and the drug, which, besides its own characteristics and constraints, are linked and impact each other.

2.2 Target/Antigen for ADC

The target/antigen is the starting point to build an ADC. It first determines which tumor indication will be targeted by the ADC and potentially impacts the choice of the conjugated drug. In addition, the target will also drive the criteria which will be defined for the selection of the targeted patient population within the tumor indication.

Many targets have been evaluated for an ADC approach across the years (for a review, *see* ref. 5), showing that a high variety of targets, either single or multiple transmembrane domains proteins or glycosylphosphatidylinositol (GPI)-anchored, can lead to ADC internalization and subsequent tumor growth delay and regression in preclinical mouse models.

The basis for the selection of the antigen is a high expression level in tumor tissues and a restricted normal tissue distribution, in order to limit on-target toxicity of the future ADC. However, tumor-specific antigens with no expression in normal tissues are rare, and most of the time, the antigen is expressed at the surface of epithelial cells in a subset of normal tissues/organs. The type of organ expressing the antigen (vital organs vs. reproductive organs, for example), the cellular subtype and cell-cycle status (dividing cells vs. differentiated quiescent cells), and the differential of expression between normal antigen-positive cells and tumor cells are to be considered for selection of the target.

It is important to notice that expression in normal organs may not always mean subsequent toxicity in clinical trials. Several ADC with normal tissue cross-reactivity have been well tolerated in patients, causing minimal or manageable and reversible toxicities, namely, cantuzumab mertansine/IMGN242 (targeting CanAg antigen, a glycotope on Mucin-like protein [6, 7]), BT-062 (targeting CD138; see below), or CDX-011 (targeting gpNMB;

Table 2
Discontinued ADC

Product name	Target name	Drug/linker	Reasons for discontinuation	Year	References
BAY79-4620	CAIX	MMAE/vc	Not disclosed	2011	Press release
IMGN388	Integrinαvβ3	DM4/SPDB	Change in business strategy	2011	Press release
MEDI547	EphA2	MMAF/mc	Safety issues: bleeding and coagulation events	2012	[122]
Mylotarg	CD33	Calicheamicin/ hydrazone	Failure to demonstrate clinical benefit	2010	[4]
BIIB015	Cryptol	DM4/SPDB	Not disclosed	2010	
IMGN242	CanAg	DM4/SPDB	Not disclosed	2009	Press release
AVE9633	CD33	DM4/SPDB	Lack of clinical efficacy	2008	[12]
MLN2704	PSMA	DM1/SPP	Not disclosed	2006	[94, 123], Press release
CMD-193	Le^Y carbohydrate	Calicheamicin/ hydrazone	Not disclosed	2006	ClinicalTrials. gov
Bivatuzumab mertansine	CD44v6	DM1/SPP	Safety issues: fatal case of toxic epidermal necrolysis	2006	[9, 11]
SGN-15	Le^Y carbohydrate	Doxorubicin/ hydrazone	Change in business strategy	2005	Press release
CMB-401	MUC1	Calicheamicin/ hydrazone	Lack of clinical efficacy	1999	[124, 125]

see below). Inversely it has clearly been demonstrated in the case of bivatuzumab mertansine (targeting CD44v6), whose trial was prematurely stopped in phase I (cf. Table 2), that the expression of the CD44v6 target in skin keratinocytes [8] led to severe skin toxicity, including a fatal case of toxic epidermal necrolysis [9–11].

While expression of the target should remain limited and at low level in normal tissues, on the contrary, the level of expression (antigen density) at the surface of cancer cells should be high and combined to the ability of the antigen/antibody complex to internalize and be processed in the right subcellular compartments, in order to release enough quantity of the active drug in the cytosol. The use of tumor models mimicking the target expression pattern and level found in patient biopsies is a very critical element to translate preclinical data into clinical efficacy. AVE9633, an immunoconjugate targeting CD33 antigen, did not show clinical efficacy in phase I [12] in part because of too limited antigen expression on the malignant cell population, suggesting an insufficient delivery of molecules in the cytoplasm to achieve cell death. In contrast, preclinical models showed good response to AVE9633 [13] but displayed a much higher CD33 antigen level than the one measured in patient biopsies (unpublished internal data, sanofi, 2009).

2.3 Drugs and Linkers

Many conventional therapeutic agents have been conjugated to antibodies, but it soon became clear that they were not potent enough, when conjugated, to achieve antitumor activity in the clinic [14–16]. Efforts have then been turned towards natural small cytotoxic molecules with higher potency but which have been found too toxic as free drug in clinical trials. Currently, only few highly potent natural cytotoxics, derivatives, or synthetic analogues have been conjugated to antibodies and progressed to the clinic. They fall into the following two classes: microtubule destabilizing agents (auristatin derivatives, MMAE and MMAF and maytansinoid derivatives, DM1 and DM4) and DNA minor groove binders (calicheamicin and duocarmycin derivatives). Both classes are extremely potent towards proliferating tumor cell lines [16]. IC_{50} of proliferation/viability of tumor cell lines are in the range of 10^{-10}–10^{-12} M for DM1/DM4 maytansinoid derivatives [17, 18], 10^{-7}–10^{-10} M for MMAF/MMAE auristatin derivatives [19], around 10^{-10} M for *N*-acetyl-γ calicheamicin DMH [20], and 10^{-11}–10^{-12} M for DC1 and CC-1065 duocarmycin precursors [14, 21].

Importantly, the engineered linker connecting the cytotoxic molecule to the antibody has been deeply studied as it is considered to be an important parameter for preclinical, clinical efficacy and safety of ADC: linkers must be stable enough in circulation since release of the cytotoxic payload may be associated with undesired and untargeted toxicities, but they must also be able to efficiently release cytotoxics in their active form in the cytosol of the target cell following internalization and trafficking in specific subcellular compartments [16, 22, 23]. Indeed, upon binding of the ADC to its target, and subsequent internalization of the antigen/ADC complex by receptor-mediated endocytosis, the ADC is trafficked in acidifying endosomal and then in lysosomal vesicles, a compartment rich in proteolytic enzymes. Due to the chemical environment or to the metabolic properties of these intracellular compartments, the ADC is activated/metabolized. This metabolization depends on the type of linker connected to the drug:

- The acid labile hydrazone linkers are relatively stable at neutral pH (pH 7.3–7.5, pH of the bloodstream) but undergo hydrolysis once the ADC is internalized into acidic endosomes (pH 5–6.5) and lysosomes (pH 4.5–5). They have been conjugated to doxorubicin, calicheamicin, and auristatin. Their relative stability depends on the antibody part attached, but they have been associated with high nonspecific release of the drug in circulation in preclinical studies [24].

- The disulfide-based linkers have been combined with DM1 and DM4 maytansinoids. The corresponding ADC is activated by lysosomal degradation of the antibody part, resulting in metabolites consisting of intact maytansinoid drug and linker attached to lysines [23, 25]. Linkers are subsequently reduced with more or less efficiency, depending on the level of steric hindrance at carbon atoms adjacent to the disulfide linkage, optimized linkers being the best compromise between high ADC plasma stability and efficient metabolization/release of the metabolites in tumor cells [26].
- The peptide-based linkers, already used for a number of years with doxorubicin, mitomycin C, camptothecin, and talysomycin [16], have been designed for the auristatin and the duocarmycin derivatives. The type of linker which has been progressed to clinical stage is composed of a valine–citrulline dipeptide selectively hydrolized by cathepsin B and plasmin enzymes, a self immolative spacer that spatially separates the drug from the site of enzymatic cleavage, and the auristatin E microtubule disruptive agent or duocarmycin prodrug derivative. In the case of an auristatin E conjugate, the membrane-permeable monomethyl auristatin E accounts for the only detectable metabolite found in antigen-positive cells [27].
- Contrary to the above linker types, which are considered as "cleavable," thioether bond containing linkers are considered as "non-cleavable," and the corresponding ADC have been clinically tested with DM1 and MMAF cytotoxics. In this case, the degradation of the mAb component into the lysosomes releases the drug still attached to the linker via a Lys or Cys residue of the antibody. These charged entities are not able to cross membranes with high efficiency, by contrast to metabolites of maytansine and auristatin ADC conjugated to "cleavable" linkers. In this case, the diffusion of metabolites induces killing of surrounding cells, a property named "bystander effect" [27–29].

2.4 Antibody Selection

All ADC currently in oncology clinical trials are canonical (i.e., full length) IgG molecules, mostly of the IgG1 isotype. They are either chimeric, humanized, or fully human antibodies (cf. Table 1). The generation of an immune response to these ADC has remained very limited, highlighting the benefit of antibody engineering technologies over the last decades, as well as the fact that small molecule cytotoxics, contrary to natural toxins, are not immunogenic.

Attention has also been focused on drug conjugation technologies on the selected antibodies. On top of the fact that drug conjugation should not disturb antigen/antibody interaction, the localization, the number, and the nature of the attachment between linker and antibody have been shown to influence pharmacokinetics, tumor exposure, and ADC plasma stability [30, 31]. So far, the two conjugation technologies which progressed to clinical trials are based on the following two principles: either conjugation through Lysine side chain amines (with drugs such as DM1, DM4, or calicheamicin) or conjugation through cysteine sulfhydryl groups activated by reducing interchain disulfide bonds (with drugs such as MMAE, MMAF, or duocarmycin) of the antibody. Both processes give more or less heterogeneous mixtures of ADC with variable drug load per antibody and variable sites of conjugation to the protein. This heterogeneous mixture is defined by an average drug–antibody ratio (DAR) and is challenging from a development point of view, although robust analytical technologies and processes are available to ensure constant quality control of the final product [32].

3 Current Clinical Results of Antibody–Drug Conjugates

A total of 27 ADC are currently in clinical trials, 20 in phase I, 5 in phase II, 2 in phase III, and 1 launched ADC (cf. Table 1). A total of 12 ADC have been stopped and are listed in Table 2.

3.1 Brentuximab Vedotin (Adcetris®) Clinical Overview

CD30, a type II transmembrane protein belonging to the TNF (tumor necrosis factor) superfamily, is abundantly and selectively expressed on the surface of Hodgkin's lymphoma (HL), Reed–Sternberg (RS) cells, anaplastic large cell lymphomas (ALCL), and other lymphoid malignancies as well as on several nonlymphoid malignancies [33]. RS cells and ALCL cells express high levels of CD30, but the downstream signalling of CD30 may differ between both diseases [34, 35]. In non-pathological conditions, CD30 expression is highly regulated and restricted to activated B and T lymphocytes and NK cells, low expression being also noticed in monocytes and eosinophils (for review, *see* refs. 34, 36), making it a good candidate target for an ADC strategy.

HL is considered as one of the most curable cancers, with a 5-year survival rate of above 85 % although up to 20 % of patients are refractory and advanced-stage patients often relapse [37]. In frontline systemic ALCL treatment, disease recurs in 40–65 % of patients [38].

Clinical trials have been reported for unconjugated anti-CD30 antibodies [39]. Acceptable safety profile but modest antitumor clinical activity precluded further development as naked but supported exploration and development of a conjugated version: SGN-35. SGN-35 (Adcetris®, brentuximab vedotin) is an ADC comprised of a chimeric anti-CD30 antibody (cAC10) conjugated through interchain disulfide bonds to monomethyl auristatin E (MMAE) via a valine–citrulline dipeptide cleavable linker, with an average DAR of 4 [40].

Based on preclinical data showing good efficacy of SGN-35 at low doses in lymphoma models [40], a phase I study was conducted in 2006. Forty-five patients (42 HL, 3 ALCL) were enrolled, in a dose escalation study ranging from 0.2 to 3.6 mg/kg with intravenous (IV) administration once every 3 weeks (q3w) [41]. The maximum tolerated dose (MTD) was found to be 1.8 mg/kg, and drug-related dose-limiting toxicities (DLT) were febrile neutropenia and hyperglycemia. At the MTD, objective clinical responses were observed, with an objective response rate (ORR) of 38 %, including 4 complete responses (CR) and 2 partial responses (PR) out of 12 patients. In terms of pharmacokinetics (PK), terminal half-life of the ADC and MMAE, at 1.8 mg/kg, was estimated to be 4–6 and 3–4 days, respectively [41]. In a second phase I study, enrolling 44 patients, a more frequent regimen was investigated, at doses ranging from 0.4 to 1.4 mg/kg administered weekly for 3 out of 4 weeks, for a total of four cycles. The MTD was 1.2 mg/kg and the ORR was 59 %, with 34 % CR. Most common grade 3 adverse events (AE) were peripheral sensory neuropathy (14 %), anemia (9 %), neutropenia (7 %), peripheral motor neuropathy (7 %), and hyperglycemia, diarrhea, and vomiting (5 % each). Overall, 32 patients (73 %) experienced one or more events of peripheral neuropathy. Compared to the q3w schedule, there was a marked increase in neuropathy which led to the adoption of the q3w schedule for further clinical studies [42].

In a phase II study, 102 heavily pretreated relapsed or refractory HL patients were treated at the dose of 1.8 mg/kg in a q3w schedule [43]. The ORR was 75 % including 34 % CR and 40 % PR. The more severe AE were grade 3 neutropenia (14 %), peripheral sensory neuropathy (5 %), fatigue and hyperglycemia (3 % each), grade 4 hematological toxicities (neutropenia 4 %; thrombocytopenia 1 %), and pulmonary embolism and abdominal pain (1 % each). In a second phase II trial, 58 patients with relapsed systemic ALCL were treated with 1.8 mg/kg of with a q3w schedule [38]. The ORR was 86 % with 53 % achieving CR. Grade 3–4 AE were similar to the previous studies.

Based on these outstanding data, SGN-35 has been granted accelerated approval by the FDA in August 2011 for the treatment of HL that had relapsed after autologous stem cell transplant (ASCT) and for the management of relapsed ALCL, making it the first approved drug over 30 years in HL. In July 2012, a positive opinion was issued in the EU, recommending conditional marketing authorization for treatment of adults with relapsed or refractory CD30-positive HL following ASCT or following at least two prior therapies when ASCT or multi-agent chemotherapy is not a treatment option as well as for the treatment of adults with relapsed or refractory systemic ALCL. SGN-35 is currently evaluated in a phase III randomized, double-blind, placebo-controlled study (AETHERA) in HL patients following autologous stem cell transplant [35]. Interim results show that 75 % of patients responded to the drug, including 34 and 40 % achieving CR and PR, respectively [44]. Future results of the AETHERA trial expected to be completed in June 2013 will form the basis for full FDA approval. Other trials are ongoing, including another phase III trial evaluating SGN-35 versus methotrexate or bexarotene in patients with CD30-positive cutaneous T cell lymphomas [44].

3.2 Trastuzumab-DM1 (T-DM1) Clinical Overview

ErbB2/neu/HER2 is a member of the ErbB receptor tyrosine kinase family which is involved in cell growth, survival, and differentiation [45]. Breast cancer accounts for 28 % of all new cases of cancer in women, and 15–25 % of these new cases contain gene amplification or overexpression of HER2 [46]. The humanized anti-HER2 monoclonal antibody trastuzumab (Herceptin®; Genentech), and the dual epidermal growth factor EGFR/HER2 tyrosine kinase inhibitor lapatinib (Tykerb®, GSK), in combination with chemotherapy, prolongs survival of HER2-positive breast cancer patients in metastatic and adjuvant settings. However, a significant portion of these patients relapse and finally die from their cancer, highlighting the need for new therapeutic approaches [47, 48].

T-DM1 (trastuzumab emtansine) is an ADC comprised of trastuzumab conjugated through lysines to DM1, via a non-cleavable thioether linker (*N*-succinimidyl 4-(*N*-maleimidomethyl) cyclohexane-1-carboxylate, SMCC), with an average DAR of 3.5 [49].

Preclinical studies of T-DM1 suggested that the ADC retained all activities of unconjugated trastuzumab, inhibition of PI3K/AKT signalling, inhibition of HER2 shedding, and Fcγ receptor engagement triggering ADCC [50]. Moreover, T-DM1 showed a strong growth inhibitory effect on trastuzumab-resistant breast cancer cell lines in vitro, as well as a significant inhibition of tumor growth when administered in trastuzumab and lapatinib resistant tumor-bearing mice [49, 51].

Four phase I/II studies evaluated T-DM1 as single agent for the treatment of HER2-positive refractory/relapsed metastatic breast cancer. In 2006, 24 patients were enrolled in a phase I dose escalation study, with doses ranging from 0.3 to 4.8 mg/kg, in a q3w schedule [52]. T-DM1 MTD was identified at 3.6 mg/kg without cardiotoxicity or neuropathy. Transient grade 4 thrombocytopenia was the most common adverse event and was defined as the DLT [52]. Encouraging antitumor activity was observed: out of 15 patients enrolled in the 3.6 mg/kg group, four had a confirmed objective partial response. One confirmed PR was also observed in the 2.4 mg/kg group [52]. A phase I weekly dosing [53] reported MTD at 2.4 mg/kg, with thrombocytopenia being also the DLT and showing the same range of activity. Different phase II studies evaluated T-DM1 at 3.6 mg/kg, q3w (for review, *see* refs. 54, 56). In one study [57] a median of seven doses was administered to 112 patients with HER2-positive metastatic breast cancer previously treated with chemotherapy and progressed under trastuzumab therapy. The ORR evaluated by independent review was 25.9 %, all PR. Interestingly, in the group of tumors confirmed HER2-positive in a retrospective central testing by immunohistochemistry (IHC) or fluorescence in situ hybridization (FISH), the ORR was 33.8 % versus 4.8 % for the group of tumors with normal HER2 expression. The most common grade 3 or 4 AE were hypokalemia (8.9 %), thrombocytopenia (8.0 %), and fatigue (4.5 %). PK parameters showed a terminal half-life of T-DM1 of around 4 days, which was found to be lower than the total trastuzumab half-life. No accumulation of T-DM1 was reported [57]. In a second study, T-DM1 was administered in 110 patients with metastatic breast cancer previously treated with an anthracycline, a taxane, and capecitabine, as well as lapatinib and trastuzumab [58]. The ORR by independent review was 34.5 % without CR and again rose to 41.3 % for patients with tumors centrally confirmed for HER2-positivity (FISH and IHC) compared to 20 % in the patient group displaying HER2-normal expression levels. The most common grade 3 and 4 AE were thrombocytopenia (9.1 %), fatigue (4.5 %), and cellulitis (3.6 %). In the different studies, thrombocytopenia was one of the most reported grade 3 or 4 abnormalities, but the decrease in platelets was generally reversible and not associated with serious hemorrhage [56–58]. Increased serum concentrations of hepatic enzymes was observed [56]. T-DM1 exposure did not correlate with clinical responses, grade 3 thrombocytopenia or grade 3 increase in hepatic enzymes serum concentrations [59]. The comparison of pharmacokinetics data from phase I and phase II studies, as single agent, demonstrated a positive correlation between DM1 and T-DM1 exposure with neither accumulation of T-DM1 nor DM1 [59, 60]. At the MTD, T-DM1 showed a median terminal half-life of 4.5 days which is shorter than the one from total trastuzumab (around 9 days) [59, 60]. The PK profile of T-DM1 was not affected by circulating levels of HER2 or residual trastuzumab [59, 60]. On a total of 286 patients, 4.5 % developed an antibody response to T-DM1 but no impact on PK parameters, safety or efficacy profiles were observed [59].

Interestingly a randomized phase II study was conducted to compare T-DM1 versus trastuzumab plus docetaxel [55] in the first-line treatment of HER-2-positive locally advanced or metastatic breast cancer. A total of 137 patients, with no prior chemotherapy for metastatic disease, were randomized to T-DM1 (3.6 mg/kg, q3w) or trastuzumab (8 mg/kg first cycle, then 6 mg/kg) plus docetaxel (75 or 100 mg/m^2). Assessment by investigators showed equivalent ORR of 47.8 % with T-DM1 and

41.4 % with docetaxel plus trastuzumab [61] but with improved therapeutic ratio in the case of T-DM1. Primary efficacy and update on safety results were presented at ESMO 2011 [62] with a significant improvement of progression-free survival (PFS) in the T-DM1 population (14.2 months vs. 9.2 months) and a confirmed favorable safety profile with grade 3 AE reported less frequently in the T-DM1 arm (46.4 % vs. 89.4 %). The most frequent AE were also different between the two arms, with increased level of liver enzymes, fatigue and thrombocytopenia in the T-DM1 arm versus alopecia, neutropenia, fatigue, and diarrhea in the trastuzumab/docetaxel arm.

In addition, three phase III trials (EMILIA, MARIANNE and TH3RESA) are ongoing [55]. EMILIA is a randomized trial designed to evaluate the safety and efficacy of T-DM1 in comparison to lapatinib plus capecitabine in patients with HER-2 positive, unresectable, locally advanced breast cancer or metastatic breast cancer, following prior trastuzumab and taxane containing chemotherapies. Recent publication of the first and second interim analysis of the 991 patients enrolled indicates that T-DM1 significantly improves PFS (9.6 months vs. 6.4 months) and overall survival (OS) (30.9 months vs. 25.1 months) as compared to lapatinib plus capecitabine treatment [63]. In addition, as previously shown in phase II, the safety profile of T-DM1 was different and more favorable than lapatinib plus capecitabine, as shown by the reduced incidence of grade 3 and 4 AE (40.8 % vs. 57.0 %). Thrombocytopenia (12.9 %) and elevated AST (4.3 %) were the most commonly reported AE for T-DM1, while diarrhea (20.7 %), palmar–plantar erythrodysesthesia (16.4 %), vomiting (4.5 %), and neutropenia (4.3 %) were the ones reported for lapatinib plus capecitabine [63]. On the basis of this study, a Biologics License Application (BLA) was filed in August 2012. MARIANNE is a randomized trial of T-DM1 with or without pertuzumab compared with trastuzumab plus taxane for first-line treatment of HER2-positive, progressive, or recurrent locally advanced or metastatic breast cancer. TH3RESA is a randomized trial to evaluate the efficacy of T-DM1 compared with treatment of physician's choice in patients with HER2-positive metastatic breast cancer who have received at least two prior regimens of HER2-directed therapy.

3.3 CMC-544 (Inotuzumab Ozogamicin) Clinical Overview

CD22 is a glycoprotein belonging to the sialic-acid-binding immunoglobulin-like lectins (siglecs) expressed at the surface of normal immature and mature B cells but neither on hematopoietic stem cells nor on memory B cells. Its function is still unclear, but it is thought to be involved in cellular adhesion, B -cell homing, and B-cell activation [64]. CD22 has been shown to be rapidly internalized upon ligand binding, an attractive property supporting CD22 as target for ADC [65]. CD22 is expressed in more than 90 % of diffuse large B-cell non-Hodgkin lymphomas

(DLBCL) and follicular lymphomas (FL) [66]. It is also expressed in up to 100 % of mature B-cell acute lymphoblastic leukemia (B-ALL) [67].

CMC-544 (Inotuzumab ozogamicin) is an ADC comprised of a humanized anti-CD22 IgG4 monoclonal antibody (G544) conjugated through a cleavable acid-labile hydrazone linker to calicheamicin with an average DAR of 6 (73 μg calicheamicin/mg of antibody) [4]. G544 binds to CD22 with subnanomolar affinity and has no effector functions and no antitumor activity as naked monoclonal antibody [4].

Based on encouraging preclinical data [68], two phase I single agent studies were conducted in relapsed/refractory B-cell NHL. The first phase I enrolled 36 patients in the dose escalation phase with a q3w schedule and 43 patients in the expanded MTD cohort [69]. In the dose escalation phase, DLT were grade 4 thrombocytopenia and grade 4 neutropenia, and the MTD was declared 1.8 mg/m^2 (0.048 mg/kg) in a q4w schedule in order to allow platelets recovery. Among the 49 patients treated at the MTD, the common grade 3 or grade 4 AE were thrombocytopenia (63.3 %) and neutropenia (34.7 %). At MTD, the ORR was 68 % for FL and 15 % for aggressive DLBCL with CR observed [69]. Drug disposition for CMC-544 and total calicheamicin was nonlinear with dose or number of doses suggesting an accumulation of the drug, which could be explained by the decrease in CD22 target after the first dose [4]. After the first cycle, terminal half-life of CMC-544 at the MTD was 17.1 h, increasing to 34.7 h at the second cycle [69]. The second phase I dose escalation study was conducted in 13 Japanese patients with relapsed/refractory FL. The MTD was confirmed at 1.8 mg/m^2 q4w, with most common grade 3 and 4 AE being also thrombocytopenia (54 %) and neutropenia (31 %). The ORR was 80 %, CR included [70]. PK parameters were similar to what was observed previously.

Based on preclinical studies suggesting superior activities of CMC-544 with rituximab [71], several phases I/II studies have been initiated in recurrent/refractory FL or DLBCL [4, 66]. The MTD was determined at 375 mg/m^2 rituximab given on day 1 and 1.8 mg/m^2 CMC-544 given on day 2 every 28 days for four cycles [72, 73]. Pharmacokinetic and safety profile of CMC-544 were shown to be equivalent to single-agent, dose-limiting toxicities being again thrombocytopenia and neutropenia [66]. In one of the study [72, 74], enrolling 110 patients treated at the combination MTD, the ORR of relapsed FL and DLBCL were 84 and 80 %, respectively. Response to rituximab in prior treatment appeared to be a very strong prognostic of response to the combination as when rituximab-refractory patients were considered; the ORR was only 20 % [66, 72, 74]. A randomized open-label phase III trial is now recruiting, comparing rituximab plus CMC-544 to rituximab plus gemcitabine or bendamustine in relapsed/refractory aggressive B-cell NHL [4].

CMC5-44 was also explored in refractory/relapsed acute lymphoblastic leukemia (ALL) patients. The first published report evaluating CMC-544 at 1.8 mg/m^2 in a q3w schedule was promising, as the ORR was 56 % [75]. A phase II trial has therefore been undertaken in patients with refractory/relapsed ALL with the same dosing schedule [76]. A total of 49 patients were treated, with CD22 expressed in more than 50 % of blasts in all patients. The ORR was 57 % with 18 % complete marrow response of short duration and 39 % with no platelets or incomplete blood cell count recovery. Thrombocytopenia was, like in NHL, a notable adverse event, but based on the leukemia risk, treatment was not delayed. Grade 3–4 fever was the most common AE (31 %). Further clinical evaluation in ALL is ongoing with a weekly schedule [76].

3.4 Other ADC in Early Clinical Trials

Beside SGN-35, T-DM1, and CMC-544, 24 other ADC are currently being evaluated in phase I and II (cf. Table 1). The more advanced ones, for which efficacy data are available, are described below.

SAR3419: CD19 is a type I transmembrane glycoprotein of the immunoglobulin (Ig) superfamily, expressed from the earliest stages of pre-B-cell development until terminal B-cell differentiation into plasma cells. CD19 expression covers all types of B-lymphomas and non-T acute lymphoblastic leukemia, with moderate to high homogeneous expression [77]. SAR3419 is composed of a humanized IgG1 monoclonal anti-CD19 antibody, huB4, conjugated via a cleavable disulfide linker to DM4 (huB4-SPDB-DM4). In a first phase I study with refractory or relapsed B-cell NHL (R/R NHL) [78], SAR3419 was evaluated in a q3w schedule. The MTD was determined at 160 mg/m^2 (4.3 mg/kg), and the DLT was reversible severe blurred vision associated with microcystic epithelial corneal changes. Tumor reduction from baseline was observed in 74 % of patients bearing a variety of lymphoma subtypes including DLBCL. The ORR was of 23.5 % at MTD [78]. A second dose escalation study was performed with a weekly schedule, again in R/R NHL patients. The regimen consisting of 4 weekly doses of 55 mg/m^2 followed by four additional doses administered every 2 weeks showed a favorable safety profile and was therefore retained for further clinical studies. In particular there was no grade 3 or 4 ocular toxicity observed and hematotoxicity incidence was low, allowing potential combination of SAR3419 with other agents used to treat NHL. In addition, no dose-limiting cumulative side effects were observed in this cohort of 21 patients [79]. In this heavily pretreated patient population, antitumor activity with around 30 % ORR in both aggressive (e.g., DLBCL) and indolent (e.g., FL) subtypes of NHL was obtained. A phase II program in patients with R/R DLBCL is underway testing the drug as a single agent and also in combination with rituximab (NCT01472887 and NCT01470456, respectively) in order to confirm the clinical benefit of SAR3419 in a more homogeneous population. Based on encouraging preclinical data, the activity of SAR3419 is also explored in adult patients with R/R ALL [80].

CDX-011 (glembatumumab vedotin): gpNMB (glycoprotein nonmetastatic melanoma protein b/osteoactivin) is a type I transmembrane glycoprotein identified in melanoma cell lines and shown to be expressed in several tumor indications including melanoma and breast [81, 82]. CDX-011 is an ADC comprising a fully human IgG2 anti-gpNMB antibody conjugated to MMAE via the cleavable protease-sensitive valine–citrulline linker [83]. A phase I/II was undertaken in 117 unresectable, stage III/IV melanoma patients treated with a q3w schedule, or with more frequent dosing regimens, q2/3w and weekly. In the q3w dose escalation, DLT were grade 3 rash and desquamation [83]. The MTD were 1.88, 1.5, and 1 mg/kg, respectively [84], with most common grade 3 or 4 AE being rash (20 %) and neutropenia (15 %) across the studies. At 1.88 mg/kg q3w, the half-life of CDX-011 was around 28 h and the half-life of the total antibody was 40 h [83, 85]. At MTD, the ORR of the q3w, q2/3w, and qw were 15 % (5/34), 33 % (2/6), and 29 % (2/7), respectively, and a clear correlation of skin rash with outcome was observed [83, 84]. Another phase I/II was completed in 42 locally advanced or metastatic breast cancers. Among the 34 patients, without preselection of gpNMB expression, treated at 1.88 mg/kg q3w, ORR was 13 % [81, 83, 86]. In the subgroup of patients expressing gpNMB, the ORR reached 29 %. A phase II clinical study with breast cancer patients expressing high gpNMB measured by IHC is ongoing [81]. It is interesting to note that one of the most common treatment-related toxicities with the melanoma and breast cancer studies were dermatologic events (pruritus, rash, alopecia). The AE could be linked to the expression of gpNMB in normal melanocytes [87].

PSMA-ADC (PSMA-vc-MMAE): PSMA (prostate-specific membrane antigen) is a type II transmembrane glycoprotein displaying carboxypeptidase activity and expressed mainly in normal prostate epithelium [88, 89]. PSMA has been shown to be highly expressed at the membrane of prostate cancer cells [90–92] providing a rationale for the design of PSMA-ADC. The PSMA-vc-MMAE ADC is a fully humanized IgG1 antibody, linked to MMAE via the cleavable valine–citrulline linker [93]. It is the second PSMA ADC to be evaluated in the clinic. The first one (PSMA-SPP-DM1/MLN2704) was stopped in 2008 (Table 2). Clinical data of MLN2704 showed low efficacy and limiting peripheral neuropathy [94]. A phase I, dose escalation trial with PSMA-vc-MMAE, is being conducted in men with taxane-refractory metastatic castration-resistant prostate cancer in a q3w schedule for up to four cycles [95, 96]. As of today 26 patients have been enrolled in a dose escalation study up to 2.0 mg/kg, and the MTD has not been reached [95]. Evidence for antitumor activity, as reflected by declines in PSA, circulating tumor cells and/or bone pain, has been observed in 4 of 12 subjects treated at 1.6 or 1.8 mg/kg. Dose proportional increases in serum concentrations of PSMA ADC have been seen with half-life of around 50 h [96]. From the last EORTC update, dose escalation has been completed and 2.5 mg/kg has been identified as the MTD. DLT observed at 2.8 mg/kg were neutropenia and reversible liver function alteration [97].

BT-062: CD138 (Syndecan-1) is a member of the family of transmembrane heparan sulfate proteoglycans overexpressed in various solid tumors and hematological malignancies. In the normal human hematopoietic compartment, CD138 expression is restricted to plasma cells [98], and in malignant hematopoiesis, CD138 is expressed on the majority of multiple myeloma (MM) cells making it a good candidate antigen for this indication [99]. BT-062 is an antibody–drug conjugate, comprised of the anti-CD138 chimeric IgG4 antibody conjugated to DM4 via a cleavable disulfide linker. In a phase I trial enrolling a total of 32 MM patients, receiving 1 of 7 dose levels ranging from 0.27 to 5.4 mg/kg in a q3w schedule, the MTD was defined at 4.3 mg/kg, with mucositis and palmar–plantar erythrodysesthesia syndrome being the DLTs [100]. Mucositis side effect could be correlated with the target expression observed in stratified squamous epithelium (mucosa) of the esophagus [99]. Of the 28 patients who were evaluated for response, 4 % achieved a PR. A phase I/IIa study in MM has been initiated to further evaluate the safety and efficacy of BT-062 using a more frequent dosing regimen of three weekly doses [100]. Combination trials with lenalidomide and dexamethasone are also ongoing.

IMGN901 (lorvotuzumab mertansine): CD56 antigen, a neural cell adhesion molecule implicated in cell–cell adhesion, neurite outgrowth, and other brain functions is overexpressed in a variety of cancers including small-cell lung cancer (SCLC), neuroblastoma and other neuroendocrine malignancies, multiple myeloma, and ovarian cancers. The expression of CD56 on normal tissues is restricted to NK cells and a subset of T lymphocytes [101]. IMGN901 is an anti-CD56 IgG1 antibody conjugated to DM1 via a hindered disulfide cleavable SPP linker. It has been evaluated in several phase I trials in patients with SCLC, MM, or other neuroendocrine tumors. A phase I dose escalation trial in 32 patients with MM established the MTD at 112 mg/m^2 (3 mg/kg) when the ADC was administered weekly for 2 consecutive weeks every 3 weeks [102]. DLT was grade 3 fatigue in 2 out of 6 patients treated at 140 mg/m^2. One sustained PR was documented in a patient treated at 140 mg/m^2/week. In a small phase I trial enrolling 6 patients with Merkel cell carcinoma, the MTD was established at 75 mg/m^2 (2 mg/kg) when the ADC was administered daily for 3 consecutive days every 3 weeks [103]. In this trial,

DLTs were grade 3 myalgia, headache, and back and shoulder pain. Out of 6 patients, there was 1 CR and 1 PR. A similar schedule of administration was used during another phase I on CD56-positive solid tumors from different types [104]. The MTD was also established at 75 mg/m^2/day, and DLT were grade 3 headache, neuropathy, fatigue, and myalgia, as previously reported. Half-life of IMGN901 at MTD was 34 h. Evidence of activity was observed with 1 CR and 1 PR in MCC and 1 unconfirmed PR in SCLC. Combination trials were also initiated. Escalating doses of IMGN901, given weekly for 3 weeks in a 4-week cycle, were evaluated in combination with lenalidomide/dexamethasone at their usual doses in patients with R/R CD56-expressing MM. Among the 12 patients enrolled, all had previously been treated with chemotherapy, with 42 % having received prior lenalidomide. No DLT has been reported and no grade 4 toxicities have been observed. One serious AE and 7 grade 3 toxicities related to combination treatment have been observed in four patients. On 12 efficacy-evaluable patients, 2 had a very good PR (VGPR) [105], and 4 had a PR. A phase I/II study to assess the safety and efficacy of IMGN901 in combination with carboplatin/etoposide in patients with advanced solid tumors including extensive stage small-cell lung cancer is ongoing. The NORTH trial is the phase II portion of this trial in which the ADC is administered for 3 consecutive days every 21 days at the dose of 60 mg/m^2/day (IMGN website, clinicaltrial.gov). Another phase I/II combination study with panobinostat and carfilzomib is currently ongoing in patients with R/R multiple myeloma [106].

4 Challenges and Perspectives

ADC have made tremendous progress over the last decades as demonstrated by the outstanding clinical efficacy observed in both hematological malignancies, with Adcetris® for the treatment of Hodgkin's lymphoma, and solid tumors, with T-DM1 for the treatment of metastatic breast cancer. The conjunction of the evolution of monoclonal antibodies from murine to humanized and human versions and the technological advances in the conjugation of highly potent non-immunogenic small molecules have been the pillars of these progresses. The increasing number of ADC reaching the clinic, targeting different antigens, and bearing different linkers and cytotoxics have contributed to the learning curve and stepwise progress of ADC. Lessons learned from the past experience of successful and stopped ADCs (*see* Tables 1 and 2) highlight the major axes that shall guide the development of future ADC.

Targets are at the heart of ADC development. Through their expression in some normal organs/tissues, they can contribute to "on-target" toxicity and thereby decrease the therapeutic index and compromise clinical benefit. Although several ADC, such as IMGN242, MLN2704, and T-DM1, targeting epithelial antigens known to be expressed in some normal tissues have been well tolerated in clinical trials, with no antigen-positive related normal tissues toxicity, it has clearly been demonstrated in the case of bivatuzumab mertansine that the expression of the CD44v6 target in the skin can lead to severe toxicity. In the same direction, the skin-related AE observed for CDX-011 could be linked to the expression of gpNMB in normal melanocytes, which highlights skin as a particularly sensitive tissue to tubulin binders cytotoxics-ADC.

In parallel, targets contribute to efficacy by their level and homogeneity of expression. AVE9633, targeting CD33 antigen, was stopped in phase I due to lack of efficacy signal, in part driven by the low expression of CD33 on AML blasts. T-DM1 ORR in clinic does not correlate with exposure but is clearly linked to the level of target expression on breast cancer cells, as ORR is higher in the group of patients whose tumors have confirmed HER2 overexpression. Similarly, preliminary data show a correlation trend between gpNMB expression level in tumors and ORR for CDX-011 [86]. In addition to antigen density, the target has to be understood and documented in the context of the pathology itself, including antigen turnover and trafficking to the "right" subcellular compartments, morphological aspects of the tumor with regard to polarized versus depolarized target expression, but also, proliferation index and intrinsic sensitivity of the tumor to the selected cytotoxics. Leveraging this knowledge will help to better select future targets.

If clinical exploration of ADC directed towards epithelial antigens has proven the value of the strategy, future ADC could also be directed towards vascular, stromal, and cancer stem cell targets [107–110].

In link with target expression features, progress of future ADC will require the capacity to better define the patient population which will benefit from the treatment. The development of improved companion diagnostics for the evaluation of target expression level and distribution in human tumor biopsies will be a critical asset.

On top of the right target choice, developing and optimizing cytotoxics and linkers to improve efficacy and safety profile is mandatory but remains very complex and therefore challenging. ADC have, unlike naked antibodies, an "off-target" driven intrinsic toxicity linked to their cytotoxic moiety. Whether it is due to plasmatic release of the cytotoxic payload, modulated by the type of linker used, or to target-independent internalization (endopinocytosis, FcR-driven internalization) by normal cells, in some body compartment(s), remains to be analyzed on a case by case basis. Progress in deciphering the origin of observed AE, like the recently published data demonstrating the impact of T-DM1 on platelet production inhibition, leading to the observed thrombocytopenia toxicity in patients [111], will help improving the design of future ADC.

Other explorations in preclinical studies include:

1. Deciphering metabolite properties: increasing metabolite accumulation in tumor cells to improve efficacy, like the design of PEGylated linkers to decrease multidrug-resistance recognition of metabolites [112]. On the same note, the chemical nature of the linker will influence not only the plasma pharmacokinetics and biodistribution of the ADC but also the type and properties of the metabolites within the tumor and the liver [113–115]. As an example, bystander effect may be wished to amplify the tumor response, although it may also bring more toxicity on normal organs.
2. Decreasing the heterogeneity of current ADC by better controlling the DAR. ADC are produced as complex mixtures whether they arise from lysine or cysteine conjugation. The different components of these mixtures might behave differently. Indeed, it has been shown that the level of cytotoxics attached to the antibody impact pharmacokinetics, efficacy, and safety [30]. Since few years, different options are explored to better monitor the DAR, like introduction in the antibody backbone of defined sites for conjugation. For example, cysteine engineering has been developed by different groups, and some thiomab-ADC have demonstrated equivalent if not better preclinical in vivo efficacy and tolerability [116, 117]. No clinical data using thiomabs has yet been published.
3. Improving physicochemical properties of the ADC, including solubility [112, 118] and capacity to aggregate. These modifications may concern the antibody backbone, as well as the linker and the drug itself.
4. Developing novel cytotoxics with different mechanisms of action, like the recently published alpha-amanitin-ADC [119]. This might help to improve therapeutic index and certainly offers new options of treatment for a larger panel of tumor indications.
5. Improving tumor penetration by using antibody fragments or protein scaffolds. Preclinical studies with anti-CD30 diabodies conjugated to auristatin demonstrated efficacy in tumor models [120]. But the balance between size, affinity, and pharmacokinetics properties has to be carefully explored to achieve optimal accumulation in tumors [121], and today no clinical exploration of ADCs with backbone different from IgG has been started.

Finally, ADC being a prodrug, understanding ADC metabolism/catabolism and properties and fate of metabolites is also essential to modulate efficacy and toxicity [59, 113–115]. Integrating quantitative and predictive understanding of PK/PD relationship will surely contribute to the optimization of all three components of the ADC in relation to target/disease properties, as well as administration regimen [115].

ADC design will be based on thoughtful combination of antibody, linker, and drugs in the context of a target and a defined cancer indication and a thorough understanding of the behavior of each ADC, with the ultimate goal to kill cancers while improving patients quality of life.

Acknowledgements

The authors would like to thank Anne Bousseau and Laurent Ducry for their helpful suggestions and critical reading of the manuscript.

References

1. Reichert JM (2012) Marketed therapeutic antibodies compendium. MAbs 4:413–415
2. Larson RA, Sievers EL, Stadtmauer EA et al (2005) Final report of the efficacy and safety of gemtuzumab ozogamicin (Mylotarg) in patients with CD33-positive acute myeloid leukemia in first recurrence. Cancer 104:1442–1452
3. Sievers EL, Larson RA, Stadtmauer EA et al (2001) Efficacy and safety of gemtuzumab ozogamicin in patients with CD33-positive acute myeloid leukemia in first relapse. J Clin Oncol J Am Soc Clin Oncol 19:3244–3254
4. Ricart AD (2011) Antibody–drug conjugates of calicheamicin derivative: gemtuzumab ozogamicin and inotuzumab ozogamicin. Clin Cancer Res J Am Assoc Cancer Res 17:6417–6427
5. Teicher BA (2009) Antibody–drug conjugate targets. Curr Cancer Drug Targets 9:982–1004
6. Helft PR, Schilsky RL, Hoke FJ et al (2004) A phase I study of cantuzumab mertansine administered as a single intravenous infusion once weekly in patients with advanced solid tumors. Clin Cancer Res J Am Assoc Cancer Res 10:4363–4368
7. Tolcher AW, Ochoa L, Hammond LA et al (2003) Cantuzumab mertansine, a maytansinoid immunoconjugate directed to the CanAg antigen: a phase I, pharmacokinetic, and biologic correlative study. J Clin Oncol J Am Soc Clin Oncol 21:211–222
8. Heider K, Kuthan H, Stehle G et al (2004) CD44v6: a target for antibody-based cancer therapy. Cancer Immunol Immunother CII 53:567–579
9. Riechelmann H, Sauter A, Golze W et al (2008) Phase I trial with the CD44v6-targeting immunoconjugate bivatuzumab mertansine in head and neck squamous cell carcinoma. Oral Oncol 44:823–829
10. Sauter A, Kloft C, Gronau S et al (2007) Pharmacokinetics, immunogenicity and safety of bivatuzumab mertansine, a novel CD44v6-targeting immunoconjugate, in patients with squamous cell carcinoma of the head and neck. Int J Oncol 30:927–935
11. Tijink BM, Buter J, Bree R et al (2006) A phase I dose escalation study with anti-CD44v6 bivatuzumab mertansine in patients with incurable squamous cell carcinoma of the head and neck or esophagus. Clin Cancer Res J Am Assoc Cancer Res 12:6064–6072
12. Lapusan S, Vidriales MB, Thomas X et al (2012) Phase I studies of AVE9633, an anti-CD33 antibody-maytansinoid conjugate, in adult patients with relapsed/refractory acute myeloid leukemia. Invest New Drugs 30:1121–1131
13. Chari R, Xie H, Leece B (2005) Preclinical evaluation of an anti-CD33-maytansinoid immunoconjugate, huMy9-6-DM4 (AVE9633) for the

targeted therapy of acute myeloid leukemia. Am Assoc Cancer Res, Abstract LB–287

14. Chari RV (2008) Targeted cancer therapy: conferring specificity to cytotoxic drugs. Acc Chem Res 41:98–107
15. Kratz F, Ajaj KA, Warnecke A (2007) Anticancer carrier-linked prodrugs in clinical trials. Expert Opin Investig Drugs 16:1037–1058
16. Senter PD (2009) Potent antibody drug conjugates for cancer therapy. Curr Opin Chem Biol 13:235–244
17. Chari RV, Martell BA, Gross JL et al (1992) Immunoconjugates containing novel maytansinoids: promising anticancer drugs. Cancer Res 52:127–131
18. Widdison WC, Wilhelm SD, Cavanagh EE et al (2006) Semisynthetic maytansine analogues for the targeted treatment of cancer. J Med Chem 49:4392–4408
19. Doronina SO, Mendelsohn BA, Bovee TD et al (2006) Enhanced activity of monomethylauristatin F through monoclonal antibody delivery: effects of linker technology on efficacy and toxicity. Bioconjug Chem 17:114–124
20. Hamann PR, Hinman LM, Beyer CF et al (2002) An anti-CD33 antibody–calicheamicin conjugate for treatment of acute myeloid leukemia. Choice of linker. Bioconjug Chem 13:40–46
21. Tietze LF, Krewer B (2009) Novel analogues of CC-1065 and the duocarmycins for the use in targeted tumour therapies. Anticancer Agent Med Chem 9:304–325
22. Ducry L, Stump B (2010) Antibody–drug conjugates: linking cytotoxic payloads to monoclonal antibodies. Bioconjug Chem 21:5–13
23. Erickson HK, Park PU, Widdison WC, Kovtun YV, Garrett LM, Hoffman K, Lutz RJ, Goldmacher VS, Blättler WA (2006) Antibody–maytansinoid conjugates are activated in targeted cancer cells by lysosomal degradation and linker-dependent intracellular processing. Cancer Res 66:4426–4433
24. Doronina SO, Toki BE, Torgov MY et al (2003) Development of potent monoclonal antibody auristatin conjugates for cancer therapy. Nat Biotechnol 21:778–784
25. Erickson HK, Widdison WC, Mayo MF et al (2010) Tumor delivery and in vivo processing of disulfide-linked and thioether-linked antibody–maytansinoid conjugates. Bioconjug Chem 21:84–92
26. Kellogg BA, Garrett L, Kovtun Y et al (2011) Disulfide-linked antibody–maytansinoid conjugates: optimization of in vivo activity by varying the steric hindrance at carbon atoms adjacent to the disulfide linkage. Bioconjug Chem 22:717–727
27. Okeley NM, Miyamoto JB, Zhang X et al (2010) Intracellular activation of SGN-35, a potent anti-CD30 antibody–drug conjugate. Clin Cancer Res J Am Assoc Cancer Res 16:888–897
28. Kovtun YV, Audette CA, Ye Y et al (2006) Antibody–drug conjugates designed to eradicate tumors with homogeneous and heterogeneous expression of the target antigen. Cancer Res 66:3214–3221
29. Sanderson RJ, Hering MA, James SF et al (2005) In vivo drug-linker stability of an anti-CD30 dipeptide-linked auristatin immunoconjugate. Clin Cancer Res J Am Assoc Cancer Res 11:843–852
30. Hamblett KJ, Senter PD, Chace DF et al (2004) Effects of drug loading on the antitumor activity of a monoclonal antibody drug conjugate. Clin Cancer Res J Am Assoc Cancer Res 10:7063–7070
31. Shen B, Xu K, Liu L et al (2012) Conjugation site modulates the in vivo stability and therapeutic activity of antibody–drug conjugates. Nat Biotechnol 30:184–189
32. Wakankar A, Chen Y, Gokarn Y et al (2011) Analytical methods for physicochemical characterization of antibody drug conjugates. MAbs 3:161–172
33. Deutsch YE, Tadmor T, Podack ER et al (2011) CD30: an important new target in hematologic malignancies. Leuk Lymphoma 52:1641–1654
34. Gerber H (2010) Emerging immunotherapies targeting CD30 in Hodgkin's lymphoma. Biochem Pharmacol 79:1544–1552
35. Katz J, Janik JE, Younes A (2011) Brentuximab vedotin (SGN-35). Clin Cancer Res J Am Assoc Cancer Res 17:6428–6436
36. Younes A (2011) CD30-targeted antibody therapy. Curr Opin Oncol 23:587–593
37. Furtado M, Rule S (2012) Emerging pharmacotherapy for relapsed or refractory Hodgkin's lymphoma: focus on brentuximab vedotin. Clin Med Insight Oncol 6:31–39
38. Pro B, Advani R, Brice P et al (2012) Brentuximab vedotin (SGN-35) in patients with relapsed or refractory systemic anaplastic large-cell lymphoma: results of a phase II study. J Clin Oncol J Am Soc Clin Oncol 30:2190–2196
39. Senter PD, Sievers EL (2012) The discovery and development of brentuximab vedotin for

use in relapsed Hodgkin lymphoma and systemic anaplastic large cell lymphoma. Nat Biotechnol 30:631–637

40. Francisco JA, Cerveny CG, Meyer DL et al (2003) cAC10-vcMMAE, an anti-CD30-monomethyl auristatin E conjugate with potent and selective antitumor activity. Blood 102:1458–1465
41. Younes A, Bartlett NL, Leonard JP et al (2010) Brentuximab vedotin (SGN-35) for relapsed CD30-positive lymphomas. N Engl J Med 363:1812–1821
42. Fanale MA, Forero-Torres A, Rosenblatt JD et al (2012) A phase I weekly dosing study of brentuximab vedotin in patients with relapsed/refractory CD30-positive hematologic malignancies. Clin Cancer Res J Am Assoc Cancer Res 18:248–255
43. Younes A, Gopal AK, Smith SE et al (2012) Results of a pivotal phase II study of brentuximab vedotin for patients with relapsed or refractory Hodgkin and other lymphoma. J Clin Oncol J Am Soc Clin Oncol 30:2183–2189
44. Minich SS (2012) Brentuximab vedotin: a new age in the treatment of Hodgkin lymphoma and anaplastic large cell lymphoma. Ann Pharmacother 46:377–383
45. Hynes NE, Stern DF (1994) The biology of erbB-2/neu/HER-2 and its role in cancer. Biochim Biophys Acta 1198:165–184
46. Dawood S, Broglio K, Buzdar AU et al (2010) Prognosis of women with metastatic breast cancer by HER2 status and trastuzumab treatment: an institutional-based review. J Clin Oncol J Am Soc Clin Oncol 28:92–98
47. Arteaga CL, Sliwkowski MX, Osborne CK et al (2012) Treatment of HER2-positive breast cancer: current status and future perspectives. Nat Rev Clin Oncol 9:16–32
48. Tsang RY, Finn RS (2012) Beyond trastuzumab: novel therapeutic strategies in HER2-positive metastatic breast cancer. Br J Cancer 106:6–13
49. Phillips GD, Li G, Dugger DL et al (2008) Targeting HER2-positive breast cancer with trastuzumab-DM1, an antibody–cytotoxic drug conjugate. Cancer Res 68:9280–9290
50. Junttila TT, Li G, Parsons K et al (2011) Trastuzumab-DM1 (T-DM1) retains all the mechanisms of action of trastuzumab and efficiently inhibits growth of lapatinib insensitive breast cancer. Breast Cancer Res Treat 128:347–356
51. Barok M, Tanner M, Koninki K et al (2011) Trastuzumab-DM1 causes tumour growth inhibition by mitotic catastrophe in trastuzumab-resistant breast cancer cells in vivo. Breast Cancer Res BCR 13:R46
52. Krop IE, Beeram M, Modi S et al (2010) Phase I study of trastuzumab-DM1, an HER2 antibody-drug conjugate, given every 3 weeks to patients with HER2-positive metastatic breast cancer. J Clin Oncol J Am Soc Clin Oncol 28:2698–2704
53. Beeram M, Krop IE, Burris HA et al (2012) A phase 1 study of weekly dosing of trastuzumab emtansine (T-DM1) in patients with advanced human epidermal growth factor 2-positive breast cancer. Cancer 118:5733–5740
54. Burris HA, Tibbitts J, Holden SN et al (2011) Trastuzumab emtansine (T-DM1): a novel agent for targeting HER2+ breast cancer. Clin Breast Cancer 11:275–282
55. Mathew J, Perez EA (2011) Trastuzumab emtansine in human epidermal growth factor receptor 2-positive breast cancer: a review. Curr Opin Oncol 23:594–600
56. Lorusso PM, Weiss D, Guardino E et al (2011) Trastuzumab emtansine: a unique antibody–drug conjugate in development for human epidermal growth factor receptor 2-positive cancer. Clin Cancer Res J Am Assoc Cancer Res 17:6437–6447
57. Burris HA, Rugo HS, Vukelja SJ et al (2011) Phase II study of the antibody drug conjugate trastuzumab-DM1 for the treatment of human epidermal growth factor receptor 2 (HER2)-positive breast cancer after prior HER2-directed therapy. J Clin Oncol J Am Soc Clin Oncol 29:398–405
58. Krop IE, Lorusso P, Miller KD et al (2012) A phase II study of trastuzumab emtansine in patients with human epidermal growth factor receptor 2-positive metastatic breast cancer who were previously treated with trastuzumab, lapatinib, an anthracycline, a taxane, and capecitabine. J Clin Oncol J Am Soc Clin Oncol 30:3234–3241
59. Girish S, Gupta M, Wang B et al (2012) Clinical pharmacology of trastuzumab emtansine (T-DM1): an antibody–drug conjugate in development for the treatment of HER2-positive cancer. Cancer Chemother Pharmacol 69:1229–1240
60. Gupta M, Lorusso PM, Wang B et al (2012) Clinical implications of pathophysiological and demographic covariates on the population pharmacokinetics of trastuzumab emtansine, a HER2-targeted antibody–drug conjugate, in patients with HER2-positive metastatic breast cancer. J Clin Pharmacol 52:691–703

61. Perez E, Dirix L, Kocsis J et al (2010) Efficacy and safety of trastuzumab-DM1 versus trastuzumab plus docetaxel in HER2-positive metastatic breast cancer patients with no prior chemotherapy for metastatic disease: preliminary results of a randomized, multicenter, open-label phase 2 study (TDM4450g). Ann Oncol 21(Suppl 8):viii2, Abstract LBA3
62. Hurvitz S, Dirix L, Kocsis J et al (2011) Trastuzumab emtansine (T-DM1) vs trastuzumab plus docetaxel (H + T) in previously-untreated HER2-positive metastatic breast cancer (MBC): primary results of a randomized, multicenter, open-label phase II study (TDM4450g/B021976). Eur J Cancer 47:ECCO–ESMO, Abstract 5001
63. Verma S, Miles D, Gianni L et al (2012) Trastuzumab emtansine for HER2-positive advanced breast cancer. N Engl J Med 367:1783–1791
64. Tedder TF, Poe JC, Haas KM (2005) CD22: a multifunctional receptor that regulates B lymphocyte survival and signal transduction. Adv Immunol 88:1–50
65. Shan D, Press OW (1995) Constitutive endocytosis and degradation of CD22 by human B cells. J Immunol 154:4466–4475
66. Wong BY, Dang NH (2010) Inotuzumab ozogamicin as novel therapy in lymphomas. Expert Opin Biol Ther 10:1251–1258
67. Thomas X (2012) Inotuzumab ozogamicin in the treatment of B-cell acute lymphoblastic leukemia. Expert Opin Investig Drugs 21:871–878
68. DiJoseph JF, Goad ME, Dougher MM et al (2004) Potent and specific antitumor efficacy of CMC-544, a CD22-targeted immunoconjugate of calicheamicin, against systemically disseminated B-cell lymphoma. Clin Cancer Res J Am Assoc Cancer Res 10:8620–8629
69. Advani A, Coiffier B, Czuczman MS et al (2010) Safety, pharmacokinetics, and preliminary clinical activity of inotuzumab ozogamicin, a novel immunoconjugate for the treatment of B-cell non-Hodgkin and other lymphoma: results of a phase I study. J Clin Oncol J Am Soc Clin Oncol 28:2085–2093
70. Ogura M, Tobinai K, Hatake K et al (2010) Phase I study of inotuzumab ozogamicin (CMC-544) in Japanese patients with follicular lymphoma pretreated with rituximab-based therapy. Cancer Sci 101:1840–1845
71. DiJoseph JF, Dougher MM, Kalyandrug LB et al (2006) Antitumor efficacy of a combination of CMC-544 (inotuzumab ozogamicin), a CD22-targeted cytotoxic immunoconjugate of calicheamicin, and rituximab against non-Hodgkin's B-cell lymphoma. Clin Cancer Res J Am Assoc Cancer Res 12:242–249
72. Dang N, Smith M, Offner F et al (2009) Anti-CD22 immunoconjugate inotuzumab ozogamicin (CMC-544) + rituximab: clinical activity including survival in patients with recurrent/refractory follicular or "aggressive" lymphoma. Blood 114, Abstract 584
73. Fayad L, Patel H, Verhoef G et al (2008) Safety and clinical activity of the anti-CD22 immunoconjugate inotuzumab ozogamicin (CMC-544) in combination with rituximab in follicular lymphoma or diffuse large B-cell lymphoma: preliminary report of a phase 1/2 study. Blood 112, Abstract 266
74. Verhoef G, Dang N, Smith M et al (2010) Anti-CD22 immunoconjugate inotuzumab ozogamicin (CMC-544) + rituximab: clinical activity in patients with relapsed/refractory follicular or aggressive lymphomas. Haematologica 95, Abstract 0573
75. Jabbour E, O'Brien S, Thomas DA, Ravandi F et al (2011) Inotuzumab ozogamicin (IO; CMC544), a CD22 monoclonal antibody attached to calicheamycin, produces complete response (CR) plus complete marrow response (mCR) of greater than 50 % in refractory relapse (R–R) acute lymphocytic leukemia (ALL). J Clin Oncol 29, Abstract 6507
76. Kantarjian H, Thomas D, Jorgensen J et al (2012) Inotuzumab ozogamicin, an anti-CD22-calecheamicin conjugate, for refractory and relapsed acute lymphocytic leukaemia: a phase 2 study. Lancet Oncol 13:403–411
77. Blanc V, Bousseau A, Caron A et al (2011) SAR3419: an anti-CD19-maytansinoid immunoconjugate for the treatment of B-cell malignancies. Clin Cancer Res J Am Assoc Cancer Res 17:6448–6458
78. Younes A, Kim S, Romaguera J et al (2012) Phase I multidose-escalation study of the anti-CD19 maytansinoid immunoconjugate SAR3419 administered by intravenous infusion every 3 weeks to patients with relapsed/refractory B-cell lymphoma. J Clin Oncol J Am Soc Clin Oncol 30:2776–2782
79. Coiffier B, Morschhauser F, Dupuis J et al (2012) Phase I study cohort evaluating an optimized administration schedule of SAR3419, an anti-CD19 DM4-loaded antibody drug conjugate (ADC), in patients (pts) with CD19 positive relapsed/refractory b-cell non-Hodgkin's lymphoma (NCT00796731). J Clin Oncol 30, Abstract 8057
80. Hammer O (2012) CD19 as an attractive target for antibody-based therapy. MAbs 4:571–577

81. Keir CH, Vahdat LT (2012) The use of an antibody drug conjugate, glembatumumab vedotin (CDX-011), for the treatment of breast cancer. Expert Opin Biol Ther 12:259–263
82. Tse KF, Jeffers M, Pollack VA et al (2006) CR011, a fully human monoclonal antibody–auristatin E conjugate, for the treatment of melanoma. Clin Cancer Res J Am Assoc Cancer Res 12:1373–1382
83. Naumovski L, Junutula JR (2010) Glembatumumab vedotin, a conjugate of an anti-glycoprotein non-metastatic melanoma protein B mAb and monomethyl auristatin E for the treatment of melanoma and breast cancer. Curr Opin Mol Ther 12:248–257
84. Hamid O, Sznol M, Pavlick A et al (2010) Frequent dosing and GPNMB expression with CDX-011 (CR011-vcMMAE), an antibody–drug conjugate (ADC), in patients with advanced melanoma. J Clin Oncol 28, Abstract 8525
85. Szol M, Hamid O, Hwu P et al (2009) Pharmacokinetics of CR011-vcMMAE, an antibody–drug conjugate, in a phase I study of patients with advanced melanoma. J Clin Oncol 27, Abstract 9063
86. Saleh M, Bendell J, Rose et al (2010) Correlation of GPNMB expression with outcome in breast cancer (BC) patients treated with the antibody–drug conjugate (ADC), CDX-011 (CR011-vcMMAE). J Clin Oncol 28, Abstract 1095
87. Hoashi T, Sato S, Yamaguchi Y et al (2010) Glycoprotein nonmetastatic melanoma protein b, a melanocytic cell marker, is a melanosome-specific and proteolytically released protein. FASEB J 24:1616–1629
88. Akhtar NH, Pail O, Saran A et al (2012) Prostate-specific membrane antigen-based therapeutics. Adv Urol 2012:973820
89. Ghosh A, Heston WD (2004) Tumor target prostate specific membrane antigen (PSMA) and its regulation in prostate cancer. J Cell Biochem 91:528–539
90. Chang SS, Reuter VE, Heston WD et al (1999) Five different anti-prostate-specific membrane antigen (PSMA) antibodies confirm PSMA expression in tumor-associated neovasculature. Cancer Res 59:3192–3198
91. Minner S, Wittmer C, Graefen M et al (2011) High level PSMA expression is associated with early PSA recurrence in surgically treated prostate cancer. Prostate 71:281–288
92. Silver DA, Pellicer I, Fair WR et al (1997) Prostate-specific membrane antigen expression in normal and malignant human tissues. Clin Cancer Res J Am Assoc Cancer Res 3:81–85
93. Wang X, Ma D, Olson WC et al (2011) In vitro and in vivo responses of advanced prostate tumors to PSMA ADC, an auristatin-conjugated antibody to prostate-specific membrane antigen. Mol Cancer Ther 10:1728–1739
94. Galsky MD, Eisenberger M, Moore-Cooper S et al (2008) Phase I trial of the prostate-specific membrane antigen-directed immunoconjugate MLN2704 in patients with progressive metastatic castration-resistant prostate cancer. J Clin Oncol J Am Soc Clin Oncol 26:2147–2154
95. Petrylak D, Kantoff P, Mega-A et al (2012) Prostate-specific membrane antigen antibody drug conjugate (PSMA ADC): a phase I trial in men with prostate cancer previously treated with taxane. J Clin Oncol 30, Abstract 107
96. Petrylak D, Kantoff P, Frank R et al (2011) Prostate-specific membrane antigen antibody–drug conjugate (PSMA ADC): a phase I trial in taxane-refractory prostate cancer. J Clin Oncol 29, Abstract 4550
97. Petrylak D, Kantoff P, Mega-A et al (2012) Prostate specific membrane antigen antibody drug conjugate (PSMA ADC): a phase 1 trial in castration-resistant metastatic prostate cancer (mCRPC). EORTC-NCI-AACR 47
98. Wijdenes J, Vooijs WC, Clément C et al (1996) A plasmocyte selective monoclonal antibody (B-B4) recognizes syndecan-1. Br J Haematol 94:318–323
99. Tassone P, Goldmacher VS, Neri P et al (2004) Cytotoxic activity of the maytansinoid immunoconjugate B-B4-DM1 against CD138+ multiple myeloma cells. Blood 104:3688–3696
100. Jagannath S, Chanan-Khan A, Heffner L et al (2011) BT062, an antibody–drug conjugate directed against CD138, shows clinical activity in a phase I study in patients with relapsed or relapsed/refractory multiple myeloma. ASH Annual Meeting, Abstract 305
101. Lutz RJ, Whiteman KR (2009) Antibody--maytansinoid conjugates for the treatment of myeloma. MAbs 1:548–551
102. Chanan-Khan A, Wolf J, Gharibo M. et al (2009) Phase I study of IMGN901, used as monotherapy, in patients with heavily pre-treated CD56-positive multiple myeloma – a preliminary safety and efficacy analysis. ASH Annual Meeting, Abstract 2883
103. Woll P, Laurigan P, O'Brien M et al (2009) Clinical experience of IMGN901 (BB-10901, huN901-DM1) in patients with Merkel cell

carcinoma (MCC). Mol Cancer Ther 8, Abstract B237

104. Woll PJ, O'Brien M, Fossella F et al (2010) Phase I study of lorvotuzumab mertansine (IMGN901) in patients with CD56-positive solid tumors. Ann Oncol J Eur Soc Med Oncol ESMO, Abstract 536

105. Berdeja J, Ailawadhi S, Niesvizky R et al (2010) Phase I study of lorvotuzumab mertansine (IMGN901) used in combination with lenalidomide and dexamethasone in patients with CD56-positive multiple myeloma, a preliminary safety and efficacy analysis of the combination. ASH Annual Meeting, Abstract 1934

106. Berdeja J, Mace J, Lamar R et al (2012) A single-arm, open-label, multicenter phase I/II study of the combination of panobinostat (pan) and carfilzomib (cfz) in patients (pts) with relapsed/refractory multiple myeloma (RR MM). J Clin Oncol 30, Abstract TPS8115

107. Mao W, Tien J, Goldenberg D et al (2010) Early study on LGR5/GPR49 molecule as a potential colon cancer stem cell target for the antibody conjugated drug treatment. Annual Meeting of the AACR, Abstract 4289

108. Schliemann C, Neri D (2010) Antibody-based vascular tumor targeting. Recent Results Cancer Res 180:201–216

109. Terrett J, Devasthali V, Pan C et al (2008) Ptk7 as a direct and tumor stroma target in multiple solid malignancies. Annual Meeting of the AACR, Abstract 1526

110. Vater C, Manning C, Millar H et al (2008) Anti-tumor efficacy of the integrin-targeted immunoconjugate IMGN388 in preclinical models. EORTC-NCI-AACR, Abstract ENA–0399

111. Thon JN, Devine MT, Begonja AJ et al (2012) High-content live-cell imaging assay used to establish mechanism of trastuzumab emtansine (T-DM1)-mediated inhibition of platelet production. Blood 120:1975–1984

112. Kovtun YV, Audette CA, Mayo MF et al (2010) Antibody–maytansinoid conjugates designed to bypass multidrug resistance. Cancer Res 70:2528–2537

113. Erickson HK, Lambert JM (2012) ADME of antibody–maytansinoid conjugates. AAPS J 14:799–805

114. Erickson HK, Phillips GD, Leipold DD et al (2012) The effect of different linkers on target cell catabolism and pharmacokinetics/pharmacodynamics of trastuzumab maytansinoid conjugates. Mol Cancer Ther 11:1133–1142

115. Lin K, Tibbitts J (2012) Pharmacokinetic considerations for antibody drug conjugates. Pharm Res 29:2354–2366

116. Junutula JR, Raab H, Clark S et al (2008) Site-specific conjugation of a cytotoxic drug to an antibody improves the therapeutic index. Nat Biotechnol 26:925–932

117. McDonagh CF, Turcott E, Westendorf L et al (2006) Engineered antibody–drug conjugates with defined sites and stoichiometries of drug attachment. Protein Eng Design Select PEDS 19:299–307

118. Zhao RY, Wilhelm SD, Audette C et al (2011) Synthesis and evaluation of hydrophilic linkers for antibody–maytansinoid conjugates. J Med Chem 54:3606–3623

119. Moldenhauer G, Salnikov AV, Lüttgau AV et al (2012) Therapeutic potential of amanitin-conjugated anti-epithelial cell adhesion molecule monoclonal antibody against pancreatic carcinoma. J Natl Cancer Inst 104:622–634

120. Kim KM, McDonagh CF, Westendorf L et al (2008) Anti-CD30 diabody–drug conjugates with potent antitumor activity. Mol Cancer Ther 7:2486–2497

121. Wittrup KD, Thurber GM, Schmidt MM et al (2012) Practical theoretic guidance for the design of tumor-targeting agents. Methods Enzymol 503:255–268

122. Annunziata CM, Kohn EC, Lorusso P et al (2012) Phase 1, open-label study of MEDI-547 in patients with relapsed or refractory solid tumors. Invest New Drugs 31:77–84

123. Milowsky M, Galsky M, George M et al (2006) Phase I/II trial of the prostate-specific membrane antigen (PSMA)-targeted immunoconjugate MLN2704 in patients (pts) with progressive metastatic castration resistant prostate cancer (CRPC). J Clin Oncol 24, Abstract 4500

124. Chan SY, Gordon AN, Coleman RE et al (2003) A phase 2 study of the cytotoxic immunoconjugate CMB-401 (hCTM01-calicheamicin) in patients with platinum-sensitive recurrent epithelial ovarian carcinoma. Cancer Immunol Immunother CII 52:243–248

125. Gillespie AM, Broadhead TJ, Chan SY et al (2000) Phase I open study of the effects of ascending doses of the cytotoxic immunoconjugate CMB-401 (hCTMO1-calicheamicin) in patients with epithelial ovarian cancer. Ann Oncol J Eur Soc Med Oncol ESMO 11:735–741

Chapter 2

Antibody–Drug Conjugate Target Selection: Critical Factors

Neil H. Bander

Abstract

ADC success requires that all three components of the agent function in a near-flawless manner. Equally important is that the target be selected with stringent consideration as the target is the one factor in ADC development that is immutable and beyond the reach of the developer to refine/manipulate. This chapter reviews the critical factors of target selection that must be met if one is to succeed at ADC development.

Key words Antibody specificity, Antigen expression, Antigen internalization

1 Introduction

The concept of antibody-targeted drugs is not a new one, yet only now is this concept reaching fruition. The long gestational period, marked by many failures, is testimony to the complexity and difficulty of translating this appealingly simple and straightforward theory into practice. The lessons learned by past failures include the realization that any weakness or flaw in any one of the components—antibody, linker, or drug—spells failure for this multicomponent therapeutic agent. And while the term "antibody–drug conjugate" highlights the three component parts of the agent, it ignores the fourth and equally important component in the equation: the target. Indeed, it should be recognized and appreciated that among the four components necessary to yield a successful ADC, only the target is immutable. That is, one may refine and "tweak" the antibody for its affinity, immunogenicity, structure, etc.; the linker for its variable chemistry, cleavability, etc.; and the drug for its potency and mechanism of action, etc., but the target is determined and controlled by nature. It is beyond the drug developers' ability to tweak, and therefore, its selection must be carefully considered, for if one selects an inappropriate target, no matter how much time, effort, money, etc. are expended on the antibody, drug, and/or linker, the project is doomed to fail.

Laurent Ducry (ed.), *Antibody-Drug Conjugates*, Methods in Molecular Biology, vol. 1045,
DOI 10.1007/978-1-62703-541-5_2, © Springer Science+Business Media, LLC 2013

In this chapter, I will outline some of the most critical elements to be considered in target selection and provide an example of a target to demonstrate how it meets these requirements.

2 Critical Factors in Target Selection

2.1 Specificity

Specificity of the target is the core principle of the ADC approach. Indeed, ADCs are predicated on the principle of targeting a tumor-restricted antigen in order to avoid drug delivery to normal tissues. But tumor specificity must be viewed as a continuous variable rather than a binary one. In practice, one looks for a target with a high degree of tumor specificity where the normal tissue expression is limited in scope and/or present on expendable tissues or tissues with regenerative capacity.

In cases where the target is expressed by normal tissues, over-expression by tumor cells relative to target-positive normal tissue is a critical benefit or requirement. In addition, the accessibility of the tumor cells relative to antigen-positive normal tissue sites, as they relate to ADC biodistribution, is an important consideration. This latter point will be discussed further as well as illustrated in the example described below.

2.2 Level of Expression

Level of expression is critical in several respects. Firstly, it has a significant impact on how much ADC will bind tumor and how much ADC will be internalized into the tumor cell. While a target antigen may be very specific, if it is expressed at a low level, the delta of ADC delivered to tumor versus target-negative normal cells (via nonspecific uptake mechanisms) will be low resulting in a low therapeutic ratio. Conversely a highly expressed target can lead to uptake of cytotoxic doses of ADC and tumor death, while normal tissues that are target antigen-negative or express substantially lower amounts of target may be unaffected. Low expression level of the target, even if highly or absolutely tumor specific, simply may not enable accumulation of adequately cytotoxic doses before non-specific toxicity becomes manifest.

2.3 Internalization

Internalization is important for efficient cytotoxicity when the drug acts intracellularly. Inability of the target antigen to transport the ADC intracellularly severely compromises the efficiency and toxicity of the drug. Targeting an ADC to a non-internalizing target antigen with the expectation that extracellularly released drug will diffuse into the target cell is not a recipe for a successful ADC. While some externally released drug may, indeed, diffuse into the tumor cell, much will also diffuse away from the tumor resulting in compromised efficacy. Ideally, not only is the target antigen internalized but a rapid internalization process combined with efficient recycling or replenishment of antigen at the surface to act as a virtual pump accumulating intracellular ADC adds to the likelihood of success. One exception to the "rule" of ADC internalization is the case of ADCs armed with radioisotopes where emissions can generally reach the DNA target from the exterior of the cell. Similarly, development of agents that act extracellularly would abrogate the requirement for internalization.

2.4 Target Heterogeneity

Target heterogeneity can be viewed at the level of the tumor type as well as the level of the individual patient. In the former case, I'm referring to the proportion of cases of a given tumor type that are target antigen-positive. Consider the example of the her2 target in breast cancer where approximately 20 % of patients' tumors are her2 positive. This factor imposes limits on the patient population able to benefit from the therapy as well as a requirement for a companion diagnostic to identify the appropriate patient for treatment.

At the level of intra-patient target antigen heterogeneity, the presence of target-negative tumor cells requires a means to treat those target-negative cells that will not bind/internalize the ADC. This might dictate, for example, the use of a linker that permits release of drug from target-positive cells to reach nearby target-negative cells (so-called bystander effect). But, clearly, the greater the proportion of target-negative cells, the more tenuous the ADC target is.

2.5 Accessibility

Tumor/target accessibility is another critical factor. With respect to this issue, solid tumors represent a higher hurdle than hematogenous (or "liquid") tumors. The latter are present in blood, bone marrow, and/or lymph nodes—sites that receive high levels of circulating ADC. Conversely, it has been amply demonstrated that solid tumors pose difficulty to the penetration of drugs, ADCs, or otherwise (including small molecules) [1, 2]. The bulkier the tumor, the more necrotic and the greater the difficulty of the ADC to reach its tumor target no matter how specific or highly expressed it is.

3 Relative Factors/Considerations in Target Selection

3.1 Identifying the Appropriate Patient Population

It is fundamentally important, and becoming increasingly more practically important, in any cancer setting and with any oncologic agent, that the optimal patient population be prospectively identifiable. Regardless of the ADC target, there are likely to be patients whose tumors are target antigen negative. Her2, targeted by trastuzumab-DM1 (T-DM1), provides an excellent example where 75–85 % of breast cancer patients are her2-negative. In the absence of a means to identify appropriate patients, it would be virtually impossible to develop an acceptable therapeutic. Identification of the target-pos population is critical for the success of the therapy.

This is also true in cases where the target is expressed at widely varying levels; in such a case, it would be beneficial to identify patients whose tumors express target levels above a threshold that can be defined in early clinical trials.

3.2 Target Antigen Modulation

With some targets, more commonly described in lymphoid cells, antibody binding may lead to depletion of the target antigen for a period of time after Ab binding ("antigenic modulation"). In such cases, it will be imperative to know the kinetics of target modulation and re-expression in order to optimize dosing. It will also be important to identify if/when selection of target-negative cells occurs as a result of selection pressure from the ADC treatment. Although less likely, in some cases, it may be possible to upregulate the target. An example of the latter phenomenon will be discussed below.

4 Case Study: Prostate-Specific Membrane Antigen

Having enumerated key features of target selection, the following case study of prostate-specific membrane antigen (PSMA) presents an exemplary ADC target. I will review each of the features outlined above to demonstrate what makes PSMA a prototypical ADC target.

4.1 Specificity

Initial studies of PSMA [3, 4] reported its near-absolute prostate specificity and led to the proposed designation "prostate-specific membrane antigen." Subsequent studies have shown that PSMA is expressed by renal proximal tubules and some astrocytes and more weakly by small bowel and salivary gland (Fig. 1). As a result, PSMA resembles other highly restricted differentiation antigens that often serve as cancer targets. In general, these antigenic targets are about as tumor specific as one can get in the ADC field.

Another consideration in the realm of specificity is whether target-positive normal tissue subject to ADC binding is necessary to support/maintain life and/or whether the tissue can regenerate. Clearly, in the case of PSMA, if renal or bowel toxicity were to occur, it would be problematic; conversely, prostatic loss may not be a problem (except perhaps where fertility was important). In other cases, loss of normal cells can be tolerated particularly if they subsequently repopulate as in the case of CD20-pos normal lymphocytes.

But there is another consideration alluded to in the discussion above that is of practical importance: the precise cellular site of expression may offer some additional specificity benefit. In the case of PSMA, for example, potential ADC targeting of astrocytes is prevented by the blood–brain barrier. And in normal tissues such as the prostate, kidney, and small bowel, PSMA is expressed in

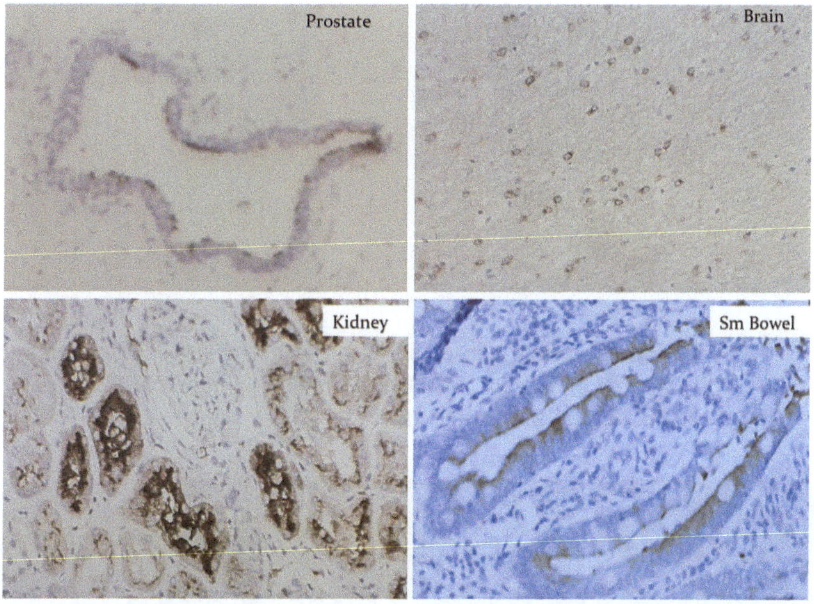

Fig. 1 Immunohistochemical demonstration of normal tissue expression of PSMA. Note that in the epithelial sites (prostate, kidney, bowel), expression is polarized and limited to the apical/luminal border

a polarized manner at the apical/luminal aspect of the cell (Fig. 1). These normal tissue sites are effectively ex vivo, and antibody access is prevented by intervening cell layers and basement membrane and by tight junctions. Based on human data of concentration gradients across such barriers, we estimate that these normal tissue sites achieve Ab concentrations of approximately 10^{-7} that of plasma.

Perhaps the lesson is that absolute tumor specificity is not a prerequisite, but a high degree of specificity is important, and there are additional considerations such as those described that can mitigate toxicity even when target expression occurs on critical normal tissues.

4.2 Level of Expression

PSMA is significantly upregulated in prostate cancer (PC) relative to its expression in other tissues including normal prostate (Fig. 2). In human PC cell lines, LNCaP, C4-2, and MDA-PCa2b express levels measured in the millions of molecules per cell [5]. Sokoloff et al. [6] used human tissue specimens and showed that PC expresses some 100- to 1,000-fold higher levels than any normal tissues.

4.3 Internalization

PSMA is rapidly and efficiently internalized [7] by an endocytic pathway (Fig. 3). In addition, it rapidly recycles back to the membrane therefore virtually pumping Ab payload (ADC) into the cell. Between high level expression and efficient internalization, high amounts of payload are efficiently internalized.

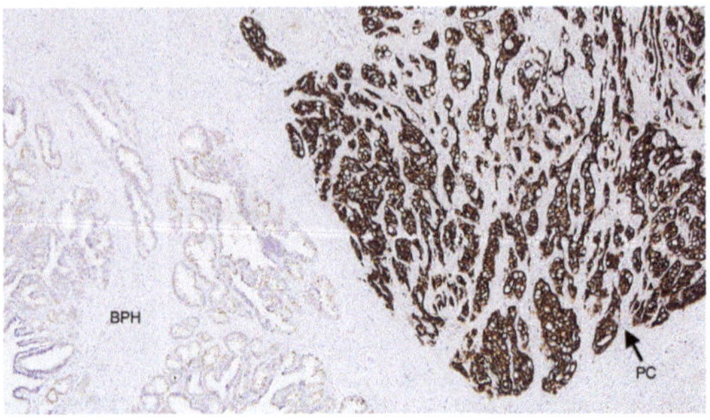

Fig. 2 Prostate cancer significantly upregulates PSMA expression relative to normal or benign prostatic hyperplasia (BPH). Note also the homogeneity of PSMA expression within the cancer

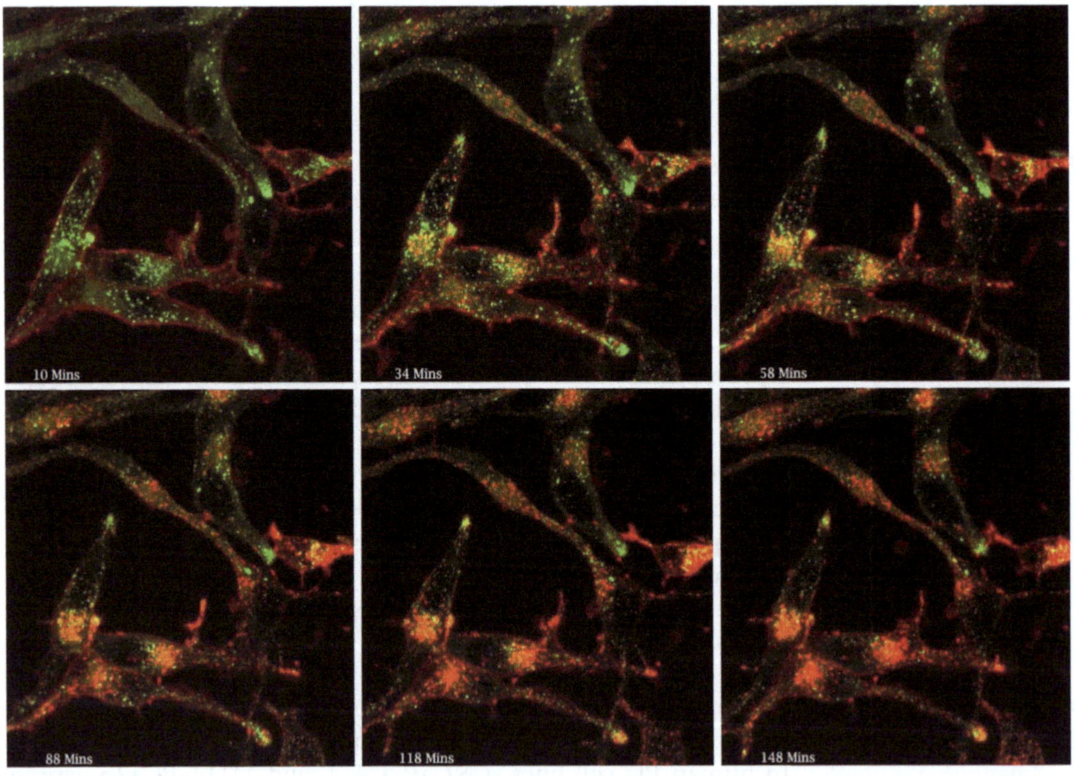

Fig. 3 Time-lapse confocal video-microscopy demonstrating internalization of J591, an anti-PSMA antibody, into viable prostate cancer cells (LNCaP). J591 is directly labeled with alexa-647 (*red*) dye; lysosomes are labeled green with LysoTracker® (Invitrogen). Incubation takes place at 4 °C and the clock starts when the cells are moved to 37 °C. Initially (10 min), the J591 (*red*) can be seen bound to the plasma membrane. Over time, an increasing amount of J591 Ab can be seen accumulating in a lysosomal compartment (*red* + *green* = *orange*) adjacent to the nucleus

4.4 Heterogeneity

As discussed above, heterogeneity should be considered at the inter-patient and the intra-patient levels. At the inter-patient level, in the case of PSMA, studies have shown that approximately 95 % of PC are PSMA positive [8–16] thus making a very high proportion of PC patients potential treatment candidates. At the intra-patient level, the literature suggests that patients with advanced, metastatic, castrate-resistant PC express high levels of PSMA in a rather homogeneous manner (*see* Fig. 2). Again, this is a favorable property for an ADC allowing greater cytotoxic efficacy.

4.5 Accessibility

Hematopoietic/liquid tumors are the most accessible to circulating ADC where the tumor cells are effectively bathed in ADC-containing plasma. It is no coincidence that the two first ADCs attaining FDA approval were CD33-pos AML (gemtuzumab ozogamicin) and CD30-pos lymphomas (brentuximab vedotin). Solid tumors present a significantly higher hurdle, but there are exceptions. For example, breast cancer, where T-DM1 is approaching regulatory approval, is a cancer that spreads predominately to lymph nodes and bone marrow—these are sites that "see" very high levels of circulating Ab, approaching those seen in plasma, due to their more porous endothelial junctions. Indeed, the same is true of PC, where the most common site of spread is bone marrow (85–90 % of patients) followed by lymph nodal disease (in 20–50 % of patients). In addition, the availability of a widely used biomarker in PC, prostate-specific antigen (PSA), provides a lead-time warning of tumor recurrence (which occurs in approximately 30 % of patients who undergo local treatment) of several years before visible on imaging studies. At the time of PSA elevation, the tumor burden is measurable in grams, substantially lower than at the time of imagable recurrence of other solid tumor types. This allows initiation of treatment at the time of a very small tumor burden when metastases are composed of small clusters of cells primarily in bone marrow (Fig. 4). As a result, ADC penetration of

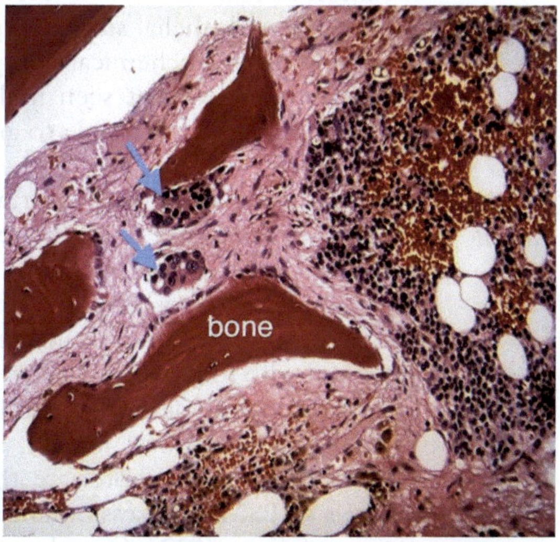

Fig. 4 A bone marrow biopsy showing two small islands of PC metastases (*arrows*) adjacent to bone spicules. These small islands of tumor cells would be very accessible to circulating Ab/ADC

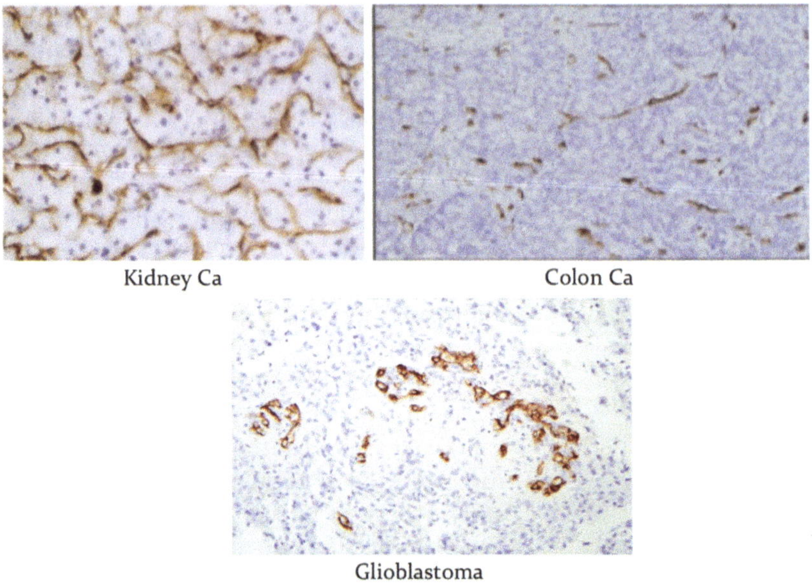

Fig. 5 Examples of three different solid tumor types demonstrating PSMA expression (*stained brown*) by neovascular endothelium

tumor in this setting approaches that of hematopoietic tumors and exceeds that of any other solid tumor. As a result, at the macro level, i.e., sites of disease, and at a micro level—tumor burden and antigen target accessibility—PC represents a very favorable target.

Another therapeutic opportunity for the PSMA target relates to its expression on the neo-vasculature of virtually all types of solid tumor, but not by normal vasculature [17–21] (Fig. 5). Expression is on the endothelial surface exposed to the circulation, and based on immunohistochemical comparisons, expression levels are in a similar range to that seen in PC. Obviously, neovascular PSMA would be highly accessible to an ADC.

4.6 Identifying the Appropriate Patient Population

We discussed above the importance of being able to identify appropriate patients and gave the example of her2-targeted therapies. In the case of PSMA, we have previously mentioned that 95 % of PC are PSMA positive. Indeed, when we began using mAbs to PSMA to target disease in clinical trials, we considered any PC patient who met the clinical criteria to be eligible. While the immunopathological data from multiple labs [8–16] covering almost 1,500 patients does, indeed, support this point, we have more recently come to appreciate that there are significantly different levels of PSMA expression among patients even when at the same state of disease [22]. Our planar imaging studies done in well >100 patients show that we can target PC, virtually flawlessly, in 90–95 % of patients (Fig. 6), consistent with the immunopathological data.

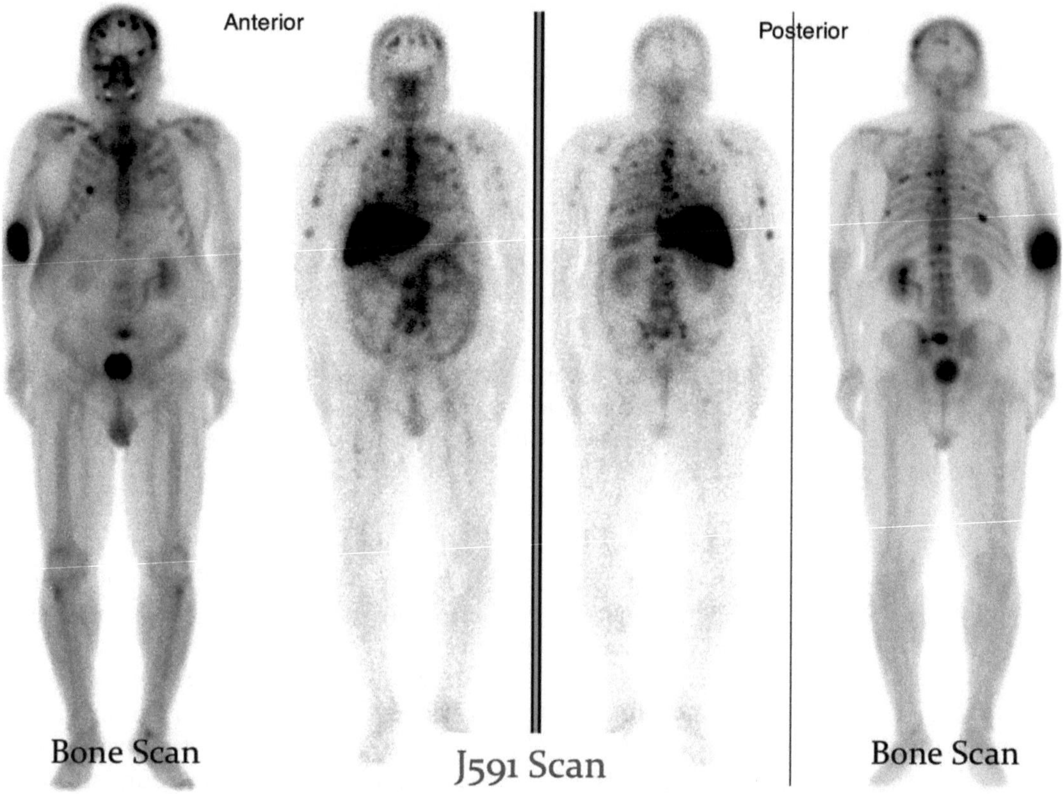

Fig. 6 Representative planar images of a patient with PC. Far *left* and far *right panels* represent anterior and posterior ^{99m}technetium methylene diphosphonate (MDP) bone scan images, respectively. *Center panels* show radiolabeled J591 mAb anterior and posterior images allowing direct comparison to bone scan. In a bone scan, the radioisotope is excreted by the urinary tract (note obstructed left kidney and bladder); in the Ab scan, the radiometal is excreted by the liver. Also apparent in the bone scan is right antecubital fossa extravasation of the isotope at the injection site. Note that every bone lesion seen on the bone scan is visible on the J591 Ab scan. In addition, the Ab scan picks up many more (true positive) lesions than the bone scan. The *midline* abdominal uptake on the anterior J591 Ab image represents retroperitoneal nodal disease that obstructed the *left* kidney

But these images, while nonquantitative, suggest that there is a wide range of expression level. Our preliminary impression suggests that there is a correlation between the image intensity (corresponding to expression level) and the likelihood of response. As a result, as our clinical trials are maturing, we have begun incorporating studies to define the small group of PC patients who are PSMA negative and exclude them, and we also plan to use quantitative analyses, either PSMA PET imaging or analysis of circulating tumor cells to define the patient subset with the highest level of expression who would be the best candidates for a PSMA ADC. Certainly, we'd anticipate that similar approaches can and will be brought to bear with other targets, and we are aware, for

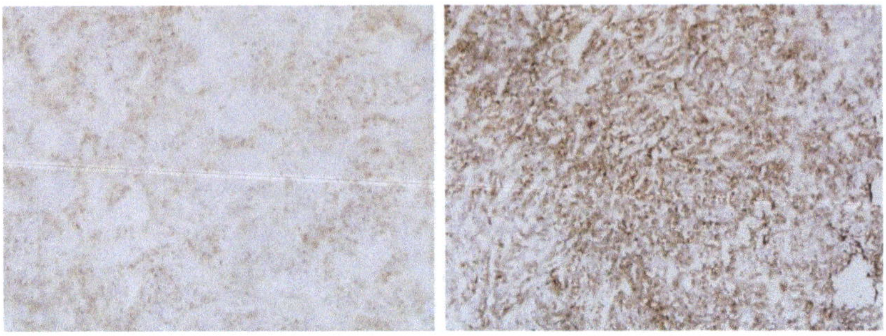

Fig. 7 Example of PC cell line (CWR22Rv1) that expresses low levels of PSMA in a non-castrate animal. After castration, PSMA expression increases considerably as demonstrated by immunohistochemistry. In vitro, this cell line increases PSMA expression by four- to fivefold after castration. The increase can also be detected by J591 PET imaging [25]

example, that effort is underway to develop PET imaging of her2 [23] which may become clinically useful in this setting as well to further improve patient selection.

In the case of neovascular expression, we have noted that PSMA is expressed by virtually every type of solid tumor yet the proportion of cases that are PSMA positive vary from one tumor type to another [22]. In addition, we have also found that the intensity of expression can also vary, again suggesting that ways to identify optimal patients will be very valuable.

4.7 Can Target Expression Be Modulated

An interesting property of PSMA is that its expression is androgen-regulated; when patients are placed on hormonal therapy, it induces upregulation of PSMA. In vitro data suggests [24] that PSMA can be upregulated by as much as 80-fold. We have also found that this upregulation occurs even in so-called "castrate-resistant" or "androgen-insensitive" PC models (Fig. 7). Using xenograft models of such a castrate-resistant tumor, we have shown that one can increase antitumor efficacy of an ADC [24]. Fortuitously, not only are antiandrogenic agents approved for use, but they also represent the cornerstone of treatment for this disease. In addition to directly enhancing tumor efficacy, this approach also improves the therapeutic window as modulating the androgen receptor (AR) and upregulation of the PSMA target occurs only in the AR-positive PC cells and not the normal tissues that express PSMA but are AR negative. This phenomenon of target upregulation, which we have termed "conditionally enhanced vulnerability/sensitivity," may be feasible in other target/tumor types. One can easily set up screens to potentially identify agents capable of upregulating the target of interest.

5 Conclusions

There is little doubt that weaving together the necessary components of an ADC requires optimal execution with respect to all of the components of the agent—antibody, linker, and drug. But it also requires a target that must meet equally stringent criteria, and the target is subject to few if any manipulations by the drug developer. Based on the criteria outlined above, it is likely that there are a relatively small number of tumor targets that would be optimal for ADC targeting. Moreover, with the requirement for high level expression in order for current cytotoxic agents to be effective, it is likely that most good targets have already been identified. Development of innovative ways to identify novel, specific, but lower level expressed targets is unlikely to yield many new targets unless more potent cytotoxics are developed, and this in turn would put further constraints of the performance of the linker.

References

1. Jain RK (1990) Physiological barriers to delivery of monoclonal antibodies and macromolecules in tumors. Cancer Res 50:814s–819s, PMID 2404582
2. Primeau AJ, Rendon A, Hedley D et al (2005) The distribution of the anticancer drug doxorubicin in relation to blood vessels in solid tumors. Clin Cancer Res 11:8782–8788, PMID 16361566
3. Horoszewicz JS, Kawinski E, Murphy GP (1987) Monoclonal antibodies to a new antigenic marker in epithelial prostatic cells and serum of prostatic cancer patients. Anticancer Res 7:927–936, PMID 2449118
4. Israeli RS, Powell CT, Fair WR et al (1994) Molecular cloning of a complementary DNA encoding a prostate-specific membrane antigen. Cancer Res 53:227–230, PMID 8417812
5. Smith-Jones PM, Vallabahajosula S, Goldsmith SJ et al (2000) In vitro characterization of radiolabeled monoclonal antibodies specific for the extracellular domain of prostate specific membrane antigen. Cancer Res 60:5237–5243, PMID 11016653
6. Israeli RS, Powell CT, Corr JG et al (1994) Expression of the prostate-specific membrane antigen. Cancer Res 54:1807–1811, PMID 7511053
7. Sokoloff RL, Norton KC, Gasior CL et al (2000) A dual-monoclonal sandwich assay for prostate-specific membrane antigen: levels in tissues, seminal fluid and urine. Prostate 43:150–157, PMID 10754531
8. Liu H, Rajasekaran AK, Moy P et al (1998) Constitutive and antibody-induced internalization of prostate-specific membrane antigen. Cancer Res 58:4055–4060, PMID 9751609
9. Wright GL Jr, Haley C, Beckett ML et al (1995) Expression of prostate-specific membrane antigen (PSMA) in normal, benign and malignant prostate tissues. Urol Oncol 1:18–28
10. Troyer JK, Beckett ML, Wright GL Jr (1995) Detection and characterization of the prostate-specific membrane antigen (PSMA) in tissue extracts and body fluids. Int J Cancer 62:552–558, PMID7665226
11. Wright GLJ, Grob BM, Haley C et al (1996) Upregulation of prostate-specific membrane antigen after androgen-deprivation therapy. Urology 48:326–334, PMID 8753752
12. Sweat SD, Pacelli A, Murphy GP et al (1998) PSMA expression is greatest in prostate adenocarcinoma and lymph node metastases. Urology 52:637–640, PMID 8763054
13. Bostwick DG, Pacelli A, Blute M et al (1998) Prostate specific membrane antigen expression in prostatic intraepithelial neoplasia and adenocarcinoma: a study of 184 cases. Cancer 82:2256–2261, PMID 9610707
14. Mannweiler S, Amersdorfer P, Trajanoski S et al (2009) Heterogeneity of prostate-specific membrane antigen (PSMA) expression in prostate carcinoma with distant metastasis. Pathol Oncol Res 15(2):167–172, PMID 18802790

15. Kusumi T, Koie T, Tanaka M et al (2008) Immunohistochemical detection of carcinoma in radical prostatectomy specimens following hormone therapy. Pathol Int 58:687–694, PMID 18844933
16. Ananias HJ, van den Heuvel MC, Helfrich W et al (2009) Expression of the gastrin-releasing peptide receptor, the prostate stem cell antigen and the prostate-specific membrane antigen in lymph node and bone metastases of prostate cancer. Prostate 69:1101–1108, PMID 19343734
17. Liu H, Moy P, Kim S et al (1997) Monoclonal antibodies to the extracellular domain of prostate specific membrane antigen also react with tumor vascular endothelium. Cancer Res 57:3629–3634, PMID 9288760
18. Silver DA, Pellicer I, Fair WR et al (1997) Prostate-specific membrane antigen expression in normal and malignant human tissues. Clin Cancer Res 3:81–85, PMID 9815541
19. Chang SS, Reuter VE, Heston WD et al (1999) Five different anti-prostate-specific membrane antigen (PSMA) antibodies confirm PSMA expression in tumor-associated neovasculature. Cancer Res 59:3192–3198, PMID 10397265
20. Chang SS, O'Keefe DS, Bacich DJ et al (1999) Prostate-specific membrane antigen is produced in tumor-associated neovasculature. Clin Cancer Res 5:2674–2681, PMID 10537328
21. Al-Ahmadie HA, Olgac S, Gregor PD et al (2008) Expression of prostate-specific membrane antigen in renal cortical tumors. Mod Pathol 21:727–732, PMID 18344976
22. Dijkers EC, Oude Munnink TH, Kosterink JG et al (2010) Biodistribution of ^{89}Zr-trastuzumab and PET imaging of HER2-positive lesions in patients with metastatic breast cancer. Clin Pharmacol Ther 87:586–592, PMID 20357763
23. Haffner MC, Kronberger IE, Ross JS et al (2009) Prostate specific membrane antigen expression in the neovasculature of gastric and colorectal cancers. Hum Pathol 40:1754–1761, PMID 19716160
24. Kuroda K, Liu H, Li M et al. Androgen suppression, prostate-specific membrane antigen and the concept of conditionally enhanced vulnerability. Manusc Submitted
25. Evans MJ, Smith-Jones PM, Wongvipat J et al (2011) Non-invasive measurement of androgen receptor signaling with ^{64}Cu-J591, a positron emitting radiopharmaceutical that targets prostate-specific membrane antigen. Proc Natl Acad Sci U S A 108:9578–9582

Chapter 3

Selecting an Optimal Antibody for Antibody–Drug Conjugate Therapy: Internalization and Intracellular Localization

Jay Harper, Shenlan Mao, Patrick Strout, and Adeela Kamal

Abstract

Antibody–drug conjugates (ADCs) combine the selectivity of a monoclonal antibody with the killing potency of a cytotoxic drug. For an antibody to function as a successful component of an ADC, it needs to bind to the target antigen on the surface of tumor cells and then be internalized by the cell. Following internalization, the ADC has to be transported to the lysosome where subsequent intracellular processing of the ADC will release the biologically active drug to exert its cytotoxic effects on tumor cells. This chapter describes some of the techniques that are currently used to determine internalization and proper intracellular trafficking of antibodies in order to select an optimal antibody for ADC therapeutics.

Key words Antibodies, Antibody–drug conjugate, Internalization, Flow cytometry, Confocal microscopy

1 Introduction

ADCs are composed of an antibody that has a drug (commonly referred to as a warhead) conjugated to it through either a cleavable or a non-cleavable linker [1]. Typically these warheads are very potent cytotoxic agents that cannot be used as a stand-alone chemotherapy because of severe dose-limiting toxicities associated with killing normal cells. However, coupling these highly potent agents with a targeting molecule, in this case an antibody, can successfully deliver these drugs directly to the tumor with decreased off-target toxicities, a strategy that is clinically validated with the recent approvals of brentuximab vedotin (Adcetris) [2] and trastuzumab emtansine (Kadcyla [3]). The key is to identify the right antibody that will help deliver the drug to the tumor while maintaining the ability of the drug to be effective.

In order for an antibody to be successful as an ADC, it not only needs to bind specifically to the surface of antigen-positive cells in the tumor, but that antigen–antibody interaction generally has to result in internalization of the ADC [4, 5]. Following internalization,

Laurent Ducry (ed.), *Antibody-Drug Conjugates*, Methods in Molecular Biology, vol. 1045,
DOI 10.1007/978-1-62703-541-5_3, © Springer Science+Business Media, LLC 2013

the ADC needs to be shuttled into the proper intracellular compartment, typically the lysosome, for subsequent degradation of the ADC and release of the toxic compound to elicit killing of these cells. Therefore three parameters need to be considered when screening antibodies for use in an effective ADC strategy: binding, internalization, and intracellular localization of the antibody following internalization.

There are no set parameters that correlate optimal binding affinities and/or internalization rates of antibodies with maximal efficacy of an ADC; however, it is typically regarded that the tighter an antibody can bind and the faster it can be internalized, the more effective it may be as an ADC therapy [6]. However, these are merely guidelines and a good example of an outlier would be Kadcyla. This ADC is very potent at inhibiting tumor growth, and its component antibody, trastuzumab (Herceptin), has a high binding affinity but has a relatively slow internalization rate compared to other antibodies used as ADCs [7, 8]. The final key to determine if an antibody may represent a good candidate for an ADC therapy is to ensure that the antibody, following internalization, is transported to the correct intracellular compartment for subsequent processing and release of the warhead, and this can be accomplished through colocalization experiments via confocal microscopy.

Several modalities such as Biacore analysis are available to determine affinities of antibodies, but this chapter will detail some of the techniques commonly used to determine relative rates of internalization of antibodies and those used to determine localization of antibodies following internalization. These can be used to screen for optimal antibodies to be used as an ADC therapeutic; however, it should be noted that an antibody that has a high affinity for a target and good internalization kinetics may still not be effective as an ADC [9]. Changes to the antibody following conjugation of a payload could alter the properties of the antibody and interfere with any of the three critical aspects described above. Therefore, while these assays could help improve the process for selecting an ideal antibody for an ADC, the final test would be to determine cytotoxicity of that ADC in in vitro and in vivo models. Subsequently, these assays can be utilized to determine if an ineffective ADC is nonfunctional due to losing the ability to bind, internalize, and/or localize properly once warheads have been conjugated to the antibody.

Internalization of an ADC is critical to its efficacy, and several methods of measuring internalization are routinely used, including confocal microscopy, assays with radiolabeled antibodies/ADCs, and flow cytometry. The first protocol described here represents a flow cytometry-based assay developed for measuring the internalization of purified antibody without the need to label the antibody directly with fluorophores or radiolabels.

Following internalization of an ADC, particularly ones with protease-labile linkers, they need to be transported to the proper intracellular compartment, typically the lysosome, for processing to release the drug. An assay is provided that can be utilized to determine colocalization of internalized antibodies to the lysosome to help select candidate antibodies for ADC therapeutics.

2 Materials

2.1 Flow-Based Internalization Assay Components

Store all reagents at 4 °C (unless indicated otherwise). Adhere to local waste disposal regulations when disposing of waste materials.

1. Phosphate-buffered saline (PBS), pH 7.2 (Invitrogen).
2. 0.25 % trypsin–EDTA (Invitrogen).
3. FACS staining buffer: PBS supplemented with 2 % heat-inactivated fetal bovine serum (Invitrogen).
4. Purified candidate antibodies.
5. Secondary antibody labeled with fluorescence: e.g., Alexa Fluor 488 Goat Anti-Human IgG (H + L) antibody (Invitrogen).
6. Polystyrene round-bottom 12 mm × 75 mm tubes (Falcon).
7. 15 or 50 ml conical centrifuge tubes (VWR).
8. Pipettes and tips (VWR).
9. Ice bucket with wet ice.
10. Refrigerated centrifuge.
11. Flow cytometer: e.g., FACSCalibur with CellQuest analysis software (BD Biosciences).
12. Vortex mixer (e.g., Fisher Scientific).

2.2 Intracellular Localization Assay Components

1. Phosphate-buffered saline (PBS), pH 7.2 (Invitrogen).
2. Slides: Lab-Tek™ Chamber Slide™ system (NUNC) (*see* **Note 1**).
3. Paraformaldehyde: 32 % paraformaldehyde diluted to 3.7 % working concentration (Electron Microscopy Sciences).
4. Blocking solution: 2 % FBS (Invitrogen) in PBS pH 7.2.
5. Permeabilization solution: 10 % Triton X-100, diluted to 0.5 % working concentration (G-Biosciences).
6. Slide mounting media: ProLong® Gold Antifade Reagent with DAPI (Invitrogen).
7. Coverslips (VWR).
8. Antibodies.
   (a) Candidate antibodies.
   (b) Mouse antihuman LAMP1 primary antibody (BD Biosciences).

(c) Alexa Fluor 488 Goat Anti-Human IgG (H + L) secondary antibody (Invitrogen) (*see* **Note 2**).

(d) Alexa Fluor 647 Goat Anti-Mouse IgG (H + L) secondary antibody (Invitrogen).

3 Methods

3.1 Flow-Based Internalization Assay

Carry out all procedures on ice or at 4 °C and use ice cold reagents unless otherwise specified.

1. Harvest cells: For cells that grow in suspension, decant the cells into a conical centrifuge tube. For adherent cells, use trypsin–EDTA buffer (*see* **Note 3**) to detach cells from culture flask or dish, and place cells into a conical centrifuge tube. Measure viability of cells via trypan blue exclusion (*see* **Note 4**) and pellet the cells by centrifugation at 300 × *g* at 4 °C for 5 min. Add FACS staining buffer to wash once. Centrifuge cells and resuspend in an appropriate volume of FACS staining buffer so that the final cell concentration is 2×10^7/ml.
2. Prepare cells for staining: Aliquot 50 μl (1×10^6) of cell suspension to each tube (*see* **Notes 5** and **6**). Ideally, samples should be run in duplicate or triplicate to ensure accuracy of results.
3. Cell surface binding of antibody (*see* **Note 7**): Combine the recommended quantity (final concentration 1–20 μg/ml; *see* **Note 8**) of each unlabeled primary antibody in an appropriate volume of FACS staining buffer so that the final staining volume is 100 μl (i.e., 50 μl of cell sample + 50 μl of antibody) and add to cells. Gently pulse vortex to mix and incubate for 60 min on ice.
4. Wash unbound antibody: Wash the cells by adding 2 ml of FACS staining buffer to remove unbound antibody. Pellet the cells by centrifugation at 300 × *g* at 4 °C for 5 min. Repeat for a total of two washes, discarding supernatants between washes (*see* **Note 9**).
5. Internalization of bound antibody at 37 °C: Add 200 μl of FACS staining buffer into each tube, and incubate each tube of cells at 37 °C for various time points from 15 min to 2 h to internalize surface-bound antibody. For each time point, incubate another tube of cells at 4 °C as a negative control without internalization. At specified time points, transfer appropriate tubes of cells incubating at 37 °C to ice and add 2 ml ice cold FACS staining buffer to terminate internalization. Also add 2 ml of ice cold FACS staining buffer to control tube incubated at 4 °C for the same duration. Pellet the cells by centrifugation at 300 × *g* at 4 °C for 5 min.

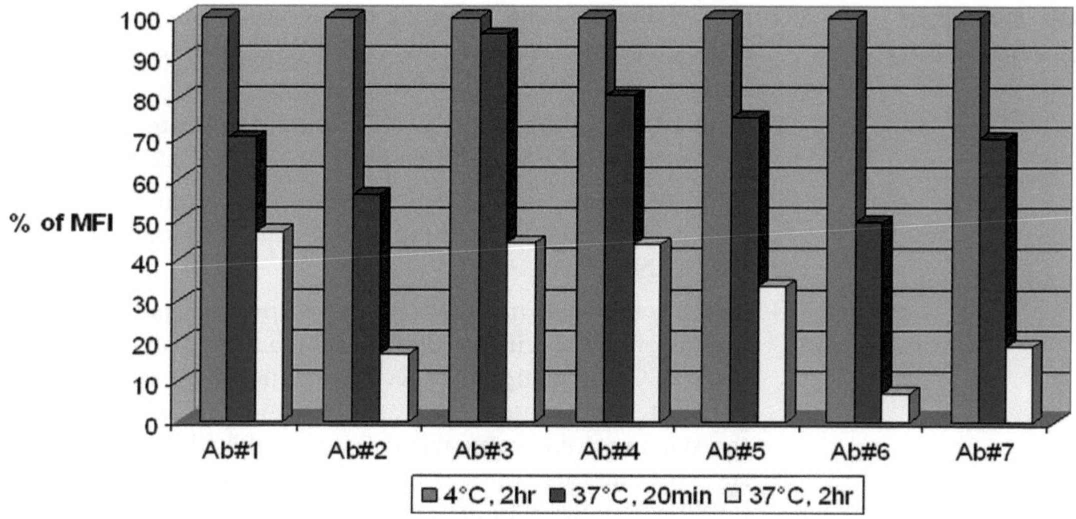

Fig. 1 Internalization of seven candidate antibodies. Prostate cancer cells were treated with 10 μg/ml of candidate antibodies at 4 °C for 1 h. After washing, the cells were incubated at 37 °C to allow for internalization. At 20 min and 2 h time points, cell samples were taken and stained with a FITC-labeled secondary antibody at 4 °C. The results show that prostate cancer cells internalized between ca. 53 % (Ab#1) and ca. 92 % (Ab#6) of cell surface-bound antibodies within 2 h

6. Stain cells with a fluorescently labeled secondary antibody to detect surface-bound antibody: Add 20 μl of Alexa Fluor 488 Goat Anti-Human IgG (H + L) antibody (or any appropriate amount of anti-mouse or antihuman IgG fluorescence-labeled secondary antibody; *see* **Note 8**) into tubes and incubate 30 min at 4 °C in the dark.
7. Wash unbound secondary antibody: Add 2 ml of FACS staining buffer into each tube. Pellet the cells by centrifugation at 300 × *g* at 4 °C for 5 min. Repeat for a total of two washes, discarding supernatants between washes. Resuspend stained cells in 500 μl ice cold PBS (*see* **Note 10**).
8. Measure the fluorescence intensity on the cell surface via flow cytometry. For best results, analyze the cells on the flow cytometer as soon as possible (*see* **Note 11**).
9. The degree of internalization of cell surface-bound antibody is determined by the percentage decrease of mean fluorescence intensity (MFI) of samples incubated at 37 °C compared to control samples incubated at 4 °C (Fig. 1). The formulas for calculating the internalization percentage and the percentage of cell surface-bound antibodies (% of MFI) after incubation at 37 °C at each time point (t_x) compared with control samples incubated at 4 °C are:
   (a) % of MFI t_x = MFI of sample incubated at 37 °C/MFI of control sample incubated at 4 °C × 100.
   (b) Internalization percentage (% t_x) of cell surface-bound antibodies = 100 − % of MFI t_x.

3.2 Intracellular Localization Assay

1. Plate 100,000 cells per well into 4-well chamber slides in cell-specific media containing 10 % FBS. Allow cells to culture 48 h.
2. After a 48 h culture, remove cells from the incubator, rinse each well once with PBS, and then place on wet ice (*see* **Note 12**).
3. Add 10 μg of total conjugated or unconjugated antibody to each well, diluted into 250 μl of PBS. Incubate on wet ice for 1 h (*see* **Note 13**).
4. Aspirate the supernatant from the chambers, and add up to 500 μl of cell-specific media to each chamber, and place in a 37 °C CO_2 incubator for specific time points to observe antibody internalization, typically 30 min and 1, 4, and 24 h. For the starting point comparator, a "Time 0" slide, aspirate the supernatant, rinse once with cold PBS, and keep on wet ice until you are ready to fix (*see* **Note 14**).
5. At each selected time point, remove slide or slides from the incubator, and rinse once with cold PBS. To fix cells, add 250 μl of freshly prepared 3.7 % paraformaldehyde at room temperature (*see* **Note 15**). Allow cells to fix for 20 min and then wash cells twice with room temperature PBS (*see* **Note 16**).
6. To permeabilize cells, add 250 μl of 0.5 % Triton X-100 to each chamber, and allow cells to sit at room temperature for 5 min. Again, wash cells twice with PBS after this permeabilization step.
7. To probe for primary antibody, add 2 μg of fluorophore-conjugated secondary antibody against the primary host species (e.g., in this case a goat antihuman secondary antibody is used) in 250 μl of blocking solution (as described in Subheading 2) and incubate for 1 h at room temperature. Conduct two washes with PBS following incubation with the secondary antibody.
8. To probe for lysosomes, add primary LAMP1 antibody to slides at a 1:50 dilution for 1 h at room temperature. Wash slides twice with PBS after primary antibody incubation.
9. To probe for primary LAMP1 antibody, incubate slides with 2 μg of total fluorophore-conjugated secondary antibody against the host species, in this case goat anti-mouse secondary antibody. Prepare dilution, and add 250 μl of diluted secondary antibody to each chamber. Allow to incubate at room temperature for 1 h. Wash slides twice in PBS.
10. Aspirate off remaining PBS from wash steps, and remove plastic chamber and silicon gasket from slide. Mount slides using ProLong® Gold Antifade Reagent with DAPI, and follow manufacturer's instructions for the setting and preservation of slides.
11. Colocalization can be visualized using a fluorescent microscope (*see* **Note 17**), preferably a confocal microscope (Fig. 2).

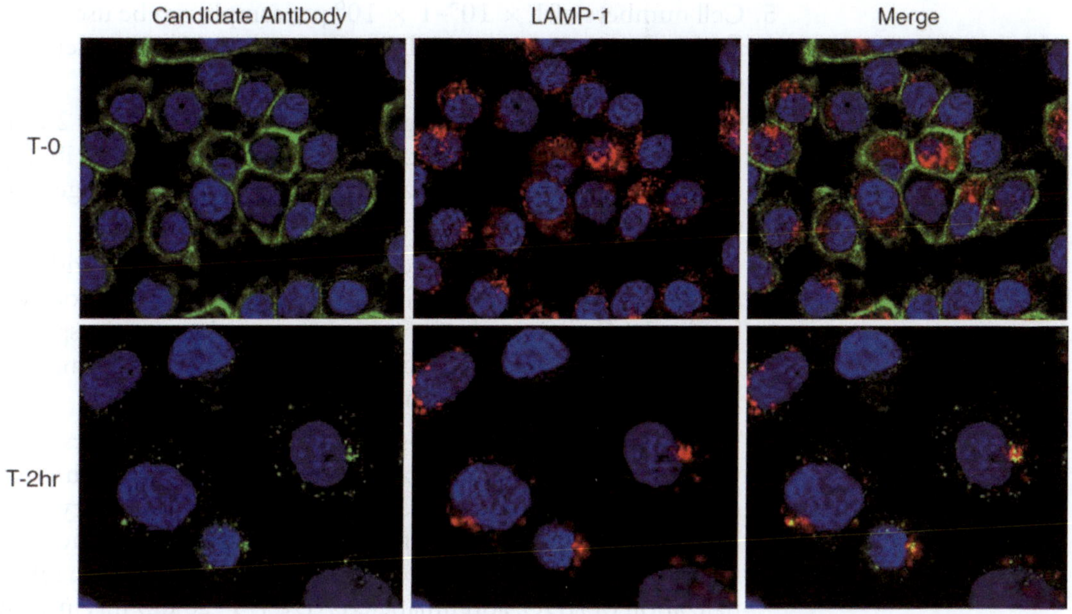

Fig. 2 Internalization and subcellular localization of primary antibody into antigen-positive cells. Confocal fluorescence microscopy was used to image primary antibody (*green*) and LAMP-1 (*red*). Primary antibody was incubated with cells for 1 h on ice, and then antibody was allowed to internalize into cells for the indicated time points. Cells were immediately fixed, permeabilized, and probed for primary antibody and LAMP-1 with fluorescent-conjugated secondary antibodies. The *left image* depicts the location of the primary antibody; the *center image* depicts the location of LAMP-1, a lysosome marker; and the *far right images* are a merge of the *left* and *center images*

4 Notes

1. Chamber slides are available in both chambered soda lime glass and plastic (Permanox™). In our hands, we have observed that using the plastic chamber slides improved cell adherence, without increasing background fluorescence, which also maximized the available cells to be imaged after fixation, permeabilization, and staining.
2. The secondary antibody that you choose will be dependent on the species from which your candidate antibody is derived, typically either human or mouse.
3. The adherent cell can be dissociated with trypsin–EDTA or other cell dissociation buffer without trypsin.
4. Cells should be greater than 90 % viable as determined by trypan blue exclusion using a hemocytometer or automated cell counting device (e.g., the Vi-Cell Cell Viability Analyzer by Beckman Coulter, Inc.).

5. Cell numbers of 1×10^5–1×10^6 per sample can be used, and it is preferable to use as high a cell count as possible to ensure optimal signal.
6. Cells are usually stained in polystyrene round-bottom 12 mm × 75 mm Falcon tubes. However, they can be stained in any container for which you have an appropriate centrifuge, for example, 96-well round-bottom microtiter plates.
7. As an option to further reduce nonspecific binding and Fc-mediated interactions, preincubate the cells with blocking buffer (FACS staining buffer with 1 % normal sera of the species from which the secondary antibody is derived or 0.1 mg/ml IgG of said species) for 20 min on ice prior to staining.
8. The secondary antibody chosen will depend on the species from which the candidate antibody is derived, such as human or mouse. The concentration used for primary and secondary antibodies and the incubation time with the antibodies will need to be optimized for various experiments. For measuring the internalization of ADC, add unlabeled ADCs (1–20 μg/ml) instead of purified primary antibody in **step 3** of Subheading 3.1.
9. After each centrifugation, carefully aspirate (for microwell plates or tubes) or invert and blot away (for tubes) supernatants from cell pellets. Resuspend cells with gentle vortexing.
10. For certain cell types that are sensitive to this procedure, decreasing viability may be observed. When this occurs, a dye can be added to measure viability (e.g., propidium iodide) of each sample in order to exclude dead cells from flow cytometry analysis. Also, in these cases it is highly recommended to determine the fluorescence intensity on the cells by flow cytometry as soon as possible without fixation (*see* **Note 11** below).
11. It is recommend to conduct flow cytometry analysis on the same day that cell staining is performed. For extended storage (> 4h) as well as for greater flexibility in planing time on the flow cytometer, the cells can be fixed with 1 % paraformaldehyde in PBS and stored at 4 °C in the dark after **step 7**. This can preserve them for at least several days. Unstained control cells will require fixation using the same procedure.
12. Prior to the addition of primary antibody to the cells, allow cells to sit in cold PBS on ice. In addition, only use cold PBS to prepare dilutions of primary antibody. Keep all antibody dilutions on ice prior to adding them to chamber slides.
13. Concentration of the primary antibody should be adjusted to properly image the antigen of interest. Here, 10 μg of total primary antibody is used to image a well-expressed antigen, but anywhere between 5 and 20 μg of total antibody per chamber has been used to image other antigens.

14. Aspirating media and PBS from chamber slides through the use of a trap is possible; however, we have found that simple pipette aspiration from the chambers reduces disturbance of the cells, especially through many wash steps.
15. Prepare fresh paraformaldehyde for each experiment.
16. If longer internalization time points are being explored (8–24 h), chamber slides can be fixed in paraformaldehyde, washed twice, and stored in cold PBS overnight (after **step 5** in Subheading 3.2) or until such time as it is convenient to stain all time points together.
17. We use a confocal microscope to image all slides, primarily using an oil immersion 63× objective.

References

1. Ducry L, Stump B (2010) Antibody–drug conjugates: linking cytotoxic payloads to monoclonal antibodies. Bioconjug Chem 21:5–13
2. Katz J, Janik JE, Younes A (2011) Brentuximab vedotin (SGN-35). Clin Cancer Res 17: 6428–6436
3. Verma S, Miles D, Gianni L, Krop IE, Welslau M, Baselga J, Pegram M, Oh DY, Dieras V, Guardino E, Fang L, Lu MW, Olsen S, Blackwell K (2012) Trastuzumab emtansine for HER2-positive advanced breast cancer. N Engl J Med 367:1783–1791
4. Alley SC, Okeley NM, Senter PD (2010) Antibody–drug conjugates: targeted drug delivery for cancer. Curr Opin Chem Biol 14:529–537
5. Polson AG, Calemine-Fanaux J, Chan P, Chang W, Christensen E, Clark S, de Sauvage FJ, Eaton D, Elkins K, Elliot JM, Frantz G, Fuji RN, Gray A, Harden K, Ingle GS, Kljavin NM, Koeppen H, Nelson C, Prabju S, Raab H, Ross S, Stephan J-P, Scales SJ, Spencer SD, Vandlen R, Wranik B, Yu S-F, Zheng B, Ebens A (2009) Antibody–drug conjugates for the treatment of non-Hodgkin's lymphoma: target and linker-drug selection. Cancer Res 69:2358–2364
6. Carter PJ, Senter PD (2008) Antibody–drug conjugates for cancer therapy. Cancer J 14:154–169
7. Lewis Phillips GD, Li G, Dugger DL, Crocker LM, Parsons KL, Mai E, Blättler WA, Lambert JM, Chari RVJ, Lutz RJ, Wong WLT, Jacobson FS, Koeppen H, Schwall RH, Kenkare-Mitra SR, Spencer SD, Sliwkowski MX (2008) Targeting HER2-positive breast cancer with trastuzumab-DM1, and antibody-cytotoxic drug conjugate. Cancer Res 68:9280–9290
8. Hommelgaard AM, Lerdrup M, van Deurs B (2004) Association with membrane protrusions makes ErbB2 an internalization-resistant receptor. Mol Biol Cell 15:1557–1567
9. Rudnick SI, Lou J, Shaller CC, Tang Y, Klein-Szanto AJ, Weiner LM, Marks JD, Adams GP et al (2011) Influence of affinity and antigen internalization on the uptake and penetration of anti-HER2 antibodies in solid tumors. Cancer Res 71:2250–2259

Chapter 4

Antibody–Drug Conjugate Payloads

Jan Anderl, Heinz Faulstich, Torsten Hechler, and Michael Kulke

Abstract

Toxin payloads, or drugs, are the crucial components of therapeutic antibody–drug conjugates (ADCs). This review will give an introduction on the requirements that make a toxic compound suitable to be used in an antitumoral ADC and will summarize the structural and mechanistic features of four drug families that yielded promising results in preclinical and clinical studies.

Key words Payload, Maytansine, DM1, DM4, Auristatin, MMAE, MMAF, Calicheamicin, Amatoxin, Amanitin

1 Introduction

The use of monoclonal antibodies (mAbs) as therapeutics for the treatment of malignancies has been established in clinical practice around 15 years ago [1]. Today cancer care is not imaginable without the arsenal of mAbs approved for solid tumors, leukemias, and lymphomas. Despite this success there are still limitations regarding the antitumoral efficacy of mAbs, so that attempts are ongoing to further improve the potency of antibody therapeutics. Such strategies include the conjugation of mAbs to radionuclides, fusion with protein toxins (immunotoxins), or coupling to small molecule drugs (antibody–drug conjugates, ADCs). Radionuclide-immunoconjugate strategies and the current state of immunotoxin developments are not within the scope of this article and have been reviewed in great detail elsewhere [2–4].

The rationale for ADCs is to combine the selective targeting capacity of mAbs by specifically binding to tumor-associated antigens with the cytotoxic potency of small molecule drugs or toxins [5–8]. Covalent coupling of a small molecule drug to a macromolecule such as an IgG promises toxin enrichment in tumor tissues by simultaneously sparing nontarget tissues, solubility enhancement of hydrophobic compounds, and plasma half-life elongation by prevention of renal clearance, altogether resulting in a widening of the

Laurent Ducry (ed.), *Antibody-Drug Conjugates*, Methods in Molecular Biology, vol. 1045,
DOI 10.1007/978-1-62703-541-5_4, © Springer Science+Business Media, LLC 2013

therapeutic window. There are myriads of cellular toxins known in nature and synthetic chemistry, but only a few poisonous structures and even fewer modes of actions have been found adaptable for an ADC concept, since the toxin to be used as ADC payload has to combine the following complex properties:

1. The cytotoxic potency of a payload has to be extremely high, as a limited tumor penetration of IgGs, low expression of antigens, inefficient internalization, and linker metabolization may result in very low toxin concentrations in the cell. There is data from patients that demonstrated that as little as 0.0003–0.08 % of an injected antibody dose is localized per gram of tumor, underlining the need for toxins that achieve cell killing at lowest concentrations [9]. Therefore, payloads affecting cellular targets that are involved in fundamental cell viability processes and are present in low copy numbers only will ensure high cytotoxic activity in the genetically heterogeneous environment of a tumor tissue and will prevent escape of cancer cells by any resistance mechanism.
2. The target of the payload must be located inside the cell, as most of today's ADC strategies depend on internalization of the toxin conjugates, starting with endocytosis of the ADC–antigen complex, lysosomal degradation of the antibody or the linker, and, finally, release of the payload into cytoplasm of the cell. Many of the highly potent toxins from microorganisms, plants, and animals act on cells from outside, e.g., on neuronal cells by blocking ion channels, or on disturbances of blood clotting and are thus unsuited for use as ADC payloads.
3. The molecular structure of a payload has to be small in size, thereby reducing the risk of immunogenicity; also, it should have reasonable solubility in aqueous buffers to facilitate conjugation to antibodies; finally, it should have a sufficient stability in plasma considering the long half-life of antibody drugs in circulation. Despite its limited structural possibilities, the toxin should allow the conjugation of a linker. And when used with a noncleavable linker, it should retain toxic potency even when bound to a protein fragment after antibody degradation, e.g., as lysine conjugate or as a thiol derivative after intracellular reduction of a disulfide linkage.

Facing the hurdles mentioned above, the ADCs described in literature are based on a limited number of toxic payloads targeting one of the three following cellular structures: tubulin filaments, DNA, and RNA (*see* Table 1). Not all of the toxins belonging to these three classes proved successful. In early immunoconjugates, approved chemotherapeutics like doxorubicin [10–12], vinca alkaloids [13–15], and methotrexate [16–18] actually failed to show sufficient antitumoral activity in clinical studies. On the other hand,

Table 1
Cellular targets and the corresponding toxin classes used as payloads in ADCs

Cellular target	Toxin
Tubulin filaments	Maytansinoids, auristatins, taxol derivatives [24, 25] (*vinca alkaloids*)
DNA	Calicheamicin, CC-1065 analogs [26, 27], duocarmycins [28] (*doxorubicin, methotrexate*)
RNA	Amanitin

Toxins which failed to confirm antitumoral activity as ADC payload in clinical trials are shown in italics

tubulin toxins from the group of maytansinoids [19, 20] and auristatins [21] and the DNA toxin calicheamicin [22], with potencies several orders of magnitude higher than conventional chemotherapeutics and hence without therapeutic window as free toxins, showed promising results as payloads in multiple clinical studies. ADCs based on such highly potent toxin structures gained market approval for the therapy of Hodgkin's lymphoma (Adcetris, brentuximab vedotin) and acute myelogenous leukemia AML (Mylotarg, gemtuzumab ozogamicin, withdrawn from market in 2010). The chemistry and use of maytansinoids, auristatins, and calicheamicin, along with that of amanitin [23], a transcription inhibitor studied in the authors' laboratory, will be described below.

2 Maytansinoids

Maytansinoids are a group of cytotoxins structurally similar to rifamycin, geldanamycin, and ansatrienin. The eponymous natural cytotoxic agent maytansine (**1**) is a 19-member lactam (ansa macrolide) structure originally isolated from the Ethiopian shrub *Maytenus ovatus* in 1972 (Fig. 1) [29]. The ansa macrolide is attached to a chlorinated benzene ring chromophore and contains carbinolamine, epoxide, or aryl functions [29, 30]. In the following years a variety of maytansine derivatives were isolated from bacteria (e.g., *Actinosynnema pretiosum*), mosses, and higher plants (e.g., *Colubrina texensis* or *Trewia nudiflora*), differing mainly in the C-3 position of the ester side chain [31, 32].

Maytansine and its derivatives are very potent inhibitors of microtubule assembly by binding to tubulin at or near the vinblastine-binding site [33–35], inducing mitotic arrest in the intoxicated cells, similar to the mode of action of vinblastine itself.

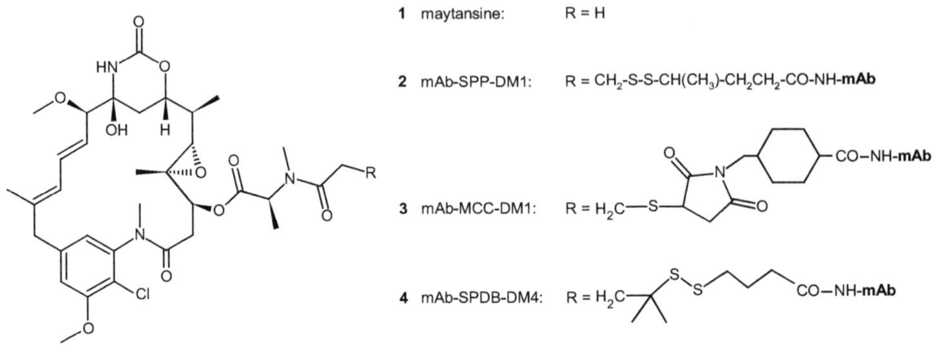

Fig. 1 Structure of maytansine (**1**) and maytansine-linker derivatives (**2–4**) used in ADCs

At low concentrations dynamic instability of microtubules and cell migration processes are suppressed, whereas at higher concentrations microtubule assembly and cell division are inhibited. The latter effect is likely a result of the generation of microtubule fragments destabilizing microtubule minus-end attachment to centrosomes and spindle poles. These effects result in an antiproliferative activity at mitosis shown to be effective in a variety of human cancer cell lines of the NIH-60 panel in vivo [32].

The antimitotic effect of maytansine at subnanomolar concentrations with an ED_{50} (effective dose) between 10^{-4} and 10^{-5} μg/ml [32] has made it an interesting candidate for anticancer drugs, and several attempts have been made to use it in clinical trials for cancer therapy [36]. Nevertheless, successful clinical use could not be established since the native substances did not elicit significant response in patients with different types of cancers. Severe side effects like neurotoxicity, gastrointestinal toxicity, weakness, nausea, vomiting, and diarrhea mainly due to the lack of tumor specificity of the toxin made its use doubtful [37]. Thus, despite of its high potency, maytansine (**1**) was ineffective in human clinical trials due to its high systemic toxicity resulting in a low therapeutic index. Nonetheless, their extremely high potency held the maytansinoids in the focus of research interest and brought them back to clinical development when the concept of ADCs arose in the early 1980s.

First attempts with antibody-conjugated maytansine derivatives have been made in the 1980s and early 1990s [38]. A variety of disulfide-containing maytansinoids were tested, all of which comprised a methyldithiopropanoyl group instead of the native *N*-acetyl group [38, 39]. It turned out very rapidly that the linker had a high influence on the usability of maytansine-based ADCs. Three types of linker comprising either a labile disulfide bond as in compound **2**, a hindered disulfide bond as in compound **4**, or a stable thioether bond as in compound **3** have been extensively tested (Fig. 1). A stabilized disulfide linker has been shown to

Table 2
Cellular targets and the corresponding toxin structures used as payloads in ADCs

Target	INN	Status (2011)
CD19	SAR4519	Clinical phase 1
CD33	AVE9633	Clinical phase 1
CD44v6	Bivatuzumab mertansine	Discontinued
CD56	IMGN901	Clinical phase 2
Her2	Trastuzumab-DM1	Clinical phase 3
MUC-1	IMGN242 cantuzumab mertansine	Clinical phase 2 discontinued
PSMA	MLN2704	Discontinued
Integrin	IMGN388	Clinical phase 1
Cripto	BIIB-015	Clinical phase 1
CD138	BT-062	Clinical phase 1/2
CA6	SAR566658	Clinical phase 1

combine several advantages since it can be modified in terms of stability during blood circulation while an efficient cleavage inside the cell can be maintained. Thus, the optimal balance between linker stability and antitumor activity can be adapted for each particular antibody [7]. For example, the prodrug-like structures *S*-methyl-DM1 and *S*-methyl-DM4, the thiomethyl derivatives of maytansine, undergo intracellular reduction by thiols like glutathione after cellular uptake while being sufficiently stable outside the cytosol. The release of membrane-permeable forms of DM1 and DM4 after cellular processing facilitates the killing of tumor cells lacking the particular epitope (bystander effect). Nevertheless, in preclinical studies with trastuzumab–maytansinoid conjugates, a stable, noncleavable, thioether linker (MCC) showed a higher efficacy and was better tolerated than conjugates with cleavable disulfide linkers, since the originally used disulfide linker (SPP) is inefficiently cleaved in the oxidizing environment of the endocytotic pathway [40, 41].

Maytansine-based ADCs entered clinical trials around the millennium turn with a set of different antibodies as carrier for the toxin (Table 2). Until now, from all promising candidates, trastuzumab-DM1 (trastuzumab emtansine, T-DM1), an ADC based on the humanized HER2 antibody, trastuzumab (Herceptin, approved by the FDA for use in metastatic breast cancer), is the most advanced substance. It entered clinical stage III in 2009 and is close to FDA approval [40, 42–45]. For T-DM1 a set of different linkers were tested. A stable non-reducible thioether linker (*N*-maleimidomethyl)cyclohexane-1-carboxylate (MCC) gave the best efficacy profile. It is believed that the drug binds to the antibody outside the cell until the whole ADC is transported via endocytosis into the cytoplasm [40]. After intracellular processing of the ADC, a lysyl-modified but still cytotoxic form of DM1 is released, resulting in antitubulin-associated cell death. This charged form of the drug is not membrane permeable and has thus no aforementioned bystander effect of killing neighboring cells not bearing the epitope [40, 46]. Nevertheless, in clinical evaluation T-DM1 has been shown to be a very promising candidate for the antibody-based targeted chemotherapy of patients with metastatic, HER2-positive breast cancer. The ADC showed a high tolerability with side effects of grade 1 and 2 concerning the elevation of the liver enzymes (AST and ALT) and thrombocytopenia. Both effects could be managed with dose reductions and seemed to be transient. Therefore T-DM1 is likely to be the first maytansine-based ADC available for the treatment of cancer and may take the leading role for the development of numerous new maytansine ADCs for diverse indications.

A general pitfall of all ADCs based on tubulin-inhibiting drugs is that the toxins unfold their cytotoxic effect mainly on proliferating cells due to their intrinsic mode of action. Nondividing and quiescent cells are likely to escape the drug mechanism, paving the way for the development of resistances to the ADC or the toxin itself. Another uncertainty in the use of maytansinoid-based ADCs is related to the hydrophobic character of the molecule. The free form of the toxin is membrane permeable and could evoke severe and uncontrollable side effects if inadvertently released in the blood or in metabolizing organs (liver, kidney). Furthermore the linkers used so far for maytansinoid-based ADCs are themselves hydrophobic, leading to an increase in conjugate aggregation or diminishing the binding capacity of the antibody especially at high drug loads [47, 48]. Another problem to consider is that the activity of ADCs can be limited by drug-resistant tumor cells, most often resulting from the increased expression or activity of drug transporters facilitating mainly the efflux of hydrophobic compounds [49, 50]. Therefore, highly water-soluble hydrophilic linkers containing either a negatively charged alpha-sulfonic acid group or a polar short polyethylene glycol (PEG) chain to increase their solubility are under development to facilitate the preparation of more hydrophilic ADCs to overcome at least some of these complications. By the use of such hydrophilic linkers, higher drug loads can be achieved, delivering the toxin in higher concentrations to the target cell. In addition these linkers theoretically generate more polar maytansinoid metabolites inside the cell, being a poor substrate for MDR efflux pumps and thus overcoming multidrug resistance [51].

In summary the development of targeted therapies using maytansinoid-based ADCs is a highly interesting approach which is expected to be validated through the approval and launch of T-DM1. Once proven to be well tolerated and effective for the treatment of cancer, maytansinoids will increasingly play an important role in the clinical development of ADCs.

3 Auristatins

In the mid-1960s, Pettit et al. started with systematic studies of marine life forms as a source for new anticancer drugs. In the late 1970s, these studies led to the discovery of lead structures extracted from the olive green (and pear-shaped) *Dolabella auricularia* (sea hare), a shell-less mollusk collected in Mauritius: dolastatins 1 and 2. Both exhibited very promising results in the P388 leukemia cell line [52]. Further work in isolating structures from the sea hare resulted in the discovery of dolastatins 3–9 [53, 54]. In the late 1980s, Pettit et al. discovered the most promising constituents, namely, dolastatins 10–15 [55–60].

Among the dolastatin family, dolastatin 10 (**5**, Fig. 2) and dolastatin 15 showed the highest cytotoxic activities against human cancer cell lines [61, 62]. In further studies, the mechanism of action responsible for these cytotoxic effects could be revealed. At the US NCI it was found that dolastatin 10 powerfully binds to tubulin, thus inhibiting polymerization mediated through the binding to the vinca alkaloid binding domain, and causes cell to accumulate in metaphase arrest [63, 64]. Applying higher concentrations of dolastatin 10 resulted in a complete disappearance of intracellular microtubules [65]. Comparable results were obtained with dolastatin 15 [66].

Dolastatin 10 entered several phase I clinical trials in the 1990s [67] and successfully progressed to phase II trials. Due to accompanying side effects, with ~40 % of patients developing moderate peripheral neuropathy, and insignificant activity in patients with hormone refractory metastatic adenocarcinoma, dolastatin 10 was withdrawn from clinical trials as a single agent [68]. Nonetheless, the high potency and positive therapeutic index in preclinical models led to the development of water-soluble dolastatin analogs: the auristatins.

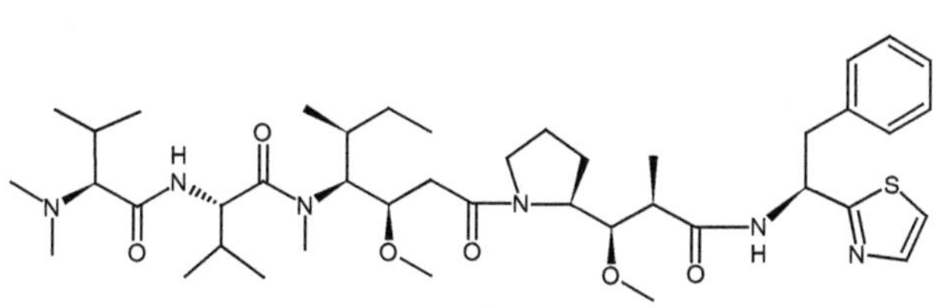

5

Fig. 2 Chemical structure of dolastatin 10 (**5**)

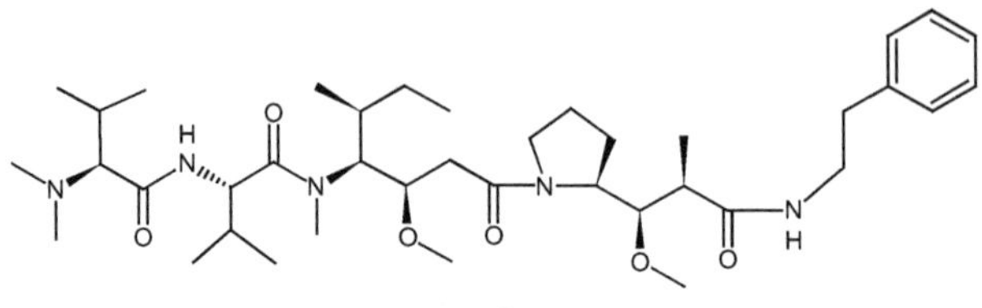

6

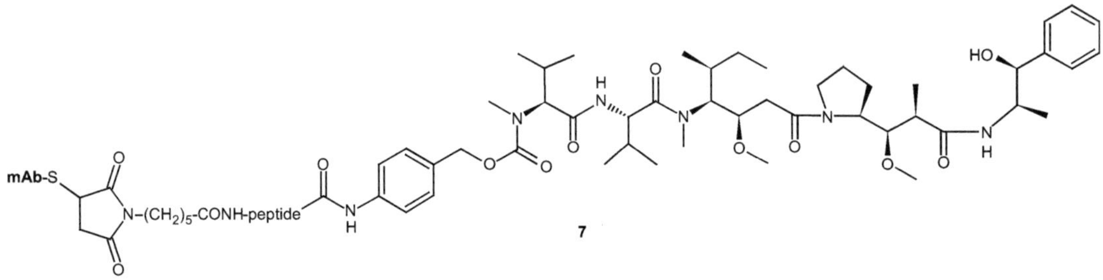

7

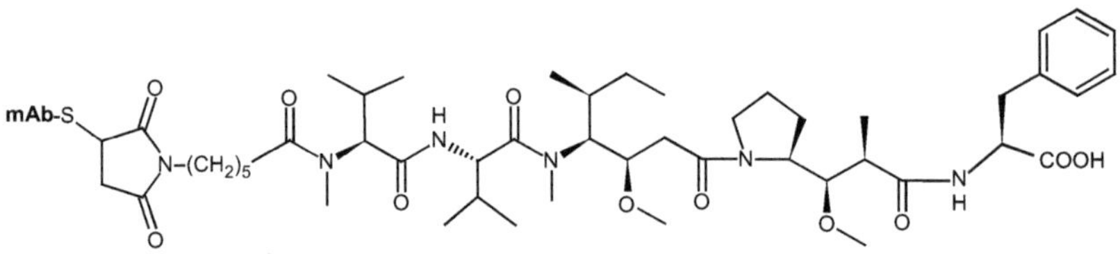

8

Fig. 3 Chemical structure of auristatin PE (**6**) and the antibody conjugates of MMAE (**7**) and MMAF (**8**)

The first described synthetic analog of dolastatin 10 was auristatin PE (**6**, also called TZT-1027 or soblidotin) [69]. Auristatin PE differs structurally in the absence of the thiazole ring from the original dolaphenine residue, resulting in a terminal benzylamine moiety (Fig. 3).

Auristatin PE entered phase I and phase II clinical trials but finally failed to show any anticancer activity in patients with advanced non-small cell lung cancer following treatment with platinum-based chemotherapy [70] or to demonstrate any confirmed response in patients with advanced or metastatic soft tissue sarcomas with prior exposure to anthracycline-based chemotherapy [71]. To our knowledge no further clinical trial is ongoing with this drug.

As a further attempt to increase in vivo efficacy, new auristatin derivatives were developed: monomethyl auristatin-E (**7**, MMAE) [5] and monomethyl auristatin-F (**8**, MMAF) [72] (Fig. 3). To avoid the adverse events seen in previous clinical trials with auristatins and therefore to increase the therapeutic index, the idea was in this case to combine the high cytotoxic potential of auristatins with the target specificity of monoclonal antibodies resulting in an antibody–drug conjugate (ADC) [5]. It should be noted that MMAE and MMAF are fully synthetic drugs, which may confer them a price advantage compared to other ADC payloads. Besides, their peptide-like structure may limit the impact conjugation on the physical properties of the mAb.

Conjugates of various auristatin derivatives have been evaluated [5], especially MMAE, and MMAF are noteworthy [72, 73]. The major difference between MMAE and MMAF is that MMAF possesses a phenylalanine at the C-terminus, contributing to membrane impermeability. It was possible to derivatize MMAF at the amine terminus with a noncleavable linker without any loss of activity, which was not the case for the MMAE analog. The ADC SGN-35 (brentuximab vedotin) composed of MMAE which is bound to a chimeric anti-CD30 monoclonal antibody through a cleavable valine–citruline linker had good clinical results in multiple phase I, II, and III clinical trials [74]. On 19 August 2011, the US Food and Drug Administration (FDA) granted accelerated approval for the use of brentuximab vedotin in relapsed Hodgkin lymphoma and relapsed systemic anaplastic large cell lymphoma under the brand name Adcetris. Currently, brentuximab vedotin is the only FDA-approved ADC and the first approved drug for treating Hodgkin lymphoma in 30 years [21].

The other promising auristatin derivative MMAF entered as a MMAF-ADC by now at least three phase I clinical trials: in subjects with renal cell carcinoma (RCC) of clear cell or papillary histology (AGS-16C3F, AGS-16M8F) [28, 75] and in subjects with CD70-positive non-Hodgkin lymphoma or RCC (SGN-75) [76].

4 Calicheamicin

The calicheamicins, identified in the mid-1980s by the Lederle Laboratories (American Cyanamid Co.) during a search for new fermentation-derived antitumor antibiotics, are a group of DNA-cleaving agents produced by prokaryotic microorganisms [77, 78]. A culture-designated LL-E33288 was isolated from a chalky (caliche) soil sample in Texas (Kerrville) and showed from macromorphological, chemotaxonomic, and physiological studies a close relation to the actinomycete genus *Micromonospora* and was subsequently considered as a new subspecies *M. echinospora* ssp. *calichensis* [79]. The calicheamicins, extracted from the whole fermentation broth with ethyl acetate, exhibited significant antimicrobial activity against Gram-positive and Gram-negative bacteria and demonstrated antitumor activity in mice against P388 leukemia and B16 melanoma. The calicheamicins were identified as members of a new class of potent enediyne containing agents which are related structurally to other enediynes like esperamicins, neocarzinostatin, C-1027, dynemicins, kedarcidin, maduropeptin, namenamicin, and shishijimicin [80–85].

Calicheamicin γ_1^{I} (**9**), the most intensively studied of the calicheamicins, is a structural and stereochemical complex structure consisting of an aglycon containing a unprecedented bicyclo[7.3.1]tridec-9-ene-2,6-diyne system with a labile methyl

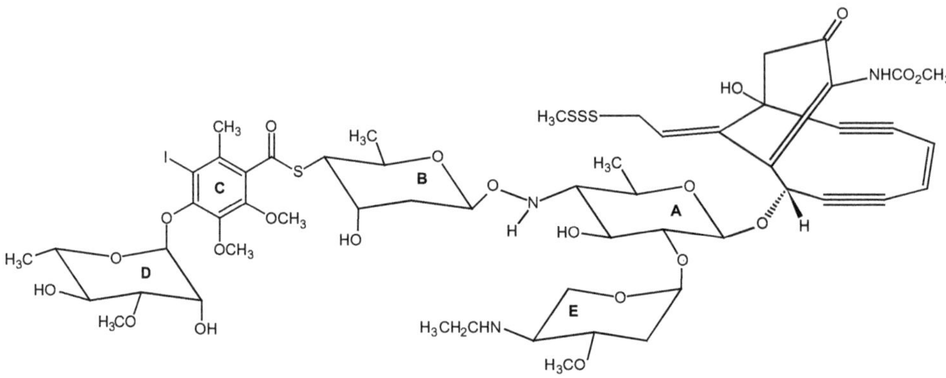

9

Fig. 4 Chemical structure of calicheamicin γ_1^{I} (**9**)

trisulfide grouping and an aryltetrasaccharide chain (Fig. 4). The aryltetrasaccharide chain is made up of linked elements involving a hydroxylamino sugar (ring A) and a thio sugar (ring B), both conjugated by a rare *N*-*O*-glycosidic linkage; a hexasubsituted iodothiobenzoate (ring C); and a rhamnose sugar (ring D). An ethylamino sugar (ring E) is connected to sugar A through a glycosidic linkage.

Beside calicheamicin γ_1^{I}, four other iodinated (α_2^{I}, α_3^{I}, β_1^{I}, δ_1^{I}) and two bromine-containing (β_1^{Br}, γ_1^{Br}) analogs have been identified in *M. echinospora* ssp. *calichensis* fermentation broth, whereupon the production of each analog was depending on the composition of the culture medium [86]. Calicheamicin γ_1^{I} (hereafter called calicheamicin) showed favorable fermentation yields and demonstrated the highest cytotoxicity of the seven analogs. Furthermore a high potency in the biochemical assay of prophage induction (active at picogram per milliliter concentrations) suggested that its activity was due to its ability to damage DNA [87]. In detail a DNA double-strand cleavage is initiated by a nucleophilic attack at the allylic trisulfide linkage leading to a thiol, which can undergo an intramolecular hetero-Michael addition to form a triggered calicheamicin, characterized by a dihydrothiophene tricyclic headgroup. The dihydrothiophene undergoes a Bergman cycloaromatization via a transient 1,4-dehydrobenzene-diradical that initiates oxidative double-strand scission by abstraction of proximal hydrogen atoms from opposite strands of the DNA's deoxyribose backbone. Furthermore, the cutting site of the DNA sequence was found to be well defined, since chemical footprinting studies revealed that the aryltetrasaccharide tail of calicheamicin makes it a highly site-specific DNA-cleaving agent, binding preferentially to the minor groove of oligopurine–oligopyrimidine tetranucleotide stretches with the highest affinity for TCCT-AGGA sites [88–90]. As shown by gel-shift experiments and NMR deuterium transfer experiments, the almost exclusive site of abstraction by the 1,4-dehydrobenzene-diradical is the 5′-hydrogen from deoxyribose of a 5′-cytosine in the TCCT site and the 4′-hydrogen at a nucleotide three bases to the 3′ side of the complementary 3′-NNNAGGA tract. Beside TCCT other sites such as GCCT, TCCG, TCCC, CTCT, TCTC, ACCT, TCCA, and their complementary sites were also cleaved in the same fashion, with the extent of cleavage apparently depending on the flanking sequences. The structural and conformational features relevant for DNA cleavage activity and thereby the antitumoral potency of calicheamicin have been published recently in an excellent review by George A. Ellestad [91].

Despite promising initial experiments, further evaluation of calicheamicins in models of preclinical oncology revealed an insufficient therapeutic window and thus prevented their use in a clinical setting. However, the extreme cytotoxic potency, the small molecular size, and the mechanism of action turned calicheamicins into a promising toxic payload for the emerging field of ADC technology. In first attempts by the Lederle Laboratories, a series of calicheamicin analogs were conjugated to CT-M-01, an antibody binding the MUC1 antigen expressed on a number of solid tumor types and characterized by a high internalization rate after antibody binding [92]. Beside calicheamicin γ_1^I, the analogs α_2^I (absence of the rhamnose sugar), α_3^I (absence of the amino sugar), PSAG (missing both rhamnose and amino sugar), and *N*-acetyl-γ_1^I (acetylation of the amino sugar) were coupled to CT-M-01 containing periodate-oxidized sugars by a disulfide–hydrazide cleavable linkage positioned at the enediyne bicyclic "warhead." Interestingly, the structural variations in the drug had a profound effect on the therapeutic efficacy of their conjugates which were not necessarily aligned with the activity of the drugs as single agents. Conjugates of α_3^I and *N*-acetyl-γ_1^I, analogs without amino sugar or with modified amino sugar, showed a clear therapeutic advantage over γ_1^I, α_2^I, and PSAG conjugates in mouse xenograft models. In addition a stabilization of the disulfide–hydrazide linker by introduction of a steric bulk (dimethyl group) adjacent to the thiol further improved the therapeutic potential, resulting in CT-M-01 calicheamicin conjugates with a therapeutic ratio >6. Based on these findings, a clinical development of calicheamicin *N*-acetyl-γ_1^I conjugated to CT-M-01 by attachment to lysine residues (amide–disulfide linker) was initiated. The conjugate, designated CMB-401, had an acceptable toxicity profile [93] but failed to show effectivity as monotherapy in the treatment of recurrent platinum-sensitive epithelial ovarian carcinoma in a phase II trial [94].

Most data has been generated with gemtuzumab ozogamicin (**10**, Mylotarg), where the 1,2-dimethyl hydrazine of calicheamicin *N*-acetyl-γ_1^I is attached to the IgG4 antibody hP67.6 through covalent linkage of a bifunctional linker, 4-(4-acetylphenoxy)butanoic acid, to lysine residues (Fig. 5) [22]. Thereby the linker between calicheamicin and hP67.6 incorporates two labile bonds, a hydrazone and a sterically hindered disulfide, one allowing

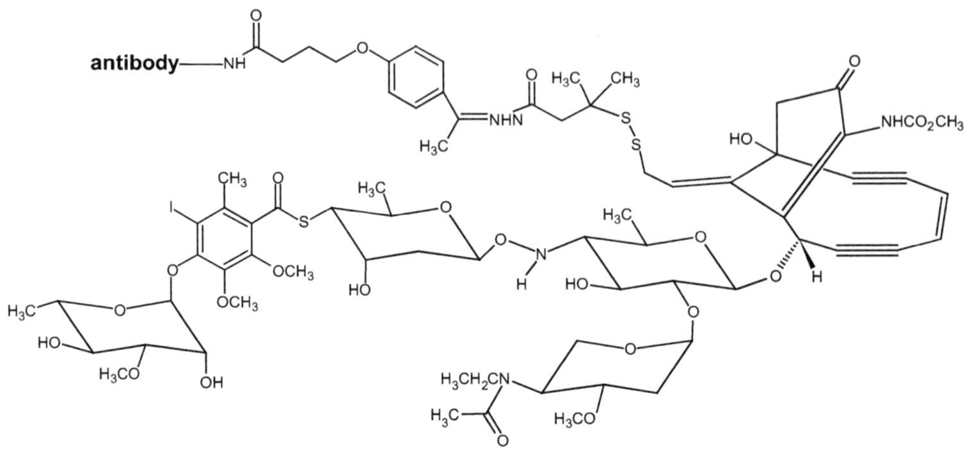

10

Fig. 5 Antibody conjugate of calicheamicin *N*-acetyl-γ_1^{I} (**10**) with linker moiety as used in gemtuzumab ozogamicin and inotuzumab ozogamicin

efficient release of toxin in the lysosomes (pH ~4) and the other ensuring activation of the enediyne warhead in the bioreductive milieu of the cytoplasm. The hP67.6 antibody binds the sialic-acid-binding immunoglobulin-like lectin CD33 (siglec-3), identified as marker of myeloid leukemias and B-cell lymphomas. Based on the efficacy and safety data of three open-label trials, the FDA granted market approval for Mylotarg, the first ADC approved at all, under the accelerated approval regulations in May 2000 for the treatment of acute myeloid leukemia (AML). However, required post-approval studies failed to confirm benefit, so that Mylotarg was withdrawn from the US and European markets in 2010. The reasons for the failure of Mylotarg in the treatment of AML are unclear but may depend on insufficient linker stability and resistance of leukemia cells to calicheamicin by drug resistance mechanisms [95] or because of a narrow therapeutic window resulting in fatal adverse events at higher doses, e.g., by ADC catabolism in non-tumor cells [96].

Currently the most advanced calicheamicin ADC in clinics is inotuzumab ozogamicin (CMC-544), an IgG4 conjugate sharing the linker structure with gemtuzumab ozogamicin **10** and specifically binding CD22, expressed on approximately 60–90 % of B-lymphoid malignancies [22]. CMC-544 shows promise as a treatment for refractory and relapsed acute lymphocytic leukemia (ALL) as demonstrated in a phase II clinical trial conducted by Pfizer [97].

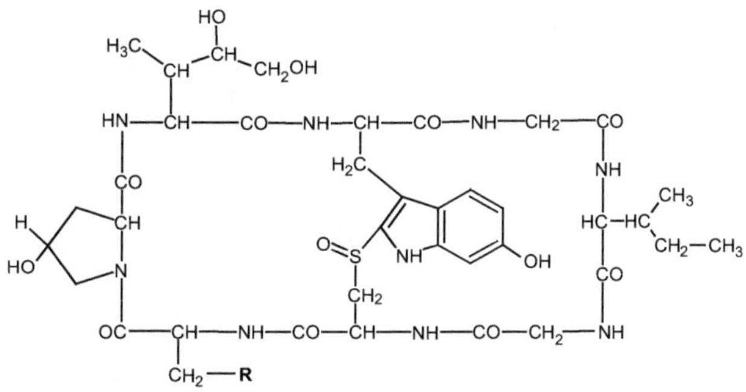

11 R = $CONH_2$ (α-amanitin)

12 R = COOH (β-amanitin)

Fig. 6 Structures of the bicyclic octapeptide toxins α-amanitin (**11**) and β-amanitin (**12**)

5 Amatoxins

The use of transcription inhibitors like amatoxins is a new approach in the field of ADC technology. Amatoxins are a family of highly toxic cyclopeptides produced by mushrooms, particularly of the genus *Amanita*. For one of these, the green death cap (*Amanita phalloides*), reports of casualties date back far to the past, while today this mushroom still causes 95 % of all fatal mushroom poisonings worldwide. Amatoxins accidently consumed with mushroom dishes are preferentially taken up into liver cells due to the presence of a transporting protein OATP1B3 on hepatocytes [98]. They cause death of the patients from liver failure, and up till now this liver toxicity discouraged any medical use of the amatoxins.

The structure of the amatoxins was elucidated in the 1960s by Wieland [99]. The nine naturally occurring amatoxins known so far share the same skeletal structure, a ring of eight L-configurated amino acids, bridged between a tryptophan and a cysteine residue by a sulfoxide moiety. Three of the side chains in the amatoxins are hydroxylated, the OH groups being responsible for pronounced water solubility and, at least partly, for binding to the target molecule. Two of the peptides, α-amanitin (**11**) and β-amanitin (**12**, Fig. 6), account for ca. 90 % of all amatoxins.

In 1966, Stirpe and Fiume [100] first described that α-amanitin inhibits RNA synthesis in mouse liver nuclei. Following investigations [101, 102] confirmed that RNA polymerase II, the enzyme transcribing DNA into precursors of messenger RNA, is the target of amatoxins. The complex between RNA polymerase II and amatoxins is very tight. For the calf thymus enzyme, the equilibrium dissociation constant K_D was determined as 3×10^{-9} M [103]. Since amatoxins form a 1:1 complex and the concentration of the enzyme in a cell is low (10^{-8} M, corresponding to ca. 22,000 copies per cell), the amatoxin concentration in cytoplasm required to stall transcription is likewise very low (ca. 10^{-8} M) [104]. Structural

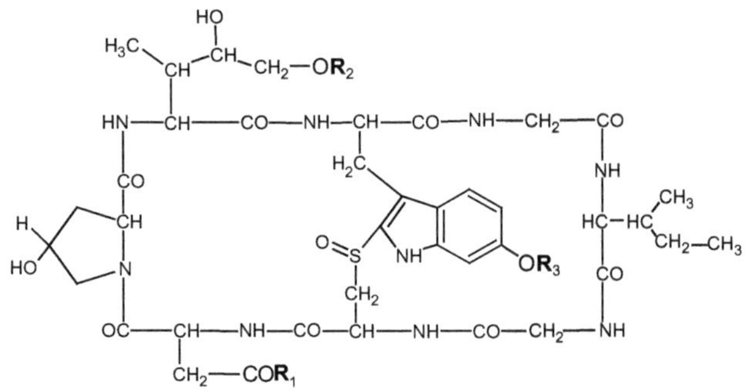

13 e.g. R_1 = -NH-mAb

14 e.g. R_2 = -CO-$(CH_2)_3$-CONH-mAb

15 e.g. R_3 **a** = -$(CH_2)_4$-NHCO-$(CH_2)_8$-CONH-mAb

16 R_3 **b** = -$(CH_2)_4$-NHCO-$(CH_2)_2$-S-S-$(CH_2)_2$-CONH-mAb

17 R_3 **c** = -$(CH_2)_5$-CONH-mAb

Fig. 7 Conjugation sites in amatoxins for coupling to antibodies

details of the toxin complex and the molecular inhibition mechanism became known recently by an X-ray analysis of the α-amanitin complex of yeast RNA polymerase II [105].

Early amatoxin conjugates with proteins, e.g., with albumin or fetuin aiming at the production of amatoxin-specific antibodies in rats and rabbits employed the carboxy group in β-amanitin (**13**, Fig. 7) for coupling with ε-amino groups of lysine in the proteins [106]. By the same reaction of the first immunoglobulin, a MUC1-specific antibody was coupled to β-amanitin and shown to develop specific cytotoxicity against T47D cells [107]. Disadvantage of this coupling site comes from the fact that the carboxy group is part of an intramolecular hydrogen bond and is located very close to the backbone of the peptide resulting in poor coupling yields. Therefore, more recent coupling reactions preferred the primary hydroxy group of the dihydroxylated isoleucine moiety in α-amanitin (**14**, Fig. 7) which can be esterified with dicarbonic acid anhydrides creating a carboxy group that can be activated and reacted with immunoglobulins [108], leaving the two secondary hydroxy groups located on proline and dihydroxyisoleucine unsubstituted. However, as primary esters, such amanitin conjugates showed poor stability in plasma leading to partial loss of the payload before arriving at the tumor cells. In a third approach it was shown that ether derivatives of the phenolic hydroxy group in 6′-position of tryptophan (**15–17**) provide high stability in plasma combined with the widest choice of coupling reactions for immunoglobulins. Attachment to the 6′-OH of tryptophan now represents the standard procedure for amanitin-supported ADCs [109]. Other structural elements of the amatoxin molecule, such as the glycyl-isoleucyl-glycyl part or the cysteine moiety, failed as attachment sites because they are chemically inert or regarded as part of the contact site with RNA polymerase II [110].

As with all ADCs, the amatoxin immunoglobulin conjugates are supposed to be taken up by tumor cells via endocytosis. Lysosomal enzymes will break down the protein carrier and release the toxin, or the toxin derivative, in a way depending on the chemistry used for the linker. Native α-amanitin with the known toxic activity is probably released from ester derivatives of type R_2 after cleavage by lysosomal esterases or proteases. In contrast, β-amanitin derivatives of type R_1 are likely to be released as ε-lysyl derivatives, which when prepared synthetically were shown to exhibit toxic activities comparable to native amanitin. Little information is available on linkers of the type R_3. The ether bond is unlikely to be cleaved under cellular conditions, and only for the type R_3 b, we can presume that the toxin species released is a thiol derivative formed after reduction of the disulfide bridge. ADCs with linkers of the types R_3 a and R_3 c may release the toxin with intact linkers attached to the lysine residue of the protein they had been coupled to, eventually even bound to the neighboring amino acids in the protein backbone. On the other hand, ADCs of these types developed high cytoxicities in cells suggesting that the amatoxin fragments released, though unknown in structure, are highly active. Concerning the toxin itself, the peptide probably remains unchanged under the conditions of proteolytic processing, since all experiments performed thus far to find a protease that might cleave one of the amide bonds present in the cyclic peptide failed.

Of great advantage for amatoxins as warheads in ADCs is their hydrophilic nature. Firstly, the high solubility in aqueous medium facilitates the coupling reaction. Secondly, it is unlikely that amatoxin molecules coupled to immunoglobulins will cause an aggregation of the ADC molecules as sometimes reported for conjugates with hydrophobic warheads. Thirdly, the toxin species released from disintegrated tumor cells are of low mwt. and unlikely to accumulate in other tissues but will be excreted in urine very quickly. This is expected from clearance values of native amatoxins (i.e., the time required to excrete 50 % of an amatoxin dose by urine), which is 30 min only [111]. Finally, the hydrophilic nature makes amatoxins and their low mwt. derivatives poor substrates of MDR processes. Indeed, experiments have shown that conjugates of amatoxins are highly active also in MDR-expressing tumor cells [109].

References

1. Scott AM, Wolchok JD, Old LJ (2012) Antibody therapy of cancer. Nat Rev Cancer 12:278–287
2. Steiner M, Neri D (2011) Antibody–radionuclide conjugates for cancer therapy: historical considerations and new trends. Clin Cancer Res 17:6406–6416
3. Kreitman RJ, Pastan I (2011) Antibody fusion proteins: anti-CD22 recombinant immunotoxin moxetumomab pasudotox. Clin Cancer Res 17:6398–6405
4. Choudhary S, Mathew M, Verma RS (2011) Therapeutic potential of anticancer immunotoxins. Drug Discov Today 16:495–503

5. Carter PJ, Senter PD (2008) Antibody–drug conjugates for cancer therapy. Cancer J 14:154–169
6. Kovtun YV, Goldmacher VS (2007) Cell killing by antibody–drug conjugates. Cancer Lett 255:232–240
7. Chari RVJ (2008) Targeted cancer therapy: conferring specificity to cytotoxic drugs. Acc Chem Res 41:98–107
8. Schrama D, Reisfeld RA, Becker JC (2006) Antibody targeted drugs as cancer therapeutics. Nat Rev Drug Discov 5:147–159
9. Sedlacek HH, Seemann G, Hoffmann D (1992) Antibodies as carriers of cytotoxicity, 1st edn. S. Karger Publishing, Basel, Switzerland
10. Tolcher AW (2000) BR96-doxorubicin: been there, done that! J Clin Oncol 18:4000
11. Saleh MN, Sugarman S, Murray J et al (2000) Phase I trial of the anti-Lewis Y drug immunoconjugate BR96-doxorubicin in patients with lewis Y-expressing epithelial tumors. J Clin Oncol 18:2282–2292
12. Tolcher AW, Sugarman S, Gelmon KA et al (1999) Randomized phase II study of BR96–doxorubicin conjugate in patients with metastatic breast cancer. J Clin Oncol 17:478–484
13. Laguzza BC, Nichols CL, Briggs SL et al (1989) New antitumor monoclonal antibody–vinca conjugates LY203725 and related compounds: design, preparation, and representative in vivo activity. J Med Chem 32:548–555
14. Apelgren LD, Zimmerman DL, Briggs SL et al (1990) Antitumor activity of the monoclonal antibody–vinca alkaloid immunoconjugate LY203725 (KS1/4-4-desacetylvinblastine-3-carboxhydrazide) in a nude mouse model of human ovarian cancer. Cancer Res 50: 3540–3544
15. Petersen BH, DeHerdt SV, Schneck DW et al (1991) The human immune response to KS1/4-desacetylvinblastine (LY256787) and KS1/4-desacetylvinblastine hydrazide (LY203728) in single and multiple dose clinical studies. Cancer Res 51:2286–2290
16. Uadia P, Blair AH, Ghose T (1984) Tumor and tissue distribution of a methotrexate–anti-EL4 immunoglobulin conjugate in EL4 lymphoma-bearing mice. Cancer Res 44:4263–4266
17. Kulkarni PN, Blair AH, Ghose T et al (1985) Conjugation of methotrexate to IgG antibodies and their F(ab)2 fragments and the effect of conjugated methotrexate on tumor growth in vivo. Cancer Immunol Immunother 19:211–214
18. Elias DJ, Kline LE, Robbins BA et al (1994) Monoclonal antibody KS1/4-methotrexate immunoconjugate studies in non-small cell lung carcinoma. Am J Respir Crit Care Med 150:1114–1122
19. LoRusso PM, Weiss D, Guardino E et al (2011) Trastuzumab emtansine: a unique antibody–drug conjugate in development for human epidermal growth factor receptor 2-positive cancer. Clin Cancer Res 17:6437–6447
20. Guha M (2012) T-DM1 impresses at ASCO. Nat Biotechnol 30:728
21. Senter PD, Sievers EL (2012) The discovery and development of brentuximab vedotin for use in relapsed Hodgkin lymphoma and systemic anaplastic large cell lymphoma. Nat Biotechnol 30:631–637
22. Ricart AD (2011) Antibody–drug conjugates of calicheamicin derivative: gemtuzumab ozogamicin and inotuzumab ozogamicin. Clin Cancer Res 17:6417–6427
23. Vetter J (1998) Toxins of amanita phalloides. Toxicon 36:13–24
24. Safavy A, Bonner JA, Waksal HW et al (2003) Synthesis and biological evaluation of paclitaxel-C225 conjugate as a model for targeted drug delivery. Bioconjug Chem 14:302–310
25. Ojima I (2008) Guided molecular missiles for tumor-targeting chemotherapy – case studies using the second-generation taxoids as warheads. Acc Chem Res 41:108–119
26. Chari RV, Jackel KA, Bourret LA et al (1995) Enhancement of the selectivity and antitumor efficacy of a CC-1065 analogue through immunoconjugate formation. Cancer Res 55:4079–4084
27. Zhao RY, Erickson HK, Leece BA et al (2012) Synthesis and biological evaluation of antibody conjugates of phosphate prodrugs of cytotoxic DNA alkylators for the targeted treatment of cancer. J Med Chem 55:766–782
28. Beck A, Lambert J, Sun M et al. (2012) Fourth world antibody–drug conjugate summit: Feb 29–Mar 1 2012, Frankfurt, Germany. MAbs 4
29. Kupchan SM, Komoda Y, Court WA et al (1972) Maytansine, a novel antileukemic ansa macrolide from *Maytenus ovatus*. J Am Chem Soc 94:1354–1356
30. Kupchan SM, Komoda Y, Branfman AR et al (1977) The maytansinoids. Isolation, structural elucidation, and chemical interrelation of novel ansa macrolides. J Org Chem 42:2349–2357

31. Rinehart KL, Shield LS (1976) Chemistry of the ansamycin antibiotics. Fortschr Chem Org Naturst 33:231–307
32. Cassady JM, Chan KK, Floss HG et al (2004) Recent developments in the maytansinoid antitumor agents. Chem Pharm Bull 52:1–26
33. Remillard S, Rebhun LI, Howie GA et al (1975) Antimitotic activity of the potent tumor inhibitor maytansine. Science 189:1002–1005
34. Mandelbaum-Shavit F, Wolpert-DeFilippes MK, Johns DG (1976) Binding of maytansine to rat brain tubulin. Biochem Biophys Res Commun 72:47–54
35. Bhattacharyya B, Wolff J (1977) Maytansine binding to the vinblastine sites of tubulin. FEBS Lett 75:159–162
36. Ravry MJ, Omura GA, Birch R (1985) Phase II evaluation of maytansine (NSC 153858) in advanced cancer. A Southeastern Cancer Study Group trial. Am J Clin Oncol 8:148–150
37. Issell BF, Crooke ST (1978) Maytansine. Cancer Treat Rev 5:199–207
38. Chari RV, Martell BA, Gross JL et al (1992) Immunoconjugates containing novel maytansinoids: promising anticancer drugs. Cancer Res 52:127–131
39. Widdison WC, Wilhelm SD, Cavanagh EE et al (2006) Semisynthetic maytansine analogues for the targeted treatment of cancer. J Med Chem 49:4392–4408
40. Lewis Phillips GD, Li G, Dugger DL et al (2008) Targeting HER2-positive breast cancer with trastuzumab-DM1, an antibody–cytotoxic drug conjugate. Cancer Res 68:9280–9290
41. Austin CD, Wen X, Gazzard L et al (2005) Oxidizing potential of endosomes and lysosomes limits intracellular cleavage of disulfide-based antibody-drug conjugates. Proc Natl Acad Sci U S A 102:17987–17992
42. Lambert JM (2005) Drug-conjugated monoclonal antibodies for the treatment of cancer. Curr Opin Pharmacol 5:543–549
43. Helft PR, Schilsky RL, Hoke FJ et al (2004) A phase I study of cantuzumab mertansine administered as a single intravenous infusion once weekly in patients with advanced solid tumors. Clin Cancer Res 10:4363–4368
44. Tijink BM, Buter J, de Bree R et al (2006) A phase I dose escalation study with anti-CD44v6 bivatuzumab mertansine in patients with incurable squamous cell carcinoma of the head and neck or esophagus. Clin Cancer Res 12:6064–6072
45. Tolcher AW, Ochoa L, Hammond LA et al (2003) Cantuzumab mertansine, a maytansinoid immunoconjugate directed to the CanAg antigen: a phase I, pharmacokinetic, and biologic correlative study. J Clin Oncol 21:211–222
46. Kovtun YV, Audette CA, Ye Y et al (2006) Antibody–drug conjugates designed to eradicate tumors with homogeneous and heterogeneous expression of the target antigen. Cancer Res 66:3214–3221
47. Chari RV (1998) Targeted delivery of chemotherapeutics: tumor-activated prodrug therapy. Adv Drug Deliv Rev 31:89–104
48. Hollander I, Kunz A, Hamann PR (2008) Selection of reaction additives used in the preparation of monomeric antibody–calicheamicin conjugates. Bioconjug Chem 19:358–361
49. Takeshita A, Shinjo K, Yamakage N et al (2009) CMC-544 (inotuzumab ozogamicin) shows less effect on multidrug resistant cells: analyses in cell lines and cells from patients with B-cell chronic lymphocytic leukaemia and lymphoma. Br J Haematol 146:34–43
50. Szakács G, Paterson JK, Ludwig JA et al (2006) Targeting multidrug resistance in cancer. Nat Rev Drug Discov 5:219–234
51. Zhao RY, Wilhelm SD, Audette C et al (2011) Synthesis and evaluation of hydrophilic linkers for antibody–maytansinoid conjugates. J Med Chem 54:3606–3623
52. Pettit GR, Kamano Y, Fujii Y et al (1981) Marine animal biosynthetic constituents for cancer chemotherapy. J Nat Prod 44:482–485
53. Pettit GR, Kamano Y, Brown P et al (1982) Antineoplastic agents. 3. Structure of the cyclic peptide dolastatin 3 from *Dolabella auricularia*. J Am Chem Soc 104:905–907
54. Pettit GR, Kamano Y, Holzapfel CW et al (1987) Antineoplastic agents. 150. The structure and synthesis of dolastatin 3. J Am Chem Soc 109:7581–7582
55. Pettit GR, Kamano Y, Herald CL et al (1987) The isolation and structure of a remarkable marine animal antineoplastic constituent: dolastatin 10. J Am Chem Soc 109:6883–6885
56. Pettit GR, Kamano Y, Herald CL et al (1993) Isolation of dolastatins 10–15 from the marine mollusc *Dolabella auricularia*. Tetrahedron 49:9151–9170
57. Pettit GR, Kamano Y, Kizu H et al (1989) Isolation and structure of the cell growth inhibitory depsipeptides dolastatins 11 and 12. Heterocycles 28:553–558
58. Pettit GR, Kamano Y, Herald CL et al (1989) Antineoplastic agent. 174. Isolation and structure of the cytostatic depsipeptide dolastatin 13 from the sea hare *Dolabella auricularia*. J Am Chem Soc 111:5015–5017

59. Pettit GR, Kamano Y, Herald CL et al (1990) Antineoplastic agents. 190. Isolation and structure of the cyclodepsipeptide dolastatin 14. J Org Chem 55:2989–2990
60. Pettit GR, Kamano Y, Dufresne C et al (1989) Isolation and structure of the cytostatic linear depsipeptide dolastatin 15. J Org Chem 54:6005–6006
61. Quentmeier H, Brauer S, Pettit GR et al (1992) Cytostatic effects of dolastatin 10 and dolastatin 15 on human leukemia cell lines. Leuk Lymphoma 6:245–250
62. Steube KG, Grunicke D, Pietsch T et al (1992) Dolastatin 10 and dolastatin 15: effects of two natural peptides on growth and differentiation of leukemia cells. Leukemia 6:1048–1053
63. Bai R, Pettit GR, Hamel E (1990) Dolastatin 10, a powerful cytostatic peptide derived from a marine animal. Inhibition of tubulin polymerization mediated through the vinca alkaloid binding domain. Biochem Pharmacol 39:1941–1949
64. Bai R, Pettit GR, Hamel E (1990) Structure-activity studies with chiral isomers and with segments of the antimitotic marine peptide dolastatin 10. Biochem Pharmacol 40:1859–1864
65. Bai R, Roach MC, Jayaram SK et al (1993) Differential effects of active isomers, segments, and analogs of dolastatin 10 on ligand interactions with tubulin. Correlation with cytotoxicity. Biochem Pharmacol 45:1503–1515
66. Bai R, Friedman SJ, Pettit GR et al (1992) Dolastatin 15, a potent antimitotic depsipeptide derived from *Dolabella auricularia*. Interaction with tubulin and effects of cellular microtubules. Biochem Pharmacol 43:2637–2645
67. Pitot HC, McElroy EA, Reid JM et al (1999) Phase I trial of dolastatin-10 (NSC 376128) in patients with advanced solid tumors. Clin Cancer Res 5:525–531
68. Banerjee S, Wang Z, Mohammad M et al (2008) Efficacy of selected natural products as therapeutic agents against cancer. J Nat Prod 71:492–496
69. Kobayashi M, Natsume T, Tamaoki S et al (1997) Antitumor activity of TZT-1027, a novel dolastatin 10 derivative. Jpn J Cancer Res 88:316–327
70. Riely GJ, Gadgeel S, Rothman I et al (2007) A phase 2 study of TZT-1027, administered weekly to patients with advanced non-small cell lung cancer following treatment with platinum-based chemotherapy. Lung Cancer 55:181–185
71. Patel S, Keohan ML, Saif MW et al (2006) Phase II study of intravenous TZT-1027 in patients with advanced or metastatic soft-tissue sarcomas with prior exposure to anthracycline-based chemotherapy. Cancer 107:2881–2887
72. Doronina SO, Mendelsohn BA, Bovee TD et al (2006) Enhanced activity of monomethylauristatin F through monoclonal antibody delivery: effects of linker technology on efficacy and toxicity. Bioconjug Chem 17:114–124
73. Doronina SO, Toki BE, Torgov MY et al (2003) Development of potent monoclonal antibody auristatin conjugates for cancer therapy. Nat Biotechnol 21:778–784
74. Anon (2011) Brentuximab vedotin: adis R&D profile. Drugs R&D 11:85–95
75. Agensys Inc. (2012) A study to assess the safety, pharmacokinetics and effectiveness of AGS-16C3F monotherapy in subjects with renal cell carcinoma (RCC) of clear cell or papillary histology. ClinicalTrials.gov, NCT01672775
76. Seattle Genetics Inc. (2009) A phase 1 dose-escalation trial of SGN-75 in CD70-positive non-Hodgkin lymphoma or renal cell carcinoma. ClinicalTrials.gov, NCT01015911
77. Lee MD, Dunne TS, Chang CC et al (1987) Calichemicins, a novel family of antitumor antibiotics. 2. Chemistry and structure of calichemicin.gamma.1I. J Am Chem Soc 109:3466–3468
78. Lee MD, Dunne TS, Siegel MM et al (1987) Calichemicins, a novel family of antitumor antibiotics. 1. Chemistry and partial structure of calichemicin.gamma.1I. J Am Chem Soc 109:3464–3466
79. Maiese WM, Lechevalier MP, Lechevalier HA et al (1989) Calicheamicins, a novel family of antitumor antibiotics: taxonomy, fermentation and biological properties. J Antibiot 42:558–563
80. Golik J, Clardy J, Dubay G et al (1987) Esperamicins, a novel class of potent antitumor antibiotics. 2. Structure of esperamicin X. J Am Chem Soc 109:3461–3462
81. Golik J, Dubay G, Groenewold G et al (1987) Esperamicins, a novel class of potent antitumor antibiotics. 3. Structures of esperamicins A1, A2, and A1b. J Am Chem Soc 109:3462–3464
82. Edo K, Akiyama-Murai Y, Saito K et al (1988) Hydrogen bromide adduct of neocarzinostatin chromophore: one of the stable derivatives of native neocarzinostatin chromophore. J Antibiot 41:1272–1274

83. Smith AL, Nicolaou KC (1996) The enediyne antibiotics. J Med Chem 39:2103–2117
84. McDonald LA, Capson TL, Krishnamurthy G et al (1996) Namenamicin, a new enediyne antitumor antibiotic from the marine ascidian Polysyncraton lithostrotum. J Am Chem Soc 118:10898–10899
85. Oku N, Matsunaga S, Fusetani N (2003) Shishijimicins A–C, novel enediyne antitumor antibiotics from the ascidian Didemnum proliferum1. J Am Chem Soc 125: 2044–2045
86. Lee MD, Dunne TS, Chang CC et al (1992) Calicheamicins, a novel family of antitumor antibiotics. 4. Structure elucidation of calicheamicins.beta.1Br, gamma.1Br, alpha.2I, alpha.3I, beta.1I, gamma.1I, and.delta.1I. J Am Chem Soc 114:985–997
87. Zein N, Poncin M, Nilakantan R et al (1989) Calicheamicin gamma 1I and DNA: molecular recognition process responsible for site-specificity. Science 244:697–699
88. Zein N, Sinha AM, McGahren WJ et al (1988) Calicheamicin gamma 1I: an antitumor antibiotic that cleaves double-stranded DNA site specifically. Science 240:1198–1201
89. De Voss JJ, Townsend CA, Ding WD et al (1990) Site-specific atom transfer from DNA to a bound ligand defines the geometry of a DNA-calicheamicin.gamma.1I complex. J Am Chem Soc 112:9669–9670
90. Mah SC, Townsend CA, Tullius TD (1994) Hydroxyl radical footprinting of calicheamicin. Relationship of DNA binding to cleavage. Biochemistry 33:614–621
91. Ellestad GA (2011) Structural and conformational features relevant to the anti-tumor activity of calicheamicin γ 1I. Chirality 23:660–671
92. Hinman LM, Hamann PR, Wallace R et al (1993) Preparation and characterization of monoclonal antibody conjugates of the calicheamicins: a novel and potent family of antitumor antibiotics. Cancer Res 53:3336–3342
93. Gillespie AM, Broadhead TJ, Chan SY et al (2000) Phase I open study of the effects of ascending doses of the cytotoxic immunoconjugate CMB-401 (hCTMO1-calicheamicin) in patients with epithelial ovarian cancer. Ann Oncol 11:735–741
94. Chan SY, Gordon AN, Coleman RE et al (2003) A phase 2 study of the cytotoxic immunoconjugate CMB-401 (hCTM01-calicheamicin) in patients with platinum-sensitive recurrent epithelial ovarian carcinoma. Cancer Immunol Immunother 52:243–248
95. Naito K, Takeshita A, Shigeno K et al (2000) Calicheamicin-conjugated humanized anti-CD33 monoclonal antibody (gemtuzumab zogamicin, CMA-676) shows cytocidal effect on CD33-positive leukemia cell lines, but is inactive on P-glycoprotein-expressing sublines. Leukemia 14:1436–1443
96. Nabhan C, Rundhaugen L, Jatoi M et al (2004) Gemtuzumab ozogamicin (MylotargTM) is infrequently associated with sinusoidal obstructive syndrome/veno-occlusive disease. Ann Oncol 15:1231–1236
97. Kantarjian H, Thomas D, Jorgensen J et al (2012) Inotuzumab ozogamicin, an anti-CD22-calecheamicin conjugate, for refractory and relapsed acute lymphocytic leukaemia: a phase 2 study. Lancet Oncol 13:403–411
98. Letschert K, Faulstich H, Keller D et al (2006) Molecular characterization and inhibition of amanitin uptake into human hepatocytes. Toxicol Sci 91:140–149
99. Wieland T (1986) Peptides of poisonous amanita mushrooms, 1st edn. Springer, New York
100. Fiume L, Stirpe F (1966) Decreased RNA content in mouse liver nuclei after intoxication with α-amanitin. Biochim Biophys Acta 123:643–645
101. Lindell TJ, Weinberg F, Morris PW et al (1970) Specific inhibition of nuclear RNA polymerase II by alpha-amanitin. Science 170:447–449
102. Kedinger C, Gniazdowski M, Mandel JL et al (1970) Alpha-amanitin: a specific inhibitor of one of two DNA-pendent RNA polymerase activities from calf thymus. Biochem Biophys Res Commun 38:165–171
103. Meihlac M, Kedinger C, Chambon P et al (1970) Amanitin binding to calf thymus RNA polymerase B. FEBS Lett 9:258–260
104. Cochet-Meilhac M, Nuret P, Courvalin JC et al (1974) Animal DNA-dependent RNA polymerases 12. Determination of the cellular number of RNA polymerase B molecules. Biochim Biophys Acta 353:185–192
105. Bushnell DA, Cramer P, Kornberg RD (2002) Structural basis of transcription: alpha-amanitin-RNA polymerase II cocrystal at 2.8 A resolution. Proc Natl Acad Sci U S A 99:1218–1222
106. Barbanti-Brodano G, Fiume L (1973) Selective killing of macrophages by amanitin–albumin conjugates. Nat New Biol 243:281–283
107. Danielczyk A, Stahn R, Faulstich D et al (2006) PankoMab: a potent new generation anti-tumour MUC1 antibody. Cancer Immunol Immunother 55:1337–1347

108. Moldenhauer G, Salnikov AV, Lüttgau S et al (2012) Therapeutic potential of amanitin-conjugated anti-epithelial cell adhesion molecule monoclonal antibody against pancreatic carcinoma. J Natl Cancer Inst 104:622–634
109. Anderl J, Mueller C, Heckl-Oestreicher B. et al. (2011) Highly potent antibody-amanitin conjugates cause tumor-selective apoptosis. AACR 102nd Annual Meeting Abstract# 3616
110. Baumann K, Zanotti G, Faulstich H (1994) A beta-turn in alpha-amanitin is the most important structural feature for binding to RNA polymerase II and three monoclonal antibodies. Protein Sci 3:750–756
111. Faulstich H, Fauser U (1978) The course of amanita intoxication in beagle dogs. In: Amanita toxins and poisoning. Gerhard Witzstrock, Baden-Baden, pp 115–123

Chapter 5

Linker Technologies for Antibody–Drug Conjugates

Birte Nolting

Abstract

Antibody–drug conjugates (ADCs), which combine the specificity, favorable pharmacokinetics, and biodistribution of a monoclonal antibody (mAb) with the cytotoxic potency of a drug, are promising new therapies for cancer. Along with the development of monoclonal antibodies (mAbs) and cytotoxic drugs, the design of the linker is of essential importance, because it impacts the efficacy and tolerability of ADCs. The linker needs to provide sufficient stability during systemic circulation but allow for the rapid and efficient release of the cytotoxic drug in an active form inside the tumor cells. This review provides an overview of linker technologies currently used for ADCs and advances that have resulted in linkers with improved properties. Also provided is a brief summary of some considerations for the conjugation of antibody and drug linker such as drug-to-antibody ratio and site of conjugation.

Key words Antibody–drug conjugate, Monoclonal antibody, Linker, Cytotoxic drug, Conjugation, Hydrazone, Disulfide, Peptide, Cleavable, Noncleavable

1 Introduction

Antibody–drug conjugates (ADCs) offer a unique-targeted therapeutic strategy combining the best features of both antibodies and small-molecule drugs to create a single moiety that is highly specific and cytotoxic. As such, they have been the subject of intense research focused on optimization to increase the therapeutic indices of ADCs. An ideal ADC should retain the favorable pharmacokinetic and functional properties of antibodies, remain intact and nontoxic in systemic circulation (blood), and become active at the target site, with the drug released in a sufficient amount to kill tumor cells; and thereby combine the cytotoxic activity of the drug with the intrinsic antigen-targeting and/or antitumor activities of the antibody.

One of the biggest challenges in the development of ADCs has been the generation of suitable linkers for the conjugation of antibody and drug. The role of the linker is fundamental because, in addition to efficient delivery of the cytotoxic drug, the stability of the drug–antibody linkage is a key factor in determining the efficacy

Laurent Ducry (ed.), *Antibody-Drug Conjugates*, Methods in Molecular Biology, vol. 1045,
DOI 10.1007/978-1-62703-541-5_5, © Springer Science+Business Media, LLC 2013

and toxicity of ADC and in doing so the ADC's therapeutic potential. There are several important considerations regarding the linker component, including the site of attachment on the antibody, the average number of attachment sites per antibody molecule, the cleavability of the linker (ability to disintegrate releasing the drug), and the polarity of the linker.

Since a key advantage of antibody-based therapeutics over most chemotherapeutic drugs is their long retention in circulation, the linker should be exceedingly stable in circulation as release of the cytotoxic payload before reaching the target would lead to nonspecific cell killing and associated toxicities. However, upon reaching the target cells, the linker must also allow for efficient release of the cytotoxic compound in an active form at the target site.

Several strategies have been employed to produce linkers that satisfy these criteria, some of which exploit differential properties between the extracellular and intracellular environments to release drug only after antigen-specific, antibody-mediated internalization of the ADC into tumor cells (receptor-mediated endocytosis) has occurred [1].

Most ADCs currently undergoing clinical evaluation contain linkers that fall into two broad categories: cleavable and noncleavable. Cleavable linkers rely on processes inside the cell to liberate the toxin, such as reduction in the cytoplasm, exposure to acidic conditions in the lysosome, or cleavage by specific proteases within the cell. Noncleavable linkages require proteolytic degradation of the antibody portion of the ADC for release of the cytotoxic molecule, which will retain the linker and the amino acid by which it was attached to the antibody.

Early generation ADCs often contained unstable linkers with short half-lives (1–2 days) such as disulfides [2–4] and hydrazones [5–7]. More recently, attention has turned toward linkers with improved stability characteristics while in the systemic circulation [8]. Included among them are peptide linkers [9, 10], glucuronides [11], and noncleavable linkers that remain covalently attached to the drug after the mAb carrier is hydrolyzed in lysosomes of target cells [8, 12].

The choice of linker is target dependent, based on the knowledge of the internalization and degradation of the antibody–target antigen complex, and a preclinical in vitro and in vivo activity comparison of conjugates. Furthermore, the choice of a linker is also influenced by which cytotoxin is used, as each molecule has different chemical constraints, and frequently the drug structure lends itself to a specific linker.

Another feature unique to ADCs that can be manipulated by the choice of linker is the bystander killing effect, which can increase the potency of these therapeutics. Some ADCs have been observed to effect killing of bystander antigen-negative cells present in the vicinity of the antigen-positive tumor cells. Studies to elucidate the mechanism of bystander cell killing by ADCs have indicated that metabolic products formed during intracellular processing of the ADCs may play a role [9, 12, 13]. Neutral cytotoxic metabolites generated by metabolism of the ADCs in antigen-positive cells can be released into the medium and can kill adjacent antigen-negative cells. Charged metabolites, however, may be prevented from diffusing across the membrane into the medium and cannot effect bystander killing [12, 14]. Manipulating the bystander killing effect through judicious use of linkers may be a valuable tool in targeting solid tumors with heterogeneous expression of the antigen.

2 Chemically Labile Linkers

Chemically labile linkers, which include hydrazone and disulfide linkers, have been designed to exploit differential properties between the plasma and some cytoplasmic compartments. The intracellular conditions to facilitate drug release for hydrazone linkers are the acidic environment of endosomes and lysosomes [15], while disulfide linkers are reduced in the cytosol [12, 13, 16], which contains high thiol concentrations (e.g., glutathione) [17]. Chemically labile linkers are often associated with limited plasma stability. However, their stability can be tuned by introducing steric hindrance using substituents near the linkage [2, 3, 18].

2.1 Acid-Labile Linkers (Hydrazones)

Acid-labile linkers, such as hydrazones, were the first to be used in early ADC constructs. These linkers are designed to remain intact during systemic circulation in the blood's neutral pH environment (pH 7.3–7.5) but to undergo hydrolysis and release drug once the ADC is internalized into mildly acidic endosomal (pH 5.0–6.5) and lysosomal (pH 4.5–5.0) compartments of the cell [15]. Although this linker technology based on a pH-dependent release mechanism has been associated with nonspecific release of the drug in clinical studies, it is still being used. Also, the stability of the hydrazone linkage, and thereby in vivo half-life, can be varied by chemical modification (e.g., substitution) allowing tuning to achieve more efficient drug release in the lysosome with a minimized loss in circulation [18].

A number of early ADC constructs used acid-labile linkages between the drug and carbohydrate residues of monoclonal antibodies. This has been accomplished via either hydrazone linkages or *cis*-aconityl. *cis*-Aconityl chemistry uses a carboxylic acid juxtaposed to an amide bond to accelerate amide hydrolysis under acidic conditions.

Daunomycin (or daunorubicin), an intercalator blocking DNA replication, was conjugated through a *cis*-aconityl linkage to carbohydrate hydroxyls groups of an anti-T-cell monoclonal antibody,

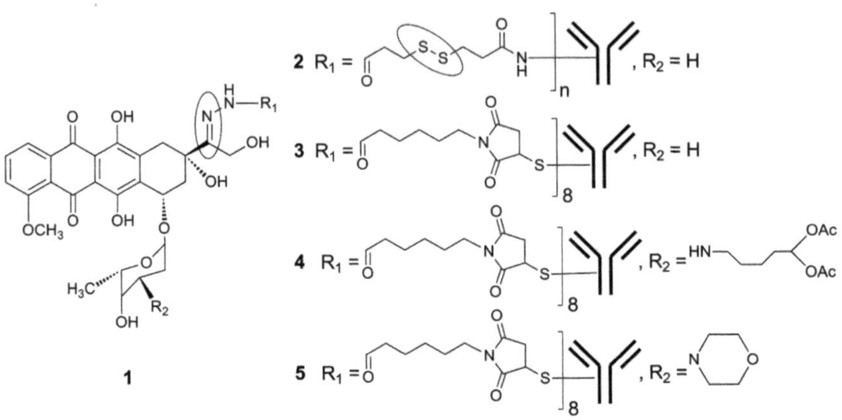

Fig. 1 Hydrazone derivatives of doxorubicin **1** and doxorubicin–antibody conjugates **2–5**

which were converted to amines prior to conjugation. The daunomycin conjugate retained cytotoxicity of the drug and showed only minimal loss of immunoreactivity, although a relatively large number of drug molecules [25–32] were attached to the antibody [19]. A *cis*-aconityl linkage was also used to conjugate doxorubicin (DOX), a member of the anthracycline antibiotics, closely related to the natural product Daunomycin, and a potent DNA intercalator, through its amino sugar moiety to an anti-melanoma monoclonal antibody via *cis*-aconitic anhydride. The anti-melanoma mAb–doxorubicin conjugates were quite effective in suppressing growth of established human melanoma xenografts in mice and increasing their life-span. This could not be achieved by either the mAb or doxorubicin alone [20]. In another example for acid-labile linkers, a hydrazide derivative of the cytotoxic vinca alkaloid vinblastine DAVLB (desacetylvinblastine), an anti-microtubule drug [21], was conjugated to a variety of murine monoclonal antibodies directed against human solid tumors. Conjugation was again achieved through the carbohydrate residues of the mAbs after periodate oxidation, which improved the therapeutic index compared to the unconjugated drug [22].

However, the main focus in the early days of ADC development remained on the use of hydrazones as acid-labile linkers, using amino acid residues on the monoclonal antibody, rather than the carbohydrate moieties, for covalent attachment. An early such doxorubicin–antibody conjugate was constructed by condensation of thiolated lysine residues of monoclonal antibodies with a 13-acylhydrazone derivative of doxorubicin. These conjugate constructs (Fig. 1, **2**) had two cleavable sites containing a disulfide linkage in addition to the hydrazone in the linker arm. Therefore, effective release of the unmodified free drug required acidic pH or disulfide reduction and acidic pH [23]. Although these conjugates were active in an antigen-specific manner, they had poor in vivo potency [24, 25].

High activity and impressive antitumor effects in preclinical studies were accomplished by using a later generation of BR96–doxorubicin ADC (Fig. 1, **3**) developed at Bristol-Myers Squibb. Trail et al. maintained the hydrazone but replaced the disulfide motif with a thioether and used (6-maleimidocaproyl)-hydrazone doxorubicin derivatives (Fig. 1, **1**) linked to the cysteine residues of BR96. BR96 is a monoclonal antibody directed against an antigen closely related to Lewis Y (LeY) and expressed on the cell surface of many human carcinomas [5]. Even though the ADC consisted of eight drugs per mAb molecule, high cumulative doses were needed for curative therapy (>100 mg/kg), presumably due to the relatively low potency of doxorubicin (IC_{50} of 0.1–0.3 μM for human carcinoma lines) [26, 27], whereas subnanomolar activities are currently typically seen. In phase I clinical trials, modest antitumor activity was obtained, and the measured half-life of systemic drug release was only 43 h [6]. Subsequently, BR96–doxorubicin was unsuccessful in a phase II trial in metastatic breast cancer (MBC) as therapeutic doses could not be reached before host toxicity [28]. Overall, BR96–doxorubicin was significantly hampered by low drug potency, insufficient stability of the hydrazone linkage, and the presence of target antigen Lewis Y (LeY) on highly sensitive non-tumor cells.

However, Bristol-Myers Squibb demonstrated the general utility of the maleimide-caproyl-hydrazone approach for other highly potent anthracyclines possessing an α,α′-dihydroxyketone side chain, such as 5-Diacetoxypentyldoxorubicin (DAPDOX) and Morpholinodoxorubicin (MorphDOX). The corresponding BR96-DAPDOX (Fig. 1, **4**) and BR96-MorphDOX (Fig. 1, **5**) conjugates were highly active and showed selective in vitro cytotoxicity when compared to the corresponding nonconjugated parent drugs. Furthermore, BR96-DAPDOX (Fig. 1, **4**) was superior in vitro by a large margin to BR96–doxorubicin (Fig. 1, **3**) [29].

The results with relatively low in vivo potency ADCs such as BR96–doxorubicin prompted significant efforts toward utilizing drugs with much higher potencies than doxorubicin. The natural product calicheamicin, an enediyne antibiotic derived from the soil bacterium *Micromonospora echinospora* ssp. *calichensis* [30] has been the subject of extensive investigation, due to its ability to bind to the minor groove and effect apoptosis with >100-fold the potency of most standard chemotherapeutics [31, 32]. As with BR96–doxorubicin (Fig. 1, **3**), an acid-labile hydrazone linker was used to attach the drug to monoclonal antibodies, providing a similar half-life for drug release from the ADC in the range of 48–72 h [7]. Pfizer's gemtuzumab ozogamicin (Mylotarg®, Fig. 2, **6**), using the hydrazone linker technology, was the first ADC to successfully complete clinical trials [33, 34] and receive regulatory approval by the US Food and Drug Administration (FDA) in 2000 [35] for use in patients over 60 suffering from relapsed acute

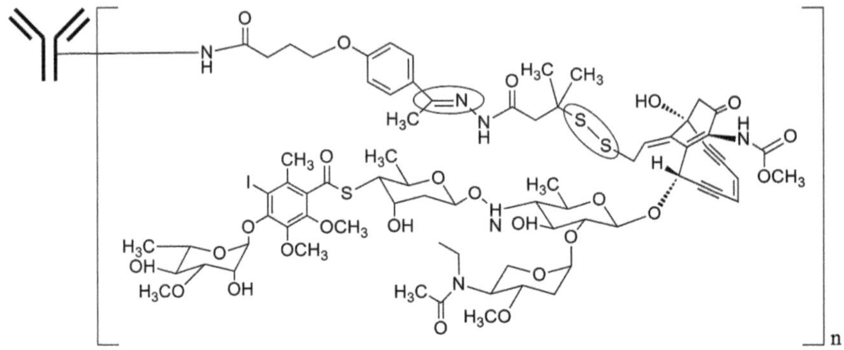

6

Fig. 2 Gemtuzumab ozogamicin **6**

myelocytic leukemia (AML), the most common form of leukemia in adults. Gemtuzumab ozogamicin (Fig. 2, **6**), more potent and selective than earlier amide and carbohydrate conjugates [36], consists of *N*-acetyl-γ-calicheamicin covalently attached to the humanized anti-CD33 (an IgG4 κ antibody) via a bifunctional linker. The 4-(4-acetylphenoxy)butanoic acid moiety provides attachment to surface-exposed lysine residues of the antibody through an amide bond and forms an acylhydrazone linkage with *N*-acetyl-γ-calicheamicin dimethylhydrazide. Calicheamicins, by the nature of their structure, also contain a disulfide bond that can serve as an additional site of release of the calicheamicin from the antibody. Typically, a drug loading of 2–3 molecules of calicheamicin per molecule of mAb is achieved [18].

Upon internalization of the ADC, the calicheamicin prodrug is released by hydrolysis of the hydrazone in the lysosomes of the CD33-positive target cells; this was observed in vitro. Indeed the hydrolysis of hydrazone linkage under physiological conditions at 37 °C for 24 h increased from 6 % at pH 7.4 (simulating neutral pH in blood) to 97 % at pH 4.5 [15]. The enediyne drug is then activated by reductive cleavage of the disulfide bond, which is stabilized by two methyl group substituents adjacent to the disulfide to prevent premature release of calicheamicin during circulation by reducing thiols, thereby leading to an improvement in the therapeutic index of the conjugate [37]. Substituents on the aromatic group adjacent to the hydrazone in calicheamicin conjugates were observed to significantly affect the rate of calicheamicin release and ADC potency [18]. Gemtuzumab ozogamicin was also able to elicit potent antitumor activity in an antigen-independent manner on solid tumors in vivo [38]. This effect was attributed to passive targeting, as nonspecific drug release through linker hydrolysis may offer a potential explanation for the activity of gemtuzumab ozogamicin in some AML patients where the cognate antigen CD33 was not detected [39].

A number of calicheamicin conjugates were prepared by reaction of an activated ester derivative with the lysine residues on the antibodies (e.g., anti-CD33 [36] and anti-CD22 [40]), which did not contain a hydrazone bond and were therefore stable to hydrolysis under physiological conditions, while still containing the disulfide bond inherent to calicheamicin. Based on the lower potency of these amide-linked conjugates, it was concluded that the disulfide alone is insufficient for efficient release of the calicheamicin from the antibody in the target cell. Additionally, the site of hydrolytic release offered by the hydrazone is essential for activity. Interestingly, with mAb CTM01 (recognizing tumor antigen PEM, a MUC1 variant present on a broad spectrum of solid tumors of epithelial origin), amide-bearing ADCs containing only the disulfide as source for drug release [41, 42], showed activities equal to or even greater than that of the corresponding hydrazone conjugate in several in vitro and in vivo tumor models [43]. Although these conjugates with CTM01 showed only limited evidence of activity in phase II clinical trials [44], this illustrates that the postulated inefficient release of the calicheamicin with disulfide alone cannot be generalized without taking target internalization properties into account.

Mylotarg® showed limited success and was withdrawn from the market in 2010 due to a narrow therapeutic window and lack of target dependence. Nonetheless, the calicheamicin ADC technology has also been successfully applied to mAbs recognizing a range of tumor antigens. Most notably CD22, a lymphoid antigen, for which the development of a humanized anti-CD22 mAb identically attached to *N*-acetyl-γ-calicheamicin dimethylhydrazide through the acid-labile 4-(4′-acetylphenoxy)butanoic acid linker, is ongoing at Pfizer with inotuzumab ozogamicin (CMC-544).

Inotuzumab ozogamicin (CMC-544) in some ways is to B cell lymphomas what Mylotarg is to leukemia [45–47]. Although this ADC is closely related to Mylotarg and using the same acid-labile linker, good stability in both human plasma and serum (rate of hydrolysis of 1.5–2 %/day over 4 days) and proven potent and specific antitumor efficacy [40, 48] led to markedly longer antitumor response in patients with refractory or relapsed indolent B cell non-Hodgkin's lymphoma (NHL) in an ongoing phase II clinical trial [49]. Other tumor antigens for conjugates using the hydrazone-linked calicheamicin include Lewis Y [50] and oncofetal protein 5T4 [51].

2.2 Disulfide Linkers

Another chemically labile linkage extensively exploited in the development of antibody–drug conjugates are disulfides. Disulfides are thermodynamically (in the absence of free sulfhydryls) stable at physiological pH and are designed to release the drug upon internalization inside cells, where the cytosol provides a significantly more reducing environment compared to the extracellular milieu [12, 17]. Since the scission of disulfide bonds requires the presence of a cytoplasmic thiol cofactor, such as (reduced) glutathione (GSH), disulfides provide reasonable stability in circulation and selective drug release in the cytosol [12, 13, 16]. Additionally, the intracellular enzyme protein disulfide isomerase, or similar enzymes capable of cleaving disulfide bonds [52], may also contribute to the preferential cleavage of disulfide bonds inside cells. GSH is reported to be present in cells in the concentration range of 0.5–10 mM [53] compared with a significantly lower concentration of GSH or cysteine, the most abundant low-molecular weight thiol, in circulation at approximately 5 μM [54]. This is especially true for tumor cells, where irregular blood flow leads to hypoxic state, resulting in enhanced activity of reductive enzymes and therefore even higher glutathione concentrations [55–57]. Furthermore, as with hydrazones, the in vivo stability of disulfide bonds—thereby more specific intracellular drug release—can be greatly enhanced through steric hindrance by introduction of substituents adjacent to the disulfide bond [2, 3].

An example of an intracellularly cleavable disulfide-based linker was already discussed for a calicheamicin amide conjugate with a fully humanized anti-MUC1 antibody containing only the disulfide linkage for release (no hydrazone linker), which showed potent antitumor effects in breast and ovarian tumor xenografts [36, 43].

Other examples are antibody conjugates of highly potent second-generation taxoids [58–60], which after conversion to the corresponding methyldisulfanyl alkanoyl derivatives were conjugated through a disulfide-bearing 4-mercapto-pentanoate linker to lysine residues on murine monoclonal antibodies recognizing the epidermal growth factor receptor (EGFR). The mAb-mediated delivery of the taxoid using tumor-selective mAbs leads to more pronounced antitumor activities than systemic drug treatment and notably good tolerability in terms of toxicity in mice [61].

However, the most important example for the use of disulfide linkers in ADCs is maytansinoid conjugates. Maytansinoids and thiol-containing maytansine analogues, widely used for ADC development, represent a class of highly potent antimitotic drugs inhibiting tubulin polymerization. Maytansinoids exhibit 100–1,000-fold higher cytotoxicity than most cancer chemotherapeutics [62]. Maytansine is easily converted to reactive thiol-containing maytansinoid derivatives by reaction with a disulfide ester, followed by reduction of the formed disulfide to yield the reactive sulfhydryl group. Thereby, maytansinoids can be linked to monoclonal antibodies via a disulfide bond in the linker in a chemically cleavable manner (or through a thioether linkage in a noncleavable fashion). Disulfide-linked antibody–maytansinoid conjugates (with about 3–4 maytansinoids per antibody molecule) were prepared by modifying lysine residues on the antibody with a bifunctional cross-linker to introduce pyridyldithio groups. Disulfide-exchange reaction of the modified antibody with a thiol-containing

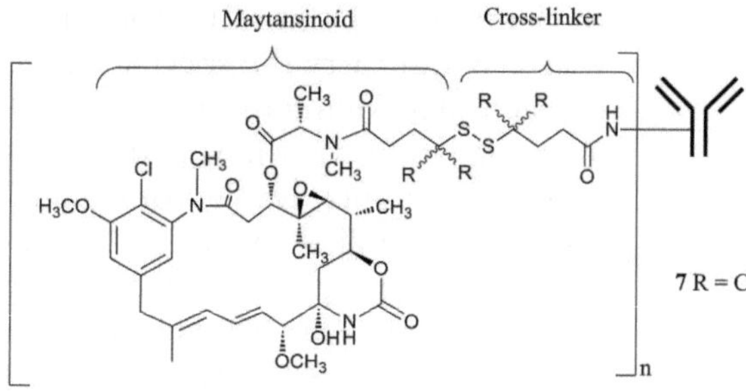

7 R = CH_3 or H

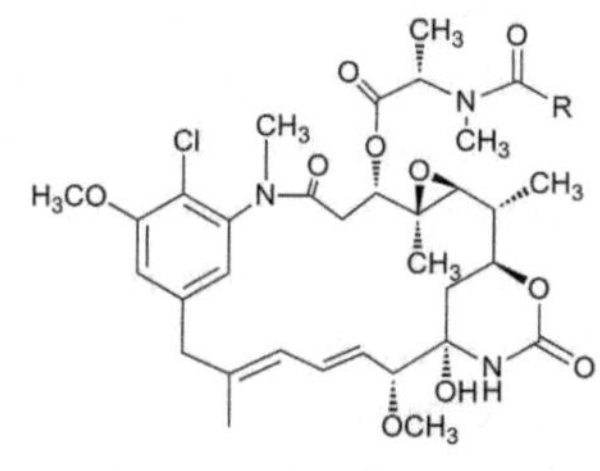

8 DM1-SMe: R = $-CH_2CH_2SSMe$
9 DM3-SMe: R = $-CH_2CH_2CH(CH_3)SSMe$
10 DM4-SMe: R = $-CH_2CH_2CH(CH_3)_2SSMe$

Fig. 3 Maytansinoid ADCs (**7**) with different degrees of methyl substitution on the carbon atoms geminal to the disulfide bond. Maytansinoid derivatives DM1, DM3, and DM4 (**8**, **9**, **10**), respectively

maytansinoid [63] leads to formation of the maytansinoid ADC. As shown with immunotoxins [2, 3], the in vivo stability of disulfide bonds (and with that the pharmacokinetic and toxicity profiles of an ADC) can be greatly enhanced through steric hindrance. It was also acknowledged that the oxidizing potential of endosomes and lysosomes may limit the intracellular cleavage of disulfide-linked ADCs [64]. To identify a balance between in vivo stability and efficient intracellular drug release, a series of maytansinoid–disulfide linker derivatives with varying degrees of steric hindrance (introduction of methyl substituents on the carbon atoms geminal to the disulfide bond) were conjugated to a monoclonal antibody. The effect of disulfide linker hindrance on the biological activity of these ADCs (Fig. 3, 7) was investigated. As control, maytansinoid derivatives were also conjugated through SMCC (succinimidyl-4-[*N*-maleimidomethyl]-cyclohexane-1-carboxylate) by forming a thioether bond (noncleavable linkage) [16, 65]. Based on results from these studies, DM1 (Fig. 3, **8**) and DM4 (Fig. 3, **10**) were selected as lead drug molecules for antibody conjugation [63].

After internalization of the ADC via antigen-mediated endocytosis and delivery to lysosomes by vesicular trafficking, the mAb is believed to be degraded to the level of amino acids [66], affording lysine derivatives linked to the maytansinoid toxin. Further intracellular modifications include cleavage of the disulfide linker through a disulfide exchange and thiol methylation presumably catalyzed by intracellular methyltransferases, generating potent metabolites of DM1 or DM4 [12]. The lipophilic *S*-methyl-maytansinoid metabolites are uncharged, facilitating their movement out of tumor cells and reentry into adjacent cells that may not carry the specific antigen, and thereby enable target-cell-activated killing of bystander cells. This bystander effect offers an explanation for the superior efficacy of disulfide-linked conjugates over noncleavable conjugates, which are degraded to the more hydrophilic—much less active—lysine-containing maytansinoid metabolites, seen in some xenograft models [12, 13, 67, 68].

One of the first maytansinoid-containing ADCs developed by ImmunoGen (using TAP (tumor-activated prodrug) conjugation technology) was C242-DM1, which targets CanAg, a tumor-selective carbohydrate epitope [69]. The clinical potential of C242-DM1 was enhanced by humanization of the antibody component to create, after conjugation with DM1, ADC huC242-DM1 (cantuzumab mertansine). Conjugate huC242-DM1 (in a similar manner as C242-DM1) had robust activity against tumors with heterogeneous antigen expression, reflecting its ability to kill bystander antigen-negative tumor cells [13]. The antibody component of huC242-DM1 had a half-life of ~100 h in mice, whereas the half-life of DM1 was about fourfold shorter [4, 70] suggesting slow release of DM1 from the ADC in circulation. Similarly, in a subsequent phase I clinical study, the terminal half-lives of the huC242-DM1 ADC and DM1 were ~100 and ~24 h, respectively [28]. The most likely mechanism for DM1 release from huC242-DM1 is by disulfide exchange with other sulfhydryls [4] (up to ~500 μM free sulfhydryls) inside cells. These sulfhydryls are likely to be almost entirely from albumin as indicated by analysis of human plasma [54]. Based on these findings, DM1 was replaced with DM4 to provide the huC242-DM4 conjugate construct, which displayed improved linker stability over huC242-DM1, resulting from increased steric hindrance around the disulfide bond, as well as improved efficacy compared to huC242-DM1 in some xenograft models [63]. Therefore, huC242-DM4 conjugate has replaced huC242-DM1 in clinical development [62].

Beyond the examples discussed above, maytansinoid ADC technology has been successfully applied to antibodies recognizing a wide range of tumor antigens, including CD19 [71], CD33 [72], CD56 [73], CD79 [74], CD138 [75], HER2 [76], PSCA [77], and PSMA [78]. Several of these ADC constructs are currently undergoing clinical testing.

3 Enzymatically Cleavable Linkers

3.1 Peptide Linkers

As mentioned, chemically labile linker, such as hydrazone [5–7] and disulfides [2–4], often suffer from limited plasma stability; therefore, peptide-based linker technologies may offer better control of drug release. Peptidic bonds are expected to have good serum stability, as lysosomal proteolytic enzymes have very low activities

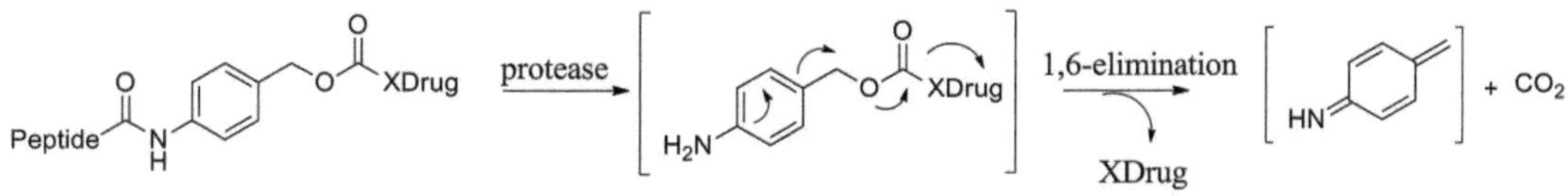

11 12

Fig. 4 Fragmentation of *p*-amidobenzyl ethers (**11**) releasing unmodified drug (**12**)

in blood due to endogenous inhibitors and the unfavorably high pH value of blood compared to lysosomes [79]. This was confirmed in preclinical in vivo studies where half-lives of 7–10 days were observed for peptide linkers [80]. Release of the drug from the mAb occurs specifically due to the action of lysosomal proteases (e.g., cathepsin and plasmin). These proteases may be present at elevated levels in certain tumor tissues [81]. So, unlike the chemically labile linkers discussed thus far, peptide linkers combine greater systemic stability with rapid enzymatic release of the drug in the target cell.

Early lysosomally cleavable peptides such as Gly-Phe-Leu-Gly [82] and Ala-Leu-Ala-Leu [83, 84] had significant potential liabilities as the drug release was relatively slow, and the hydrophobic nature of the tetrapeptides, in combination with the hydrophobicity of many cytotoxic drugs, may lead to aggregation. Therefore, optimized dipeptide-based linkers Val-Cit and Phe-Lys were developed, which were reasonably stable under physiological conditions but underwent rapid hydrolysis in the presence of lysosomal extracts and purified human cathepsin B [85, 86]. Cathepsin B is an ubiquitous cysteine protease whose properties do not differ very much from species to species [26, 27, 57, 87]. However, direct attachment of the drug to the peptide linker would result in proteolytic release of an amino acid adduct of the cytotoxic agent, thereby perhaps impairing the cytotoxic activity. In order to avoid the formation of metabolites with potentially reduced activity and any possible negative influence of the drug on the kinetics of peptide hydrolysis (drug release), a self-immolative spacer was designed to spatially separate the drug from the site of enzymatic cleavage. The subsequent collapse of the incorporated spacer allows for the elimination of the fully active, chemically unmodified drug from the conjugate upon amide bond hydrolysis. One of the most commonly used spacers is the bifunctional *p*-aminobenzyl alcohol group, which is linked to the peptide through the amino group, forming an amide bond, while amine-containing cytotoxic drugs are attached through carbamate functionalities to the benzylic hydroxyl group of the linker (PABC). The resulting prodrugs (Fig. 4, **11**) are activated upon protease-mediated cleavage, leading to a 1,6-elimination reaction releasing the unmodified drug (Fig. 4, **12**), carbon dioxide, and remnants of the linker group [88].

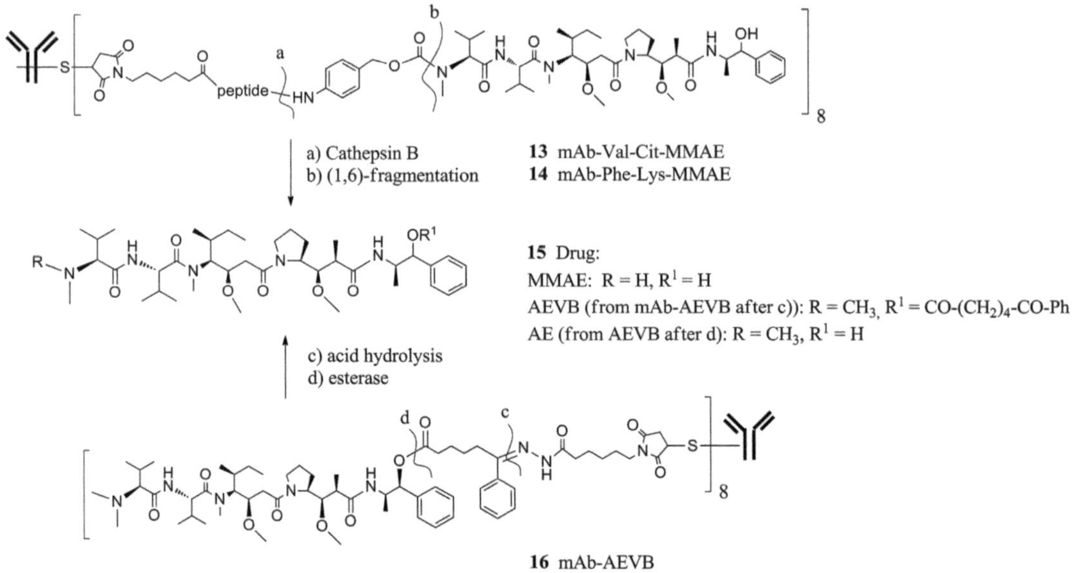

Fig. 5 Structures of auristatin drugs (**15**) and ADCs (**13**, **14**, **16**) and drug release mechanism: Drug **15** is released from peptide conjugates **12** and **13** through enzymatic hydrolysis (step a) and spontaneous fragmentation (step b) of the *p*-aminobenzylcarbamate intermediate. Drug **15** is released from mAb–AEVB conjugates **16** through hydrazone hydrolysis (step c) and hydrolysis of the ester (step d)

Antibody–drug conjugates comprised of drugs such as doxorubicin [26, 89], mitomycin C [90], camptothecin [91], tallysomycin [92], and auristatins/auristatin family members [8, 9, 93] have been prepared using cleavable peptide linkers for intracellular drug release. Of these, the auristatins are of particular interest. Auristatins are highly potent, totally synthetic, and stable and are amenable to chemical modification strategies to allow for linker attachment.

An auristatin derivative, monomethyl auristatin E (MMAE), was modified with maleimide-containing dipeptide linkers, and the resulting drug-linker derivatives were linked to cysteine residues in chimeric mAbs cBR96 (specific to Lewis Y on carcinomas) and cAC10 (specific to CD30 on hematological malignancies) [8, 9]. In vitro studies demonstrated that peptide-linked MMAE conjugates targeting CD30 on Hodgkin's lymphoma and Lewis Y on carcinomas were highly potent with 10- to 100-fold greater immunologically dependent cell kill compared with the corresponding hydrazone-linked MMAE ADCs. The peptide-linked MMAE conjugates (Fig. 5, **13** and **14**) were more stable in buffers and human plasma than the mAb conjugates with the hydrazone of 5-benzoylvaleric acid-auristatin E ester (AEVB, Fig. 5, **16**). This is shown by the half-lives of drug release from Val-Cit-linked ADCs (Fig. 5, **13** and **14**) in vivo being about threefold higher compared to the hydrazone linker (Fig. 5, **16**) (in mice, 6 days versus 2 days, respectively) [80]. Furthermore, the peptide-linked MMAE

ADCs (Fig. 5, **13** and **14**) were also less toxic than the corresponding hydrazone-linked ADC (Fig. 5, **16**). In vivo studies showed pronounced antitumor activity in xenograft models for the peptide-linked MMAE ADCs (Fig. 5, **13** and **14**), leading to cures of established tumors at very small fractions of the maximum-tolerated doses [9].

A bystander killing effect, similar to that observed with disulfide-linked maytansinoid ADCs, can also be achieved using cleavable dipeptide-linked auristatin ADCs. For example, the exposure of CD30-expressing cells to Seattle Genetics' Brentuximab Vedotin (anti-CD30 cAC10-Val-Cit-MMAE, SGN-35) resulted in lysosomal degradation and intracellular release of chemically unmodified MMAE, and the efflux of MMAE led to killing of cocultivated CD30-negative cells [14].

In addition to attaching the cleavable linker to the N-terminus of auristatins, attachment to their C-terminus was also attempted. Because of the negatively charged phenylalanine residue at the C-terminus, the potency of auristatin F (AF) and MMAF is impaired. However, their ability to kill target cells is greatly enhanced through facilitated cellular uptake by internalizing mAbs. The effects of linker technology on AF-based ADC potency, activity, and tolerability using dipeptide linkers between the C-terminal residue and the mAb carrier were investigated. While the resulting ADCs differed widely in activity, some showed significantly improved therapeutic indices compared to the N-terminally linked mAb-Val-Cit-PABC-MMAF conjugate [9, 94].

Seattle Genetics' Brentuximab Vedotin SGN-35 (Adcetris™) was granted accelerated regulatory approval by the US Food and Drug Administration (FDA) (2011) for use in relapsed or refractory Hodgkin's lymphoma and relapsed or refractory systemic anaplastic large cell lymphoma based on an unprecedented high rate of response in early clinical trials in relapsed and refractory HL and sALCL as well as tolerability and manageable toxicity [95–98]. Adcetris™ is the second antibody–drug conjugate, after Pfizer's Mylotarg® in 2000, to have received approval by regulatory agencies.

Several other ADCs containing enzymatically cleavable dipeptide-linked auristatins are currently in clinical trials, e.g., from Seattle Genetics SGN-75 (anti-CD70,Val-Cit-MMAF) (phase I) [99], from Celldex Therapeutics glembatumumab (CDX-011) (anti-NMB, Val-Cit-MMAE) (phase II) [100, 101], and from Cytogen PSMA-ADC (PSMA-ADC-1301) (phase I) (anti-PSMA, Val-Cit-MMAE) [102].

The versatility of enzyme-labile linkers was also shown by applying it for doxorubicin derivatives, which were conjugated to cysteine residues of mAbs [26, 103]. Conjugation involved the attachment of the dipeptide linker containing a PABC spacer, to the daunosamine nitrogen. With this strategy for BR96 mAb-peptide-doxorubicin conjugates, levels of cytotoxic activity with

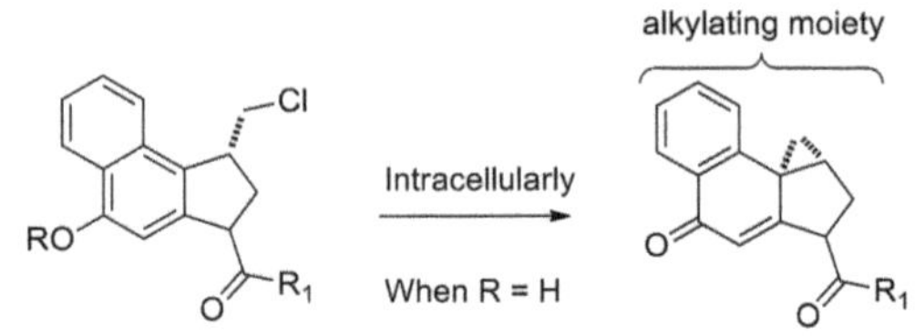

17

18

Fig. 6 Structure of the seco form of minor-groove-binding DNA-alkylating agent where R_1 is a DNA-binding moiety (**17**); intracellular processing of ADC liberates the potent drug (**18**)

immunological specificity were significantly improved compared to that of the corresponding hydrazone-based conjugates (Fig. 1). However, the potency of the conjugates was significantly less compared with the free drug, which may be attributed to the fact that passive cellular uptake of free drug may lead to higher intracellular concentrations compared to those obtained through mAb-mediated delivery [26], demonstrating not only the importance of the linker structure for the ADC properties but also that of the drug potency.

The impact of linker chemistry on stability and efficacy has also been reported for ADCs with SN-38, an active metabolite of the cancer prodrug, irinotecan. ADCs with a systemically inert, but cathepsin B sensitive, Phe-Lys linker were significantly less efficacious than those with an esterase-labile carbonate linker, independent of the internalizing rates of carrier mAbs [104], indicating that purely cellular mechanisms of drug release were inadequate for delivering therapeutic levels of free SN-38 from peptide-linked conjugates in tumor cells. The carbonate-linked SN-38 conjugates were efficacious, with good therapeutic windows, in solid and hematopoietic human tumor xenograft models [105–107]. These ADCs can be used in combination with radiolabeled mAb [108] or naked mAb [105], targeting different antigens, for enhanced therapeutic effects.

Peptide-containing linkers have also been successfully used for ADC of another very potent class of cytotoxic drugs which belong to the minor-groove-binding DNA-alkylating agents (DNA MGBA), including duocarmycins, CC-1065 and other cyclopropapyrroloind-4-one (CPI), and cyclopropabenzindol-4-one analogues (CBI). The common structural feature **17** is shown in Fig. 6 [109], where R can be a hydroxyl or an amine group and R_1 is a DNA-binding moiety. The conjugation strategy involves derivatizing the R group to include an antibody-binding group, e.g., a maleimide and cleavable peptide linker (or a glucuronidase-susceptible glucuronide). Alternatively, R could also be protected in the form of a carbamate prodrug, with the cleavable peptide and maleimide incorporated in the R_1 segment. In the latter case, the

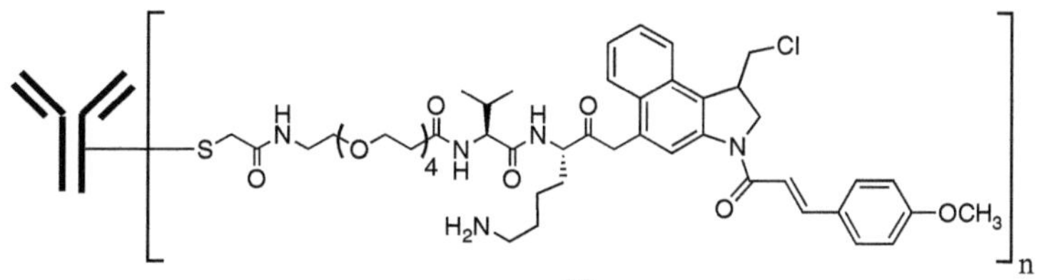

19

Fig. 7 ADCs (**19**) containing an amino-CBI payload linked through a valine–lysine peptide

prodrug form is generated in the tumor lysosomes, which must undergo human carboxylesterase-mediated cleavage to the active drug [110]. After intracellular processing, the seco form of the drug is released, which then undergoes Winstein cyclization to the potent cyclopropane-containing DNA alkylator **18** (Fig. 6).

To extend its ADC technology to drugs with a complementary mode of action, Seattle Genetics developed ADCs containing an amino-CBI and a hydroxy aza-CBI payload, respectively. Because of the hydrophobicity of this class of drugs, attention was focused on developing hydrophilic peptide-linker derivatives that prevented aggregation. This was achieved by replacing the Val-Cit linker with a more hydrophilic valine–lysine (Val-Lys) sequence, omitting the self-immolative spacer PABC and incorporating a tetra(ethylene glycol) unit (PEG_4) between the mAb and the peptide linker [111].

The direct attachment of the linker to the amine of the CBI building block prohibits the spontaneous formation of the active toxin in the plasma. Only the enzymatic cleavage of the linker after internalization of the ADC into the cancer cell triggers the release of the prodrug that is transformed into the DNA-alkylating cyclopropyl derivative via a Winstein cyclization. The resulting mAb conjugates (Fig. 7, **19**) were not prone to aggregation, and in vitro cytotoxicity assays established that the mAb-MGBA conjugates were highly cytotoxic and effected immunologically specific cell kill at subsaturating doses. This illustrates the importance of linker hydrophilicity in the design for mAb-MGBA conjugates [111].

3.2 β-Glucuronide Linkers

In an extension of the peptide-based linker strategies to provide high ADC stability, a β-glucuronic acid-based linker was developed [11]. Facile release of the active drug is realized through cleavage of the β-glucuronide glycosidic bond by the lysosomal enzyme β-glucuronidase (Fig. 8). This enzyme is abundantly present within lysosomes and is overexpressed in some tumor types [112], while the enzyme activity outside cells is low. This provides the potential for a high ADC stability in the systemic circulation and selective intracellular drug release. Furthermore, incorporating the highly hydrophilic nature of β-glucuronides may circumvent the tendency of some ADCs to undergo aggregation, especially for those with highly hydrophobic drugs (e.g., DNA minor-groove binders) [111].

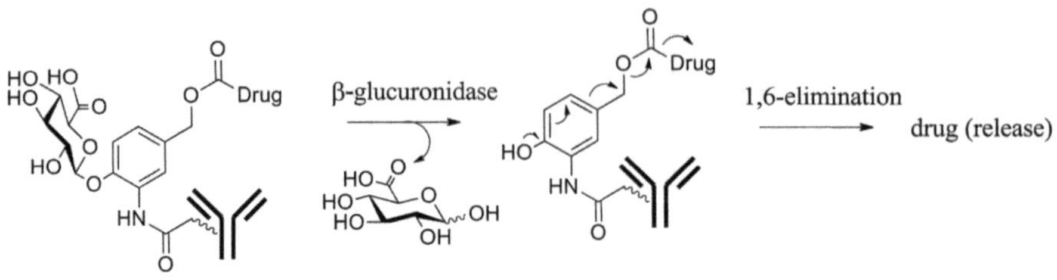

20

Fig. 8 Drug release from ADC containing β-glucuronic acid-based linker (**20**) by β-glucuronidase

For example, drug-linker moieties consisting of a β-glucuronide linked to auristatins MMAE, to MMAF, or to doxorubicin propyloxazoline (DPO) were prepared. Evaluation of the stability of the β-glucuronide-drug moieties in rat plasma showed an extrapolated half-life of 81 days for the β-glucuronide-linked MMAF compared with about 6 days for the corresponding valine–citrulline dipeptide-linked MMAF. After conjugation to mAbs (anti-CD70 c1F6 and anti-CD30 cAC10), the resulting ADCs (up to eight drug molecules per mAb) were found to be highly stable in plasma, well tolerated at high doses, and efficacious both in vitro and in vivo [11]. These results suggest that the β-glucuronide linker system may be a complementary alternative to peptide linkers. Therefore, β-glucuronide linkers have been used to prepare antibody conjugates of several drug classes, e.g., auristatins, camptothecin and doxorubicin analogues [11], CBI minor-groove binders [113], and psymberin [114].

4 Noncleavable Linkers

This class of linkers is considered noncleavable-meaning linker cleavage, and payload release does not depend on the differential properties between the plasma and some cytoplasmic compartments. Instead, the release of the cytotoxic drug is postulated to occur after internalization of the ADC via antigen-mediated endocytosis and delivery to lysosomal compartment, where the antibody is degraded to the level of amino acids through intracellular proteolytic degradation [12]. This process releases a drug derivative, which is formed by the cytotoxic drug, the linker and the amino acid residue to which the linker was covalently attached. A noncleavable linker can be successfully utilized only if the released drug metabolite functions as an active cytotoxic drug component [9, 16, 115]. A potential disadvantage maybe that ADCs incorporating noncleavable linkers are restricted to the specific tumor cell targeted and require good internalization for degradation within the cell to become active, as there is no mechanism for extracellular cleavage of the linker and subsequent permeation of the drug into the cell (passive diffusion). The amino acid–drug metabolites from conjugates with noncleavable linkers are more hydrophilic and much less membrane permeable, which leads to less bystander effects and less nonspecific toxicities compared to conjugates with a cleavable linker [12, 14]. ADCs with cleavable linkers on the other hand may also be active even when they are poorly internalized [116]. Thus, although internalization is often the common initial activation process for both cleavable and noncleavable linkers [12], ADC constructs with noncleavable linkers are more dependent on the biology of the target cell compared to cleavable linkers. Nevertheless, an advantage of these linkers is their greater stability in circulation compared to cleavable linkers. This can potentially improve the therapeutic index of a cytotoxic drug because it may be better tolerated [16, 117, 118]. Overall, the efficacy of ADCs containing noncleavable linkers and requiring antibody degradation for drug release is likely to be antibody, drug, and tumor dependent, in contrast to ADCs with cleavable linkers.

Early examples for immunoconjugates with noncleavable linkers include immunoconjugates of methotrexate [119], daunorubicin [87, 120], the vinca alkaloids [121], mitomycin C [122], idarubicin [123], and *N*-acetyl melphalan [124] via amide or succinimide spacers to different murine monoclonal antibodies. An average of 2–8 molecules per mAb were linked; and in all cases, attempts to increase the number of drug molecules linked to the antibody lead to low conjugate yield. Although mAb recognition was maintained, the full potency of the drug was not, in these ADC constructs (too stable linkages).

At this time, the most commonly used noncleavable linkages in antibody–drug conjugates are succinimide–thioether bonds, which are formed by the reaction of maleimides with thiols. This methodology has been applied to both of the two currently mostly used classes of toxic moieties, maytansinoids, and auristatins.

The evaluation of a panel of ImmunoGen's CanAg disulfide-linked huC242-maytansinoid conjugates showed that the thioether-linked huC242-MCC-DM1 control ADC, prepared by using heterobifunctional SMCC as cross-linker between lysine residues of the mAb and the thiol group of DM, had superior in vivo stability compared to that of the corresponding disulfide-linked ADC constructs of DM1 and DM4 [65]. But while huC242-MCC-DM1 was at least as potent in vitro as the selected conjugate huC242-SPDB-DM4 with a cleavable disulfide linker, it displayed significantly lower in vivo activity in multiple xenograft tumor models [125]. An evaluation of the mechanism of cell killing by the disulfide and thioether-linked maytansinoid-antibody conjugates showed that both required lysosomal degradation of the antibody component of the conjugate. The sole metabolite from thioether-linked mAb-MCC-DM1 ADCs was the lysine adduct lysine-MCC-DM1, which was only active when generated inside the tumor cell, while it had greatly diminished potency when examined separately in vitro, likely due to the charged hydrophilic nature, impairing membrane translocation capabilities and diffusion into neighboring cells [126, 127].

HER-2-targeted trastuzumab-MCC-DM1, an ADC with trastuzumab (T) antibody linked to the maytansinoid DM1, again prepared by using SMCC as cross-linker between lysine residues of the mAb and the thiol group of DM1, has been shown to be better tolerated with a more favorable pharmacokinetic and safety profile compared to the disulfide-linked maytansinoid ADC constructs. The thioether-linked trastuzumab-MCC-DM1 also displayed superior in vitro and in vivo activity compared with trastuzumab linked to other maytansinoids through disulfide linkers, suggesting that distribution and delivery of maytansinoid metabolites is sufficient in the trastuzumab-DM1/HER2 system without the need for bystander killing. Therefore, trastuzumab-MCC-DM1 was selected for clinical development [16].

The use of noncleavable linkers has thus become an important feature of ImmunoGen TAP conjugation technology. This is illustrated by the promising clinical results obtained by Genentech's Trastuzumab-DM1 (T-DM1) for HER2-positive metastatic breast cancer [128, 129] and the very recent success for the primary end point with significantly improved overall survival among metastatic patients in a phase III trial in women with advanced breast cancer, which triggered the application for approval by the regulatory agencies.

The transporter multidrug resistance protein 1 (MDR1)-mediated efflux of anticancer drugs is a frequently observed mechanism of drug resistance resulting poor response to chemotherapy, as documented for many cancer types [130, 131]. Recently, Kovtun et al. [132] described the conjugation of maytansinoid DM1 to different antibodies (anti-EpCAM, anti-EGFR, and anti-CanAg) via the maleimidyl-based hydrophilic linker PEG_4Mal, designed to evade MDR1-mediated resistance. It was found that following uptake into target cells, conjugates made with the PEG_4Mal linker (Fig. 9, **21**) were processed to a cytotoxic metabolite (lysine-PEG_4-Mal-DM1) that was retained by MDR1-expressing cells better than a metabolite (lysine-SMCC-DM1) of corresponding conjugates prepared with the nonpolar SMCC linker. The PEG_4Mal-linked conjugates (Fig. 9, **21**) were tolerated similarly as the corresponding SMCC-linked conjugates but more potent in killing MDR1-expressing cells in culture and more effective in eradicating MDR1-expressing human xenograft tumors. Antibody–maytansinoid conjugates containing the PEGylated linker (Fig. 9, **21**) showed an improved therapeutic index and were as cytotoxic to MDR1-expressing cells as they were to MDR1-negative cells. This suggests that conjugates with a short PEG oligomer in the linker are capable of evading the MDR1-mediated resistance [132].

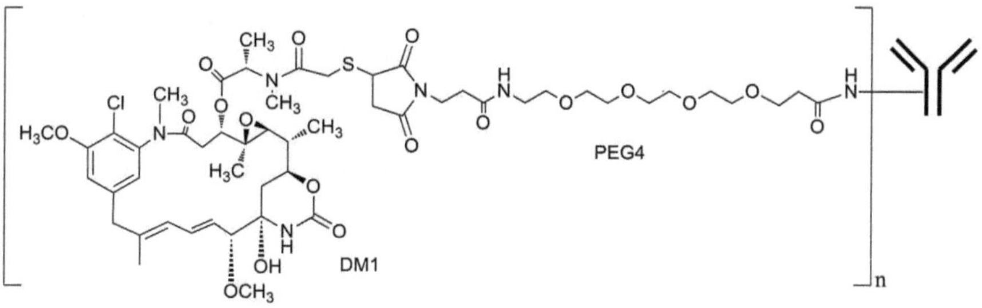

21

Fig. 9 DM1 ADC containing a PEG_4 linker (**21**)

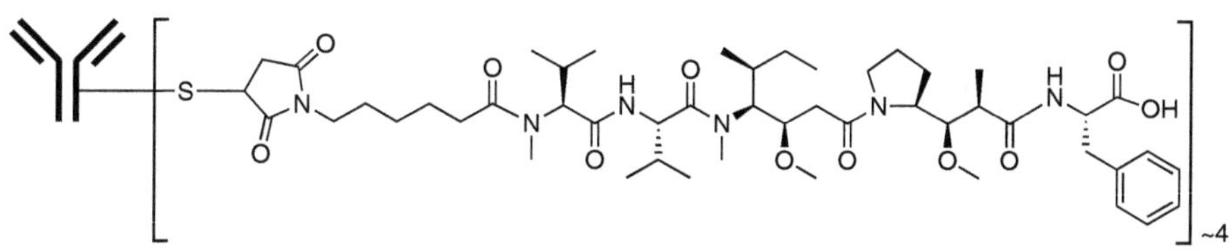

22

Fig. 10 Conjugate (**22**) linking auristatin MMAF to the antibody through a noncleavable linker (maleimidocaproyl, mc)

Noncleavable thioether linkers have also been employed to link auristatin derivatives to monoclonal antibodies. Because auristatins are synthetic, integral structural modifications can be made that significantly alter the properties of the drug. One such auristatin, MMAF, terminates with phenylalanine, a negatively charged residue that impairs cell membrane permeability [8]. Consequently, ADCs containing MMAF that facilitate drug uptake by antigen-positive cells are >2,000-fold more potent than the free drug itself.

A surprising finding with MMAF ADCs was that the cleavable dipeptide linker Val-Cit-PABC (vc-PABC) could be omitted, and highly potent (both in vitro and in vivo) ADCs were obtained by direct attachment of the drug to antibodies (anti-CD30 and anti-Lewis Y) through thioether adducts (Fig. 10, **22**) [8]. The switch from an enzymatically labile dipeptide linker to a thioether also increased the therapeutic index as the maleimidocaproyl-MMAF (mcMMAF) conjugate (Fig. 10, **22**) was equally efficacious in vivo but tolerated at significantly higher doses in rodents compared to the vc-PABC-MMAF conjugate. Mass spectrometry showed that the released drug was the cysteine adduct of the linker-MMAF derivative, presumably resulting from antibody degradation within lysosomes. The closely related auristatin, MMAE, was not active when attached in this manner, indicating that ADCs requiring antibody degradation for drug release are highly dependent on the nature of the drug for activity. MMAF can sustain significant modification to the N-terminal position and remain active, while most other drugs (e.g., MMAE, doxorubicin) are inactivated when modified in such an extensive manner [8].

In a mouse preclinical model, an anti-CD70 (h1F6) ADC with a thioether linkage to MMAF had a half-life of 7 days for drug release [133] which is similar to the 6–10 days half-life for drug release from the corresponding peptide-linked ADC [80]. The anti-CD70-mcMMAF conjugate showed potent antitumor activities in vitro and in vivo, inhibiting the growth of solid tumors in all models of renal cell carcinoma tested [134].

Using a noncleavable maleimidocaproyl linker provided potential for reduced off-target toxicity, and due to the more selective drug release following internalization into the target cancer cell, higher maximum doses were tolerated compared with the vcMMAF conjugate [8] in the context of the anti-CD70 antibody, leading to an improved therapeutic index. Therefore, a h1F6-mcMMAF conjugate (with an average of 4 mcMMAF molecules per mAb), designated as SGN-75, was selected for clinical development in solid tumor indications [134] and is currently in clinical trials for relapsed/refractory non-Hodgkin's lymphoma (NHL) and metastatic renal cell carcinoma.

Taken together, the reported findings [8, 133, 134] suggest that auristatin-based antibody–drug conjugates using a noncleavable linker may have broad utility for the treatment of human carcinomas.

5 Considerations for Conjugation

Apart from optimizing the individual components of an ADC, monoclonal antibody, drug, and linker, joining them in the conjugation step is another important factor for the therapeutic potential of an ADC. Some considerations are: the conjugation of the antibody to the drug should not alter the integrity of the antibody, binding of the antibody to the antigen, or the biological activity of the drug upon reaching the target cell (and effector functions of the selected mAb—if preserved). The pharmacodynamic properties of the ADC must resemble that of the mAb while in circulation. Therefore, progress in the area of conjugation technology is also a critical aspect in generating effective ADCs with optimal therapeutic properties. Optimization strategies have varied depending on the cytotoxic drug, linker chemistry, and antibody used.

While some earlier ADC constructs used carbohydrate moieties on antibodies as attachment sites, current conjugation technologies focus on the linking of the cytotoxic drug to amino acid residues in the antibody. Cytotoxic drugs are generally conjugated (through the linker) to antibodies either through accessible lysine side-chain amines or cysteine sulfhydryl groups, activated by reducing interchain disulfide bonds. Both of these procedures lead to heterogeneous ADCs, containing mixtures of species with different molar ratios of drug molecules attached to different sites in the antibody. Although typically approximately ten lysine residues are preferentially accessible for chemical modification, conjugation through lysine residues was shown to distribute to approximately 40 different sites, potentially resulting in $>10^6$ ADC species [135]. As there are only four inter-chain disulfide bonds in IgG_1 molecules, which are significantly more susceptible to reduction than the intra-chain disulfide bonds [136, 137], partial reduction yields eight possible conjugation sites. Therefore, conjugates generated through cysteine residues result in conjugates with less heterogeneity but could potentially comprise >100 different ADC species due to the variable stoichiometry (0–8 drugs per antibody) with several isomers at each drug substitution level [138–140].

The number of cytotoxic molecules attached to the antibody (drug-to-antibody ratio or DAR) is an important consideration that can effect the properties and pharmacokinetics of an ADC. A low DAR may result in low potency of the ADC, while increasing the number of drug molecules can potentially lead to higher concentrations of the drug at the target sites. Nevertheless, a too high degree of antibody modification may adversely affect its affinity toward the target antigen, the antibody receptor binding, and may also result in aggregation and precipitation of the antibody and potentially decrease ADC stability and faster clearance of the ADC [141]. Therefore, the optimal DAR is empirical for each antibody and must be judged on the basis of a variety of criteria such as the feasibility of conjugate synthesis and solubility of the resulting conjugate, impact on antigen-binding affinity, antigen-specific as well as non-targeted cytotoxicity of the ADC, and its behavior in animal models such as antitumor activity, pharmacokinetics, and systemic toxicity. However, for auristatin ADCs, it was found that while the in vitro activity directly correlated with the number of drug molecules, the in vivo activity of the ADCs with four and eight drug molecules per antibody was found to be equivalent. This was explained by the finding that clearance of the ADC was dependent on drug loading and that exposure is inversely correlated to the drug loading (higher loaded ADC species cleared faster leading to lower exposure). Also, 8-loaded ADC species showed increased toxicity compared to 4-loaded. Decreasing the number of drug molecules from 8 to 4 increased the therapeutic index of the ADC by twofold. This suggests that optimizing the drug-to-antibody ratio to maintain favorable pharmacokinetics, while maximizing drug payload may be a helpful tool in creating better ADCs [138, 139, 142]. Most of the conjugates currently in clinical testing (regardless of cytotoxic compound, antibody, or linker used) have 2–4 cytotoxic molecules per antibody molecule. The type of conjugation (via lysine or cysteine) can be selected and the DAR controlled by conjugation stoichiometry and conditions, an additional factor is the site of conjugation. While in some instances, it has been observed that the site of conjugation is not as important as the stoichiometry of drug attachment [139, 142], potentially unfavorable in vivo effects associated with heterogeneity of antibody–drug conjugates could compromise their promise as cancer therapeutics. Therefore, efforts to modulate the number and site of drug conjugation by site-specific conjugation are becoming a prevalent trend in the ADC design. Methods have been developed, mostly based on protein engineering, to allow cytotoxic drugs to be conjugated to antibodies with defined site and stoichiometry. In earlier efforts, one or more interchain cysteines were replaced with serine, thereby limiting available conjugation sites. These were used to create homogeneous ADC with two or four drug molecules per antibody [142]. However, removal of the hinge region interchain disulfide bonds from an IgG1 may impair antibody-dependent cellular cytotoxicity, consistent with impaired Fc–Fcγ receptor interactions, and also reduce complement-dependent cytotoxicity [143]. Current efforts include the engineering of reactive cysteine residues (usually 2 or 4) at specific sites in the antibody backbone to allow drug conjugation with defined stoichiometry and without disruption of interchain disulfide bonds, e.g., Genentech's ThioMab platform [140, 144]. Other examples for approaches to enable site-specific conjugation include the introduction of nonnatural amino acids to enable orthogonal conjugation chemistry as represented by AmbrX ReCODE™ [145, 146] and Allozyne Biociphering™ technologies [147]. Additionally, enzymes may be utilized to achieve site-specific conjugation. One example is "aldehyde tagging" (Redwood Bioscience) which includes the engineering of a specific amino acid sequence recognized by formylglycine-generating enzyme (FGE). This creates an unusual aldehyde-bearing formylglycine (FGly) residue providing a unique chemical functionality in the antibody that can be chemically conjugated in a selective manner [148]. Alternatively, the conjugation of the drug to the monoclonal antibody itself is enzyme mediated, as demonstrated, for example, by Schibli et al. using transglutaminase to covalently attach primary amine-functionalized drug moieties through specific glutamine residues in an antibody molecule [149].

6 Conclusion

One of the biggest challenges in the design and development of ADCs has been the generation of suitable linkers for the conjugation of antibody and drug. The role of the linker is fundamental in determining the therapeutic potential of an ADC: For efficient delivery of the cytotoxic drug, the stability of the drug–antibody linkage in circulation is a key factor. However, upon reaching the target cells, the linker must also allow for efficient release of the cytotoxic compound in an active form at the target site.

ADCs linkers fall into two broad categories: cleavable and noncleavable. Cleavable linkers rely on the differential properties between the plasma and cytoplasmic compartments to release the drug (e.g., low pH, reducing environment, action of lysosomal enzymes). Noncleavable linkages require internalization of the ADC and intracellular proteolytic degradation of the antibody portion of the ADC for release of the cytotoxic molecule (retaining the linker and amino acid by which it was attached to the antibody). While earlier cleavable linkers (e.g., hydrazones) have been associated with low serum stability, more recent cleavable linkers (e.g., hindered disulfides, peptide linkers) show higher stability in circulation resulting in lower nonspecific cell killing and reduced off-target toxicity. Noncleavable linkers (e.g., thioethers) have greater stability in circulation compared to cleavable linkers and can thereby improve the therapeutic index of a cytotoxic drug but are also more dependent on the biology of the target cell compared to cleavable linkers.

ADCs with noncleavable linkers are restricted to the specific-targeted tumor cell. They require good internalization for degradation within the cell to become active, as there is no mechanism for extracellular cleavage of the linker and subsequent permeation of the drug into the cell. In contrast, ADCs with cleavable linkers may be active against targets even when they are poorly internalized (passive diffusion) or effect killing of bystander antigen-negative cells present in the vicinity of the antigen-positive tumor cells (bystander effect).

Therefore, although great advances have been made in the development of the linker technology for ADCs, there is no general guideline for linker selection. It is highly dependent on the antibody, drug and tumor target, and the design and selection of the most suited linker must be evaluated based on efficacy and toxicity of an individual ADC construct.

References

1. Walter RB, Raden BW, Kamikura DM et al (2005) Influence of CD33 expression levels and ITIM-dependent internalization on gemtuzumab ozogamicin-induced cytotoxicity. Blood 105:1295–1302
2. Thorpe PE, Wallace PM, Knowles PP et al (1987) New coupling agents for the synthesis of immunotoxins containing a hindered disulfide bond with improved stability in vivo. Cancer Res 47:5924–5931
3. Thorpe PE, Wallace PM, Knowles PP et al (1988) Improved antitumor effects of immunotoxins prepared with deglycosylated ricin A-chain and hindered disulfide linkages. Cancer Res 48:6396–6403
4. Xie H, Audette C, Hoffee M et al (2004) Pharmacokinetics and biodistribution of the antitumor immunoconjugate, cantuzumab mertansine (huC242-DM1), and its two components in mice. J Pharmacol Exp Ther 308:1073–1082
5. Trail PA, Willner D, Lasch SJ et al (1993) Cure of xenografted humancarcinomas by BR96-doxorubicin immunoconjugates. Science 261:212–215
6. Saleh MN, Sugarman S, Murray J et al (2000) Phase I trial of the anti-Lewis Y drug immunoconjugate BR96-doxorubicin in patients with Lewis Y-expressing epithelial tumors. J Clin Oncol 18:2282–2292

7. Boghaert ER, Khandke KM, Sridharan L et al (2008) Determination of pharmacokinetic values of calicheamicin-antibody conjugates in mice by plasmon resonance analysis of small (5 μl) blood samples. Cancer Chemother Pharmacol 61:1027–1035
8. Doronina SO, Mendelsohn BA, Bovee TD et al (2006) Enhanced activity of monomethylauristatin F through monoclonal antibody delivery: effects of linker technology on efficacy and toxicity. Bioconjug Chem 17:114–124
9. Doronina SO, Toki BE, Torgov MY et al (2003) Development of potent monoclonal antibody auristatin conjugates for cancer therapy. Nat Biotechnol 21:778–784
10. Dubowchik GM, Walker MA (1999) Receptormediated and enzyme-dependent targeting of cytotoxic anticancer drugs. Pharmacol Ther 83:67–123
11. Jeffrey SC, Andreyka JB, Bernhardt SX et al (2006) Development and properties of beta-glucuronide linkers for monoclonal antibody–drug conjugates. Bioconjug Chem 17:831–840
12. Erickson HK, Park PU, Widdison WC et al (2006) Antibody–maytansinoid conjugates are activated in targeted cancer cells by lysosomal degradation and linker-dependent intracellular processing. Cancer Res 66:4426–4433
13. Kovtun YV, Audette CA, Ye Y et al (2006) Antibody–drug conjugates designed to eradicate tumors with homogeneous and heterogeneous expression of the target antigen. Cancer Res 66:3214–3221
14. Okeley NM, Miyamoto JB, Zhang X et al (2010) Intracellular activation of SGN-35, a potent anti-CD30 antibody–drug conjugate. Clin Cancer Res 16:888–897
15. Van der Velden VHJ, te Marvelde JG, Hoogeveen PG et al (2001) Targeting of the CD33-calicheamicin immunoconjugate Mylotarg (CMA-676) in acute myeloid leukemia: in vivo and in vitro saturation and internalization by leukemic and normal myeloid cells. Blood 97:3197–3204
16. Lewis Phillips G, Li G, Dugger DL et al (2008) Targeting HER2-positive breast cancer with trastuzumab-DM1, an antibody–cytotoxic drug conjugate. Cancer Res 68:9280–9290
17. Meister A, Anderson ME (1983) Glutathione. Annu Rev Biochem 52:711–760
18. Hamann PR, Hinman LM, Hollander I et al (2002) Gemtuzumab ozogamicin, a potent and selective anti-CD33 antibody–calicheamicin conjugate for treatment of acute myeloid leukemia. Bioconjug Chem 13:47–58
19. Dillman RO, Johnson DE, Shawler DL et al (1988) Superiority of an acid-labile daunorubicin monoclonal antibody immunoconjugate compared to free drug. Cancer Res 48:6097–6102
20. Yang HM, Reisfeld RA (1988) Doxorubicin conjugated to a monoclonal antibody directed against a melanoma-associated proteoglycan suppresses growth of established tumor xenografts in nude mice. Proc Natl Acad Sci U S A 85:1189–1193
21. Schneck D, Butler F, Dugan W et al (1990) Disposition of a murine monoclonal antibody vinca conjugate (KS1/4-DAVLB) in patients with adenocarcinomas. Clin Pharmacol Ther 47:36–41
22. Laguzza BC, Nichols CL, Briggs SL et al (1989) New antitumor monoclonal-antibody vinca conjugates LY203725 and related-compounds—design, preparation, and representative in vivo activity. J Med Chem 32:548–555
23. Greenfield RS, Kaneko T, Daues A et al (1990) Evaluation invitro of adriamycin immunoconjugates synthesized using an acid-sensitive hydrazone linker. Cancer Res 50:6600–6607
24. Trail PA, Miner DV, Lasch SJ et al (1992) Antigen-specific activity of carcinoma-reactive BR64-doxorubicin conjugates evaluated in vitro and in human tumor xenograft models. Cancer Res 52:5693–5700
25. Braslawsky GR, Edson MA, Pearce W et al (1990) Antitumor activity of adriamycin (hydrazone-linked) immunoconjugates compared with free adriamycin and specificity of tumor cell killing. Cancer Res 50:6608–6614
26. Dubowchik GM, Firestone RA, Padilla L et al (2002) Cathepsin B-labile dipeptide linkers for lysosomal release of doxorubicin from internalizing immunoconjugates: model studies of enzymatic drug release and antigen specific in vitro anticancer activity. Bioconjug Chem 13:855–869
27. King HD, Yurgaitis D, Wilner D et al (1999) Monoclonal antibody conjugates of doxorubicin prepared with branched linkers: a novel method for increasing the potency of doxorubicin immunoconjugates. Bioconjug Chem 10:279–288
28. Tolcher AW, Sugarman S, Gelmon KA (1999) Randomized phase II study of BR96-doxorubicin conjugate in patients with metastatic breast cancer. J Clin Oncol 17:478–484
29. King HD, Staab AJ, Pham-Kaplita K et al (2003) BR96 conjugates of highly potent

anthracyclines. Bioorg Med Chem Lett 13:2119–2122
30. Lee MD, Dunne TS, Siegel MM et al (1987) Calichemicins, a novel family of antitumor antibiotics. 1. Chemistry and partial structure of calichemicin y_1^I. J Am Chem Soc 109:3464–3466
31. Damle NK, Frost P (2003) Antibody-targeted chemotherapy with immunoconjugates of calicheamicin. Curr Opin Pharmacol 3:386–390
32. Damle NK (2004) Tumour-targeted chemotherapy with immunoconjugates of calicheamicin. Expert Opin Biol Ther 4:1445–1452
33. Sievers EL, Appelbaum FR, Spielberger RT et al (1999) Selective ablation of acute myeloid leukemia using antibody-targeted chemotherapy: a phase I study of an anti-CD33 calicheamicin immunoconjugate. Blood 93:3678–3684
34. Sievers EL, Larson R, Estey E et al (1999) Preliminary results of the efficacy and safety of CMA-676 in patients with AML in first relapse. Proc Am Soc Clin Oncol 18:Abstract 21
35. Bross PF, Beitz J, Chen G et al (2001) Approval summary: gemtuzumab ozogamicin in relapsed acute myeloid leukemia. Clin Cancer Res 7:1490–1496
36. Hamann PR, Hinman LM, Beyer CF et al (2002) An anti-CD33 antibodycalicheamicin conjugate for treatment of acute myeloid leukemia. Choice of linker. Bioconjug Chem 13:40–46
37. Hinman LM, Hamann PR, Upeslacis J (1995) Preparation of conjugates to monoclonal antibodies. In: Borders DB, Doyle TW (eds) Enediyne antibiotics as antitumor agents, 1st edn. Marcel Dekker, New York, pp 87–106
38. Boghaert E, Khandke K, Sridharan L et al (2006) Tumoricidal effect of calicheamicin immuno-conjugates using a passive targeting strategy. Int J Oncol 28:675–684
39. Jedema I, Barge RMY, van der Velden VHJ et al (2004) Internalization and cell cycle-dependent killing of leukemic cells by gemtuzumab ozogamicin: rationale for efficacy in CD33-negative malignancies with endocytic capacity. Leukemia 18:316–325
40. DiJoseph JF, Dougher MM, Kalyandrug LB et al (2006) Antitumor efficacy of a combination of CMC-544 (inotuzumab ozogamicin), a CD22-targeted cytotoxic immunoconjugate of calicheamicin, and rituximab against non-Hodgkin's B-cell lymphoma. Clin Cancer Res 12:242–249
41. Hinman LM, Hamann PR, Wallace R et al (1993) Preparation and characterization of monoclonal antibody conjugates of the calicheamicins: a novel and potent family of antitumor antibiotics. Cancer Res 53:3336–3342
42. Hamann PR, Hinman LM, Beyer CF et al (2005) An anti-MUCl antibodycalicheamicin conjugate for treatment of solid tumors. Choice of linker and overcoming drug resistance. Bioconjug Chem 16:346–353
43. Hamann PR, Hinman LM, Beyer CF et al (2005) A calicheamicin conjugate with a fully humanized anti-MUC1 Antibody shows potent antitumor effects in breast and ovarian tumor xenografts. Bioconjug Chem 16:354–360
44. Chan SY, Gordon AN, Coleman RE et al (2003) A phase II study of the cytotoxic immunoconjugate CMB-401(hCTM01-calicheamicin) in patients with platinum-sensitive recurrent epithelial ovarian carcinoma. Cancer Immunol Immunother 52:243–248
45. DiJoseph JF, Popplewell A, Tickle S et al (2005) Antibody-targeted chemotherapy of B-cellIymphoma using calicheamicin conjugated to murine or humanized antibody against CD22. Cancer Immunol Immunother 54:11–24
46. DiJoseph JF, Armellino DC, Boghaert ER et al (2004) Antibody-targeted chemotherapy with CMC-544: a CD22-targeted immunoconjugate of calicheamicin for the treatment of B-Iymphoid malignancies. Blood 103:1807–1814
47. DiJoseph JF, Goad ME, Dougher MM et al (2004) Potent and specific antitumor efficacy of CMC-544, a CD22-targeted immunoconjugate of calicheamicin, against systemically disseminated B-cell lymphoma. Clin Cancer Res 10:8620–8629
48. Wong BY, Dang NH (2010) Inotuzumab ozogamicin as novel therapy in lymphomas. Expert Opin Biol Ther 10:1251–1258
49. Mugundu G, Vandendries E, Boni J (2012) Reported Interim findings. Annu Meet Am Assoc Canc Res J PO.ET05.03
50. Boghaert ER, Sridharan L, Armellino DC et al (2004) Antibody-targeted chemotherapy with the calicheamicin conjugate hu3S I 93-*N*-acetyl γ calicheamicin dimethyl hydrazide targets Lewis Y and eliminates Lewis Y-positive human carcinoma cells and xenografts. Clin Cancer Res 10:4538–4549
51. Boghaert ER, Sridharan L, Khandke KM et al (2008) The oncofetal protein, 5T4, is a suitable target for antibody-guided anti-cancer chemotherapy with calicheamicin. Int J Oncol 32:221–234

52. Appenzeller-Herzog C, Ellgaard L (2008) The human PDI family: versatility packed into a single fold. Biochim Biophys Acta 1783:535–548
53. Wu G, Fang YZ, Yang S et al (2004) Glutathione metabolism and its implications for health. J Nutr 134:489–492
54. Mills BJ, Lang CA (1996) Differential distribution of free and bound glutathione and cyst (e)ine in human blood. Biochem Pharmacol 52:401–406
55. Russo A, Degraff W, Friedman N et al (1986) Selective modulation of glutathione levels in human normal versus tumor-cells and subsequent differential response to chemotherapy drugs. Cancer Res 46:2845–2848
56. Sedlacek H-H, Seemann G, Hoffmann D et al (1993) Antibodies as carriers of cytotoxicity. In: Queisser W, Scheithauer W (eds) Contributions to oncology, vol 43, 1st edn. Karger, Basel, pp 1–208
57. De Groot FMH, Damen EWP, Scheeren HW (2001) Anticancer prodrugs for application in monotherapy: targeting hypoxia, tumor-associated enzymes, and receptors. Curr Med Chem 8:1093–1122
58. Ojima I, Slater JC, Michaud E et al (1996) Syntheses and structure-activity relationships of the second generation antitumor taxoids. exceptional activity against drug-resistant cancer cells. J Med Chem 39:3889–3896
59. Ojima I, Slater JS, Kuduk SD et al (1997) Syntheses and structure-activity relationships of taxoids derived from 14β-Hydroxy-10-deacetylbaccatin III. J Med Chem 40:267–278
60. Lin S, Geng X, Qu C et al (2000) Synthesis of highly potent second-generation taxoids through effective kinetic resolution coupling of racemic β-lactams with baccatins. Chirality 12:431–441
61. Ojima I, Geng X, Wu X et al (2002) Tumor-specific novel taxoid monoclonal antibody conjugates. J Med Chem 45:5620–5623
62. Chari RVJ (2008) Targeted cancer therapy: conferring specificity to cytotoxicdrugs. Acc Chem Res 41:98–107
63. Widdison WC, Wilhelm SD, Cavanagh EE et al (2006) Semisynthetic maytansine analogues for the targeted treatment of cancer. J Med Chem 49:4392–4408
64. Austin CD, Wen X, Gazzard L et al (2005) Oxidizing potential of endosomes and lysosomes limits intracellular cleavage of disulfide-based antibody–drug conjugates. Proc Natl Acad Sci U S A 102:17987–17992
65. Kellogg BA, Garrett L, Kovtun Y et al (2011) Disulfide-linked antibody–maytansinoid conjugates: optimization of in vivo activity by varying the steric hindrance at carbon atoms adjacent to the disulfide linkage. Bioconjug Chem 22:717–727
66. Franano FN, Edwards WB, Welch MJ et al (1994) Metabolism of receptor targeted 111In-DTPA-glycoproteins: identification of 111In-DTPA-epsilonlysine as the primary metabolic and excretory product. Nucl Med Biol 21:1023–1034
67. Kovtun YV, Goldmacher VS (2007) Cell killing by antibody–drug conjugates. Cancer Lett 255:232–240
68. Erickson H, Wilhelm S, Widdison W et al (2008) Evaluation of the cytotoxic potencies of the major maytansinoid metabolites of antibody–maytansinoid conjugates detected in vitro and in preclinical mouse models. AACR Meeting Abstracts 2150
69. Tanimoto M, Scheinberg DA, Cordon-Cardo C et al (1989) Restricted expression of an early myeloid and monocytic cell surface antigen defined by monoclonal antibody M195. Leukemia 3:339–348
70. Liu C, Tadayoni BM, Bourret LA et al (1996) Eradication of large colontumor xenografts by targeted delivery of maytansinoids. Proc Natl Acad Sci U S A 93:8618–8623
71. Aboukameel A, Goustin A-S, Mohammad R et al (2007) Superior anti-tumor activity of the CD 19-directed immunotoxin, SAR3419 to rituximab in non-Hodgkin's xenograft animal models: preclinical evaluation. Blood 110:2339 (ASH Annual Meeting Abstracts)
72. Legrand O, Vidriales MB, Thomas X et al (2007) An open label, dose escalation study of AVE9633 administered as a single agent by intravenous (IV) infusion weekly for 2 weeks in 4-week cycle to patients with relapsed or refractory CD33-positive acute myeloid leukemia (AML). Blood 110:1850 (ASH Annual Meeting Abstracts)
73. Tassone P, Gozzini A, Goldmacher V et al (2004) In vitro and in vivo activity of the maytansinoid immunoconjugate huN90 I-N2′-deacetyl-N2′(3-mercapto-l-oxopropyl)-maytansine against CD56+ multiple myeloma cells. Cancer Res 64:4629–4636
74. Polson AG, Yu S-F, Elkins K et al (2007) Antibody–drug conjugates targeted to CD79 for the treatment of non-Hodgkin lymphoma. Blood 110:616–623
75. Tassone P, Goldmacher VS, Neri P et al (2004) Cytotoxic activity of the maytansinoid

immunoconjugate B-B4-DMI against CD138+ multiple myeloma cells. Blood 104:3688–3696
76. Ranson M, Sliwkowski MX (2002) Perspectives on anti-HER monoclonal antibodies. Oncology 63:17–24
77. Ross S, Spencer SD, Holcomb I et al (2002) Prostate stem cell antigen as therapy target: tissue expression and in vivo efficacy of an immunoconjugate. Cancer Res 62:2546–2553
78. Henry MD, Wen S, Silva MD et al (2004) A prostate-specific membrane antigen-targeted monoclonal antibody-chemotherapeutic conjugate designed for the treatment of prostate cancer. Cancer Res 64:7995–8001
79. Ciechanover A (2005) Intracellular protein degradation: from a vague idea through the lysosome and the ubiquitin-proteasome system and onto human diseases and drug targeting. Angew Chem Int Ed Engl 44:5944–5967
80. Sanderson RJ, Hering MA, James SF et al (2005) In vivo drug-linker stability of an anti-CD30 dipeptide-linked auristatin immunoconjugate. Clin Cancer Res 11:843–852
81. Koblinski JE, Ahram M, Sloane BF (2000) Unraveling the role of proteases in cancer. Clin Chim Acta 291:113–135
82. Kovár M, Strohalm J, Etrych T et al (2002) Star structure of antibody-targeted HPMA copolymer-bound doxorubicin: a novel type of polymeric conjugate for targeted drug delivery with potent antitumor effect. Bioconjug Chem 13:206–215
83. Versluis AJ, Rump ET, Rensen PCN et al (1998) Synthesis of a lipophilic daunorubicin derivative and its incorporation into lipidic carriers developed for LDL receptor-mediated tumor therapy. Pharm Res 15:531–537
84. Studer M, Kroger LA, DeNardo SJ et al (1992) Influence of a peptide linker on biodistribution and metabolism of antibody-conjugated benzyl EDTA. Comparison of enzymatic digestion in vitro and in vivo. Bioconjug Chem 3:424–429
85. Kirschke H, Barrett AJ, Rawlings ND (1995) Cathepsin B in protein profiles proteinases 1. In: Sheterline P (ed) Lysosomal cysteine proteinases, 1st edn. Academic Press, London, pp 1587–1643
86. Otto H-H, Schirmeister T (1997) Cysteine proteases and their inhibitors. Chem Rev 97:133–172
87. Trouet A, Masquelier M, Baurain R et al (1982) A covalent linkage between daunorubicin and proteins that is stable in serum and reversible by lysosomal hydrolases, as required for a lysosomotropic drug-carrier conjugate: in vitro and in vivo studies. Proc Natl Acad Sci U S A 79:626–629
88. Toki BE, Cerveny CG, Wahl AF et al (2002) Protease-mediated fragmentation of p-amidobenzyl ethers: a new strategy for the activation of anticancer prodrugs. J Org Chem 67:1866–1872
89. Dubowchik GM, Firestone RA (1998) Cathepsin B-sensitive dipeptide prodrugs. 1. A model study of structural requirements for efficient release of doxorubicin. Bioorg Med Chem Lett 8:3341–3346
90. Dubowchik GM, Mosure K, Knipe JO et al (1998) Cathepsin B-sensitive dipeptide prodrugs. 2. Models of anticancer drugs paclitaxel (Taxol), mitomycin C and doxorubicin. Bioorg Med Chem Lett 8:3347–3352
91. Walker MA, Dubowchik GM, Hofstead SJ et al (2002) Synthesis of an immunoconjugate of camptothecin. Bioorg Med Chem Lett 12:217–219
92. Walker M, King HD, Dalterio RA et al (2004) Monoclonal antibody mediated intracellular targeting of tallysomycin S(10b). Bioorg Med Chem Lett 14:4323–4327
93. Francisco JA, Cerveny CG, Meyer DL et al (2003) cAC10-vcMMAE, an anti-CD30-monomethylauristatin E conjugate with potent and selective antitumor activity. Blood 102:1458–1465
94. Doronina SO, Bovee TD, Meyer DW et al (2008) Novel peptide linkers for highly potent antibody–auristatin conjugate. Bioconjug Chem 19:1960–1963
95. Bartlett N, Forero-Torres A, Rosenblatt J et al (2009) Complete remissions with weekly dosing of SGN-35, a novel antibody–dug conjugate (ADC) targeting CD30, in phase I dose-escalation study in patients with relapsed or refractory Hodgkin lymphoma (HL) or systemic anaplastic large cell lymphoma (sALCL). J Clin Oncol 27:8500 (ASCO Annual Meeting Proceedings)
96. Younes A, Bartlett NL, Leonard JP et al (2010) Brentuximab vedotin (SGN-35) for relapsed CD30-positive lymphomas. N Engl J Med 363:1812–1821
97. Younes A, Gopa AK, Smith SE et al (2012) Results of a pivotal phase II study of brentuximab vedotin for patients with relapsed or refractory hodgkin's lymphoma. J Clin Oncol 30:2183–2189
98. Gualberto A (2012) Brentuximab vedotin (SGN-35), an antibody–drug conjugate for the treatment of CD30-positive malignancies. Expert Opin Investig Drugs 21:205–216

99. Thompson JA, Forero-Torres A, Heath EI et al (2011) The effect of SGN-75, a novel antibody–drug conjugate (ADC), in treatment of patients with renal cell carcinoma (RCC) or non-Hodgkin lymphoma (NHL): a phase I study. J Clin Oncol 29:3071 (ASCO Annual Meeting Proceedings)
100. Naumovski L, Junutula JR (2010) Glembatumumab vedotin, a conjugate of an anti-glycoprotein non-metastatic melanoma protein B mAb and monomethyl auristatin E for the treatment of melanoma and breast cancer. Curr Opin Mol Ther 12:248–257
101. Keir CH, Vahdat LT (2012) The use of an antibody drug conjugate, glembatumumab vedotin (CDX-011), for the treatment of breast cancer. Expert Opin Biol Ther 12:259–263
102. Ma D, Zhang H, Donovan GP et al (2007) Preclinical studies of PSMA ADC, an auristatin-conjugated fully human monoclonal antibody to prostate-specific membrane antigen. Prostate Cancer Symposium, Abstract 87
103. Jeffrey SC, Nguyen MT, Andreyka JB et al (2006) Dipeptide-based highly potent doxorubicin antibody conjugates. Bioorg Med Chem Lett 16:358–362
104. Govindan SV, Cardillo TM, Tat F et al (2012) Optimal cleavable linker for antibody–SN-38 conjugates for cancer therapy: impact of linker's stability on efficacy. Cancer Res 72:2526 (Proceedings: AACR)
105. Sharkey RM, Govindan SV, Cardillo TM et al (2012) Epratuzumab-SN-38: a new antibody–drug conjugate for the therapy of hematologic malignancies. Mol Cancer Ther 11:224–234
106. Govindan SV, Cardillo TM, Moon S-J et al (2009) CEACAM5-targeted therapy of human colonic and pancreatic cancer xenografts with potent labetuzumab-SN-38 immunoconjugates. Clin Cancer Res 15:6052–6061
107. Cardillo TM, Govindan SV, Sharkey RM et al (2011) Humanized anti-Trop-2 IgG-SN-38 conjugate for effective treatment of diverse epithelial cancers: preclinical studies in human cancer xenograft models and monkeys. Clin Cancer Res 17:3157–3169
108. Sharkey RM, Karacay H, Govindan SV et al (2011) Combination radioimmunotherapy and chemoimmunotherapy involving different or the same targets improves therapy of human pancreatic carcinoma xenograft models. Mol Cancer Ther 10:1072–1081
109. Govindan SV, Goldenberg DM (2012) Designing immunoconjugates for cancer therapy. Expert Opin Biol Ther 12:873–890
110. Derwin D, Passmore D, Sung J et al (2010) Activation of antibody drug conjugate MDX-1203 by human carboxylesterase 2. Proc Am Assoc Cancer Res 51:Abstract 2575
111. Jeffrey SC, Torgov MY, Andreyka JB et al (2005) Design, synthesis, and in vitro evaluation of dipeptide-based antibody minor groove binder conjugates. J Med Chem 48(5):1344–1358
112. Albin N, Massaad L, Toussaint C et al (1993) Main drug-metabolizing enzyme systems in human breast tumors and peritumoral tissues. Cancer Res 53:3541–3546
113. Jeffrey SC, Nguyen MT, Moser RF et al (2007) Minor groove binder antibody conjugates employing a water soluble beta-glucuronide linker. Bioorg Med Chem Lett 17:2278–2280
114. Jiang X, García-Fortanet J, de Brabander JK (2005) Synthesis and complete stereochemical assignment of psymberin/irciniastatin A. J Am Chem Soc 127:11254–11255
115. Alley SC, Zhang X, Okeley NM (2007) Effects of linker chemistry on tumor targeting by anti-CD70 antibody–drug conjugates. Proc Am Assoc Cancer Res 48
116. Polson AG, Calemine-Fenaux J, Chan P et al (2009) Antibody–drug conjugates for the treatment of non-Hodgkin's lymphoma: target and linker-drug selection. Cancer Res 69:2358–2364
117. Singh R, Erickson HK (2009) Antibody--cytotoxic agent conjugates: preparation and characterization. In: Dimitrov AS (ed) Methods in molecular biology, 1st edn. Springer, Humana Press, New York, pp 445–467
118. Polson AG, Williams M, Gray AM et al (2010) Anti-CD22-MCC-DM1: an antibody–drug conjugate with a stable linker for the treatment of non-Hodgkin's lymphoma. Leukemia 24:1566–1573
119. Endo N, Takeda Y, Kishida K et al (1987) Target-selective cytotoxicity of methotrexate conjugated with monoclonal anti-mm46 antibody. Cancer Immunol Immunother 25:1–6
120. Pimm MV, Paul MA, Ogumuyiwa Y et al (1988) Biodistribution and tumor-localization of a daunomycin monoclonal antibody conjugate in nude-mice with human-tumor xenografts. Cancer Immunol Immunother 27:267–271
121. Spearman ME, Goodwin RM, Apelgren LD et al (1987) Disposition of the monoclonal antibody–vinca alkaloid conjugate ks1/4-davlb (ly256787) and free 4-desacetylvinblastine in tumor-bearing nude-mice. J Pharmacol Exp Ther 241:695–703

122. Kato Y, Tsukada Y, Hara T et al (1983) Enhanced antitumor activity of mitomycin C conjugated with anti-alpha-fetoprotein antibody by a novel method of conjugation. J Appl Biochem 5:313–319
123. Rowland AJ, Pietersz GA, McKenzie IF (1993) Preclinical investigation of the antitumour effects of anti-CD19-idarubicin immunoconjugates. Cancer Immunol Immunother 37:195–202
124. Smyth MJ, Pietersz GA, McKenzie IF (1987) Selective enhancement of antitumor-activity of N-acetyl melphalan upon conjugation to monoclonal-antibodies. Cancer Res 47:62–69
125. Tolcher AW, Ochoa L, Hammond LA et al (2003) Cantuzumab mertansine, a maytansinoid immunoconjugate directed to the CanAg antigen: a phase I, pharmacokinetic, and biologic correlative study. J Clin Oncol 21:211–222
126. Erickson HK, Widdison WC, Mayo MF et al (2010) Tumor delivery and in vivo processing of disulfide-linked and thioether-linked antibody–maytansinoid conjugates. Bioconjug Chem 21:84–92
127. Sun X, Widdison W, Mayo M et al (2011) Design of antibody–maytansinoid conjugates allows for efficient detoxification via liver metabolism. Bioconjug Chem 22:728–735
128. Krop IE, Beeram M, Modi S et al (2010) Phase I study of Trastuzumab-DM1, an HER2 antibody–drug conjugate, given every 3 weeks to patients with HER2-positive metastatic breast cancer. J Clin Oncol 28:2698–2704
129. Vogel CL, Burris HA, Limentani S et al (2009) A phase II study of trastuzumab-DM1 (T-DM1), a HER2 antibody–drug conjugate (ADC), in patients (pts) with HER2+ metastatic breast cancer (MBC): final results. J Clin Oncol 15(Suppl):Abstract 1017
130. Takara K, Sakaeda T, Okumura K (2006) An update on overcoming MDR1-mediated multidrug resistance in cancer chemotherapy. Curr Pharm Des 12:273–286
131. Leonard GD, Fojo T, Bates SE (2003) The role of ABC transporters in clinical practice. Oncologist 8:411–424
132. Kovtun YV, Audette CA, Mayo MF et al (2010) Antibody–maytansinoid conjugates designed to bypass multidrug resistance. Cancer Res 70(6):2528–2537
133. Alley SC, Benjamin DR, Jeffrey SC et al (2008) The contribution of linker stability to the activities of anticancer immunoconjugates. Bioconjug Chem 19:759–765
134. Oflazoglu E, Stone IJ, Gordon K et al (2008) Potent anticarcinoma activity of the humanized anti-CD70 antibody h1F6 conjugated to the tubulin inhibitor auristatin via an uncleavable linker. Clin Cancer Res 14:6171–6180
135. Wang L, Amphlett G, Blättler WA et al (2005) Structural characterization of the maytansinoid-monoclonal antibody immunoconjugate, huN901–DM1, by mass spectrometry. Protein Sci 14:2436–2446
136. Willner D, Trail PA, Hofstead SJ et al (1993) (6-Maleimidocaproyl)hydrazone of doxorubicin: a new derivative for the preparation of immunoconjugates of doxorubicin. Bioconjug Chem 4:521–527
137. Schroeder DD, Tankersly DL, Lundblad JL (1981) A new preparation of modified immune serum globulin (human) suitable for intravenous administration. I. Standardization of the reduction and alkylation reaction. Vox Sang 40:373–382
138. Hamblett KJ, Senter PD, Chace DF et al (2004) Effects of drug loading on the antitumor activity of a monoclonal antibody drug conjugate. Clin Cancer Res 10:7063–7070
139. Sun MMC, Beam KS, Cerveny CG et al (2005) Reduction-alkylation strategies for the modification of specific monoclonal antibody disulfides. Bioconjug Chem 16:1282–1290
140. Junutula JR, Raab H, Clark S et al (2008) Site-specific conjugation of a cytotoxic drug to an antibody improves the therapeutic index. Nat Biotechnol 26:925–932
141. Vater CA, Goldmacher VS (2010) Antibody–cytotoxic compound conjugates for oncology. In: Reddy LH, Couvreur P (eds) Macromolecular anticancer therapeutics, 1st edn. Springer, New York, pp 331–369
142. McDonagh CF, Turcott E, Westendorf L et al (2006) Engineered antibody–drug conjugates with defined sites and stoichiometries of drug attachment. Protein Eng Des Sel 19:299–307
143. Gillies SD, Wesolowski JS (1990) Antigen binding and biological activities of engineered mutant chimeric antibodies with human tumor specificities. Hum Antibodies Hybridomas 1:47–54
144. Junutula JR, Flagella KM, Graham RA et al (2010) Engineered thio-trastuzumab-DM1 conjugate with an improved therapeutic index to target human epidermal growth factor receptor 2-positive breast cancer. Clin Cancer Res 16:4769–4778

145. Ambrx (2012) http://www.ambrx.com/wt/page/recode. Accessed 20 Sep 2012
146. Sapra P, Tchistiakova L, Dushin R et al (2012) Novel site-specific antibody drug conjugates based on novel amino acid incorporation technology have improved pharmaceutical properties over conventional antibody drug conjugates. Proc Am Assoc Cancer Res 72: Abstract 5691
147. Allozyne (2012) http://www.allozyne.com/what/platform. Accessed 20 Sep 2012
148. Redwood Bioscience (2012) http://www.redwoodbioscience.com/background/redwood-platform/; http://www.redwoodbioscience.com/background/antibody-drug-conjugates/. Accessed June 2013
149. Jeger S, Zimmermann K, Blanc A et al (2010) Site-specific and stoichiometric modification of antibodies by bacterial transglutaminase. Angew Chem Int Ed 49:9995–9997

Chapter 6

In Vivo Testing of Drug-Linker Stability

Pierre-Yves Abecassis and Céline Amara

Abstract

Antibody-drug conjugates (ADCs) are promising biotherapeutics designed to selectively deliver highly cytotoxic drugs to tumor cells while sparing normal tissues. They can be viewed as prodrugs, stable in the bloodstream in order to minimize drug release in circulation and efficiently converted into active drugs in the tumor tissues. Designing the right combination of monoclonal antibody (mAb), linker and drug, requires monitoring and understanding the behavior of all three components in the bloodstream and tumor. In particular, linkers have been shown to influence efficacy and safety profiles of ADCs, and monitoring in vivo "drug-linker stability" is therefore critical to help the linker choice and is performed by identifying the pharmacokinetics (PK) profiles. PK properties of ADCs are measured by following the profiles of three entities: (a) the conjugate (mAb entity carrying at least one drug), (b) the total antibody (mAb entity regardless of drug load), as well as (c) the free drugs and metabolites entities. This chapter focuses on the key analytical methods (ELISA immunoassays, TFC-MS/MS, and HRMS) used to support the PK profiles assessment of the three entities, allowing the characterization of ADC "drug-linker stability".

Key words Antibody-drug conjugate (ADC), Biotherapeutics, Cytotoxic, Drug-to-antibody ratio (DAR), Enzyme-linked immunosorbent assays (ELISA), High-resolution mass spectrometry (HRMS), Monoclonal antibody (mAb), Linker, Pharmacokinetic (PK), Total antibody, Turbulent flow chromatography coupled to mass spectrometry (TFC-MS/MS)

1 Introduction

Antibody-drug conjugates (ADCs) are targeted anticancer agents able to deliver highly cytotoxic payloads to tumor cells while minimizing delivery to normal tissues. ADCs are constituted of three components, a monoclonal antibody (mAb) selective for a tumor antigen attached to highly potent small molecules cytotoxic, via a linker moiety [1, 2]. After binding to the targeted antigen localized on the cell surface, the ADC undergoes internalization and trafficking through subcellular compartments to be finally chemically and/or enzymatically converted into an active drug (also considered as active metabolite(s)) able to kill the cell [3, 4]. Like an ideal prodrug, the ADC is theoretically aimed to reach the target as a

Laurent Ducry (ed.), *Antibody-Drug Conjugates*, Methods in Molecular Biology, vol. 1045,
DOI 10.1007/978-1-62703-541-5_6,

whole entity, stable in the bloodstream, in order to limit systemic drug release that could damage healthy tissues, without compromising drug delivery to tumor cells [5]. In order to ensure selective release of the drug in the cancer cell, the differences between bloodstream and intracellular compartments properties have been exploited and generated a number of options for the design of efficient linkers [6]. These linkers differ by their stability and drug-release properties, which are often considered as "cleavability" properties. They are thus divided in so-called cleavable and non-cleavable linkers. In the first group, different options have been exploited in the current ADC in development of (a) chemically labile acid-cleavable hydrazone linkers, relatively stable at neutral pH in the bloodstream while undergoing rapid hydrolysis within acidic cellular compartments like endosomes (pH 5–6.5) and lysosomes (pH 4.5–5) [7, 8]; An example of this linker is illustrated by CMC-544, (b) disulfide linkers, more or less sterically hindered in order to modulate stability in circulation whereas maintaining efficient intracellular drug release through the reduction of the disulfide bound due to high intracellular concentration of glutathione [9, 11]; Different ADCs bearing this type of linkers are in development including SAR3419 [12], nBT062 [13] and IMGN901 [14], and (c) enzyme-labile linkers, based on the cleavage of the peptide bond by lysosomal proteases such as cathepsin B. Proteases are not active in the extracellular environment due to unfavorable pH conditions and inhibition by serum protease inhibitors [15]; Different ADCs bearing this type of linkers are in development including SGN35, recently approved by the FDA for the treatment of Hodgkin and non-Hodgkin lymphoma [16, 17]. In the second group, release of the active drug is done through one single step which is the antibody proteolysis within the lysosome, producing an amino acid-linker-drug active metabolite. These types of linkers were originally designed for maximum blood stability, like the thioether [17, 18] and maleimidocaproyl moieties. An example of non-cleavable linker is represented by T-DM1 [10, 19] today FDA approved for the treatment of HER2+ breast cancers. Obviously the different linkers will generate different active drugs/metabolites which will have physicochemical properties and potentially different cell killing properties [14].

If developing a safe and effective ADC requires careful understanding of its behavior in the bloodstream, as a critical step influencing toxicity and efficacy, the interpretation of the PK profiles of the different entities is highly complex because it reflects multiple phenomena, among which (a) the linker chemistry and intrinsic properties as described above and (b) the conjugation chemistry, including both site of conjugation and drug-to-antibody ratio (DAR) generating high heterogeneity. ADCs are indeed composed of a mixture of species, due to the synthesis process itself, and this heterogeneity increases the challenge for ADC quantification and characterization. Conjugates are usually generated through cysteines or lysine residues, both processes leading to the production of mixtures of defined ADC species with different sites of conjugation. The cysteine conjugation is done through partial reduction of interchain disulfide bonds leading to ADC with zero to eight drugs per antibody for an IgG1 mAb with three different cysteine bonds [6, 20]. The lysine conjugation will react with multiple residues distributed at specific positions, across the entire antibody on heavy and light chains, depending on the mAb sequence. Reactive lysine residues of a specific mAb will be mainly located on the surface of the IgG, in areas of structural flexibility, with large solvent accessibility [21]. In addition the average DAR reached during a synthesis will also introduce variability in the species produced.

Linker type, conjugation sites, and DAR will impact the PK properties of an ADC with various effects on the ADC species. Indeed, high DAR ADC species have been shown to be cleared much more rapidly from the circulation than low DAR species [19, 22, 23]. Furthermore, the location of the conjugation site within the antibody has also been shown to influence the clearance, as exemplified by the different PK profiles of thiomAb conjugates with diverse conjugation site, within the Fab or Fc part of the antibody [22, 24]. Finally, other parameters can influence the PK properties of the ADC, as for naked antibody, including (a) their overall physicochemistry properties which will influence solubility and aggregation, (b) impact of mAb engineering on FcRn binding capacity, and (c) the target itself, through its expression level in the tumor, or as shed antigen, as well as its potential modulation during treatment [24, 26].

ADC PK profile characterization is done by key analytical methods which are (a) ELISA immunoassays measuring the conjugate and total antibody kinetic profiles, (b) TFC-MS/MS that accurately quantify free drugs/metabolites, and (c) high-resolution mass spectroscopy for DAR analysis in vivo. Two types of complementary ELISA immunoassays providing quantitative measurement of analytes are explored during discovery and preclinical and clinical development of an ADC: the first type of assay measures the *total antibody*, defined as the ADC with a DAR higher than or equal to zero. The second type of assay measures the *drug-conjugated antibody*, defined as the ADC with a DAR greater or equal to one.

For *total antibody assay*, several ELISA formats are available: (a) A direct antigen coat format is used as capture agent if the purified target protein antigen is available, followed by detection with an enzyme-conjugated anti-murine or humanized IgG; (b) When the purified antigen is not available, an alternative approach is used that takes advantage of electroluminescence detection (Meso Scale Discovery [MSD]) [27] with a goat anti-human IgG-sulfo-TAG™ tracer that emits light upon chemical stimulation.

Another strategy for mAb capture when antigen is not utilized is also to use an anti-idiotype antibody which bear the internal image of a human tumor antigen and can mimic it [28]. A standard assay, dedicated to high throughput, uses a goat anti-human IgG (Fc or $F(ab')_2$) antibody as capture and a donkey anti-human IgG antibody conjugated to HRP detection [29], or the capture is carried out by a donkey anti-human IgG-biotin, Fcγ-specific antibodies captured on streptavidin, and the detection by the use of goat anti-human IgG Alexa-tag fluorescent (GyroLab). Several assay formats are used with the potential advantage of being sensitive to drug load that result in possible binding affinity modifications and impact on ADC quantification [6, 30].

For *conjugated antibody assay*, the conventional ELISA format is based on the capture by an anti-drug antibody and the detection with the target antigen if available or an antibody anti-CDR or even an anti-IgG (anti-Fc or anti-$F(ab')_2$). This format is most commonly used but the anti-drug antibody can also be used as detection reagent. Other formats consist of coating a murine or human anti-cytotoxic monoclonal antibody as capture, and the detection can be by the use of (a) a goat antihuman IgG-sulfo-tag tracer with electroluminescence signal or (b) a biotinylated antigen followed by streptavidin-HRP reading or (c) an HRP-conjugated donkey anti-human IgG antibody or HRP-conjugated goat anti-human IgG antibodies, Fc or F(ab′). Possible discrepancies between results obtained with these different techniques reflect assay sensitivity, efficiency, or drug underestimation differences [6, 29, 30]. However, it should be reminded that since the conjugated antibody format assay detects at least one drug attached to the antibody, this assay is not suitable to monitor the drug loss from the ADC heterogeneous mixture in the bloodstream and can lead to quantification variability depending on drug number and position on the antibody [6, 29, 30]. In addition, PK profiles may vary depending on the presence of shed antigen or high levels of soluble ligand in blood [25, 26].

For the free drug/metabolites quantification assays, ELISA competition assays are used, as well as highly sensitive and specific physicochemical mass spectrometry analysis followed by solid-phase extraction of plasma protein content, precipitation, and reverse-phase liquid chromatography or high-throughput turbulent flow chromatography as described below.

For high-resolution mass spectroscopy (HRMS) assay for DAR analysis, the technique is described in Chapter 18.

The following sections detail the experimental protocols and tips carried out for the ELISA immunoassay, the TFC-MS/MS physicochemical assay for free drugs quantification and subsequent PK analysis to support in vivo characterization of an ADC.

2 Materials

All materials described below refer to the pharmacokinetics study itself, i.e., in-life phase and bioanalysis, by ELISA for conjugate and total antibody concentrations and by TFC-MS/MS for free drugs levels. HRMS assay for DAR profile is described in Chapter 18. All buffers and solutions are prepared at room temperature and stored at +4 °C unless indicated otherwise.

2.1 In-Life Phase

1. Formulation: Compound in vehicle: stock ADC solution (*see* **Note 1**) in histidine 10 mM, glycine 130 mM, sucrose 5 %, and pH 5.5 (HGS). For HGS buffer, add 146 mL of a 1 M sucrose solution (weigh 17.1 g of sucrose in a glass beaker and add 38.4 mL of water), 1.55 g of histidine, and 9.76 g of glycine in a volumetric flask. Adjust the pH with 8 mL of HCl and make up 1 L with water. Store at 4 °C. Dilute ADC in HGS buffer to the required concentration depending on selected dose (*see* **Notes 2** and **3**).
2. Animals: Female SCID mice (Charles Rivers, France), three per time point, 5–6 weeks old, weight on average 20–25 g. Mice are housed in a sterile room, under aseptic conditions in a laminar hood (*see* **Notes 4** and **5**) and they are fed ad libitum (UAR A04 pellets, delivered in paper sacks, provided by SAFE, France). Water is filtered from main water by polyetherimide bottles with stainless steel sipper tubes.
3. Consumables: Lithium heparinized glass tubes, polypropylene microtubes. Deep well 1 mL propylene 96-well plate, needle 25 Gauge.

2.2 ELISA Analysis

1. Coating buffer: Phosphate buffer solution (PBS). Dissolve one tablet into 1 L of water to yield 140 mM NaCl, 3 mM KCl, 10 mM phosphate buffer, and pH 7.4 at 25 °C. The solution is stored at +4 °C for up to 3 months.
2. Wash buffer: PBS buffer solution with 0.05 % tween 20 (PBST). Dissolve one tablet into 1 L of water to yield 140 mM NaCl, 2.7 mM KCl, 10 mM phosphate buffer, 0.05 % Tween 20, and pH 7.4 at 25 °C. The solution is stored at +4 °C for up to 3 months.
3. Blocking buffer, diluent for standards, quality Controls (QC), and first dilution of samples: PBST solution in 0.5 % BSA. Weigh 500 mg of bovine serum albumin (BSA) and dissolve in 100 mL of PBST buffer. The solution is stored for up to 1 day.
4. Assay buffer: Last dilution of sample: PBST solution with 0.5 % BSA, 1 % plasma. Dilute 60.0 μL of pool mouse lithium heparin plasma in 6.00 mL of PBST/0.5 % BSA buffer.
5. Reagents solutions: Anti-cytotoxic solution stored in low-binding polypropylene tubes at 4 °C, Ag-biotinylated stored

at −80 °C, peroxidase HRP-streptavidin used at 1:200, TMB substrate (color reagents A and B), stored at +4 °C, sulfuric acid 1 M (*see* **Note 6**). Plate costar, (Sigma Aldrich), stored at room temperature. Bovine serum albumin (BSA), water for HPLC grade, control mouse plasma collected on lithium heparin stored at −20 °C, and phosphate-buffered saline (and saline tween) tablets, stored at room temperature.

6. Consumables: Polypropylene tubes, automatic pipettes, and multipettes of various volumes.
7. Instrumentation: Analytical balance, vortex mixer, spectrophotometer plate reader Sunrise (Tecan), Microplate shaker Orbital, Microplate washer Tecan Columbus, and Multicalc software v2.7 (Perkin Elmer).

2.3 TFC-MS/MS Analysis

1. Free drug stock solution (100 μg/mL): Weigh 5.00 mg of cytotoxic (corrected for purity), dissolve and dilute into 50.0 mL volumetric flask (class A) with methanol. Process the same way for each compound if several drugs. These solutions are stored at +4 °C (*see* **Note 7**).
2. Working solutions for calibration standards (range 0.05–12.5 μg/mL) and quality controls (low 0.05 μg/mL, medium 1.25 μg/mL, and high 10 μg/mL) are prepared from initial stock solutions in volumetric flasks by dilutions in methanol (*see* **Note 8**).
3. Internal standard solution (ISW): Weigh 2.50 mg (corrected for purity) of radiolabelled drug [^{13}C4, D7]. Dissolve and dilute into 25.0 mL volumetric flask (class A) with methanol. Process the same way for any other drug. These solutions are stored at +4 °C. Transfer 0.500 mL of each solution into 10.0 mL volumetric flask (class A) to obtain IS intermediate working solution at 5.00 μg/mL in methanol. Then transfer 100 μL of the last solution into 50.0 mL volumetric flask (class A) and complete with formic acid at 1.00 % (v/v) to obtain ISW solution at 10.0 ng/mL of labelled IS to be added to plasma sample.
4. Solvents for TFC: Solvent A is prepared by diluting 1 mL of formic acid in 1 L of water. Solvent B for Quaternary pump is prepared by diluting 1 mL of formic acid in 1 L of acetonitrile. Solvent B for Binary pump is prepared by diluting 1 mL of formic acid in 1 L of methanol. Solvent D is prepared by mixing 400 mL of acetonitrile, 300 mL of acetone, and 300 mL of propanol.
5. Columns: For TFC: Turboflow™ Cyclone, 0.5 mm × 50 mm, for analysis: Chromolith RP-18e, 2 mm × 50 mm.
6. Consumables: 1 mL polypropylene deep 96-well plate, 1.5 mL polypropylene microtubes, 1.5 mL polypropylene screw cap

tubes, Combitips plus Eppendorf (1–10 mL), and Class A volumetric flask (5.00–100 mL).

7. Reagents: Chemicals and biologicals: Water, methanol, acetonitrile, acetone, propanol, and formic acid (99 %) for HPLC. Lithium heparinized mouse plasma.
8. Instrumentations: Balance Mettler Toledo, AT261 Delta Range, Centrifuge Sigma 6K15, Vortexer, Ika-Schuttler MTSZ, Pipettes, Biohit, e-line e120, e300, e1000, Pipette, Eppendorf, Multipette plus 4981, Autosampler CTC PAL (software PAL ver.2.3.6), TFC Thermo Fisher Scientific TX1 (software Aria OS ver.1.5.1.), and Mass Spectrometer Applied Biosystems API4000 (software Analyst 1.4.1).

3 Methods

In vivo testing of drug-linker stability is carried out by assessing the conjugate and total antibody PK profiles following administration to SCID female mice, species and strain used for pharmacological efficacy performed on xenograft tumor models. Linker instability, suspected by the liberation of free drug, attached or not to the linker moiety, is seen by naked antibody release and therefore profile disconnection of the two species.

Pharmacokinetics study consists of assessing these PK profiles and PK parameters of several entities (conjugated (DAR 1 to *n*) and total antibody (DAR 0 to *n*) and the free drugs) from plasma concentrations following intravenous administration to the mouse. Therefore, to focus on linker instability in the bloodstream, pharmacokinetics are designed in non-bearing tumor rather than tumor bearing mice to descriminate tumor related clearance.

Carry out all procedures at room temperature unless otherwise specified.

3.1 Pharmacokinetics Study

1. Treatment: Thirty-three animals are identified by tail vein marking and are divided as three mice per cage (per time point). Mice are dosed as single intravenous bolus (10 mL/kg) (*see* **Note 9**).
2. Blood sampling: Whole blood sample (at least 600 μL, per sampling time for each animal) is collected from cardiac puncture at selected times for up to 21 days (0.083, 0.25, 24, 72, 96, 168, 240, 336, and 504 h) into glass tubes containing lithium heparin as anticoagulant.
3. Samples processing: After blood collection, invert tube to mix with anticoagulant. Blood is then centrifuged (15 min, at 4 °C at 3,500 tr/min) and the plasma fraction is separated and collected in 1 mL 96-well plate format and stored at −80 °C until analysis.

4. Animals: They are observed throughout the study for clinical signs and mortality. Any animal in poor clinical condition, especially if death appears imminent, is anesthetized with isoflurane and euthanized by massive inhalation of CO_2 (*see* **Note 10**).

3.2 ELISA: Conjugate and Total Antibody

PK profiles of the conjugate (drug conjugate carrying at least one drug) and total antibody (drug conjugate regardless of drug load) can be measured by assessing the plasma concentration-time course using immunological detection of protein. Immunoassays take advantage of the binding specificity of the antibody with its specificity to the antigen (variable domain) on one side and on the other side, the specificity of cytotoxic molecule recognition or the specificity for protein (Fc domain), providing a convenient way of identifying the targeted immunoconjugate.

There are several ELISA (enzyme-linked immunosorbent assays) assay formats, enabling for the detection of these ADCs. The choice between the different formats is made on the grounds of convenience, cost, availability of appropriate equipment and reagents, the level of sensitivity required and the dynamic range, and the phase of development.

Conventional ELISA uses an antibody that binds the mAb component of the ADC and another antibody which recognizes the small cytotoxic molecule. Plasma concentrations are determined with an ELISA that measures any mAb linked to one or more cytotoxic molecules. Conjugate (cytotoxic-conjugated—DAR 1 to *n*): The assay is based on the capture of ADC by anti-cytotoxic monoclonal antibodies coated on the plate and its detection by the use of the Ag-biotinylated followed by streptavidin-HRP tracer before the reading by spectrophotometry.

Total antibody (conjugated and not cytotoxic-conjugated—DAR 0 to *n*): The assay is based on the capture of the ADC by goat anti-huIgG Fc antibodies coated on the plate and its detection by the use of the biotinylated anti-hulgG Fc antibodies (from different host) followed by streptavidin-HRP tracer before the reading by spectrophotometry.

The following describes an ELISA method for the ADC as used in preclinical studies. For clinical compounds, the target antigen is used to detect.

1. Calibration standards: Nine standards are prepared by first spiking lithium heparinized mouse plasma (1:10) with compound stock solution and dilutions in plasma to cover the 50–2,000 ng/mL concentration range (*see* **Note 11**).
2. Quality controls (QC): three QCs at three levels, low, medium, and high, are prepared according to same dilutions as calibration standard (QC low at 150 ng/mL, QC mid at 300 ng/mL, and QC high at 1,000 ng/mL) (*see* **Note 12**).

3. Assay procedure day 0: Coating: Prepare the anti-cytotoxic solution at 100 ng/mL in PBS buffer and immediately, dispense 60 μL of anti-cytotoxic at 100 ng/mL into each well of a microplate costar type 2592. Cover the microplate and incubate for at least 18 h at +4 °C.
4. Assay procedure: Day 1 (*see* **Note 13**): Dosage: Prepare the wash buffer as described previously. Wash the wells three times with 300 μL of wash buffer. After the washing, the microplate is inverted and tapped dry on absorbent tissue.
5. Assay procedure: Blocking step: Add 250 μL of blocking buffer to each well. Cover the microplate and incubate for 1 h at room temperature on a microplate shaker.
6. Prepare fresh calibration standards and thaw QC samples stored at −80 °C. Dilute standards, QC samples, and study samples at 1:100—as identical treatment in all of these subsets—as exampled thereafter: 5.00 μL of standards, QC, and study samples diluted in 495 μL of PBST/0.5 % BSA (*see* **Note 14**). Washing step: wash the wells three times with 300 μL of wash buffer. After the washing, the microplate is inverted and tapped dry on absorbent tissue. Dispense 50.0 μL of standards, controls, or samples per well. Cover the microplate and incubate for 1.5 h in incubator at room temperature on a microplate shaker. Wash the wells three times with 300 μL of wash buffer. After the washing, the microplate is inverted and tapped dry on absorbent tissue.
7. Add 50 μL of Ag-biotinylated at 100 ng/mL to each well. Cover the microplate and incubate for 1 h at room temperature on a microplate shaker protected from light. Wash the wells three times with 300 μL of wash buffer. After the washing, the microplate is inverted and tapped dry on absorbent tissue.
8. Add 50 μL of Streptavidin-HRP diluted 1:200 to each well. Cover the microplate and incubate for 1 h at room temperature on a microplate shaker protected from light. Wash the wells three times with 300 μL of wash buffer. After the washing, the microplate is inverted and tapped dry on absorbent tissue.
9. Add 50 μL of substrate solution (TMB) to each well. Cover the microplate and incubate for 10 min at room temperature on a microplate shaker (*see* **Note 15**).
10. Stop the reaction by addition of 50 μL of stop solution (sulfuric acid) at the same rhythm than substrate solution (*see* **Note 16**).
11. Determine the optical density of each well using a microplate reader set to 450 nm with wavelength correction set to 620 nm.
12. Data are acquired using Multicalc software v2.7. Raw data (DO) measured by the plate reader are plotted against nominal standard concentrations to construct the standard calibration curves.

13. Concentration values of standards, quality control samples, and unknown samples are interpolated from these curves using an unweighted parabolic regression fitting model with a log–log transformation of the data from 50 to 2,000 ng/mL.
14. All these calculations are done using Multicalc software v2.7. Concentration values of standards, quality controls, and study specimens are then exported into LIMS Watson (version 7.4., Thermo) (*see* **Note 17**).

3.3 TFC-MS/MS Analysis for Free Drug

Free drug in plasma can also help to characterize linker stability and is determined by a TFC-MS/MS assay (TFC: turbulent flow chromatography) (*see* **Note 18**).

1. Calibration standards, validation samples, and quality control samples are prepared in heparinized mouse plasma. In glass tubes or volumetric flasks, dilute the respective working solutions (*see* **Notes 19–21**).
2. Sample extraction: For all calibration standard, validation, QC, and blank and analytical samples: Thaw samples, Vortex mix. Centrifuge samples at approximately 4,000 × *g* for 10 min. Add 100 μL of the relevant calibration standard, validation, QC, and blank or analytical samples into a deep well. Add 100 μL of internal standard (ISW: plasma concentration 10.0 ng/mL). Seal the plate and vortex for a few seconds.
3. Sample injection: Load deep well into autosampler tray maintained at +4 °C. Inject 50.0 μL.
4. Integration/quantification: The response ratios (cytotoxic/its labelled IS) for standards are plotted against nominal standard concentrations to construct calibration curves. Concentration values of standard, validation, and quality control samples are interpolated from these curves using a calibration model (*see* **Note 22**).

3.4 Pharmacokinetics Analysis

Pharmacokinetic profiles are determined as a function of time and pharmacokinetics parameters are estimated by non-compartmental analysis using WinNonLin, version 5.2.1 (Pharsight).

1. Plasma concentrations (above limit of quantification, LOQ) are plotted against time. Concentrations below limit of quantification are reported BLQ. Concentrations above the upper limit of quantification are diluted and reanalyzed.
2. Pharmacokinetics parameters that are calculated are the following: The area under the concentration-time curve to the last observable point (AUC_{last} and to infinity, estimated by trapezoidal rule), C_0, clearance, volume of distribution, and terminal elimination half-life is obtained from the terminal linear portion of the concentration-time curve.

4 Notes

1. The appropriate vehicle used to formulate the ADC administered to mice is specific for each ADC and depends in particular on the cytotoxic and linker moieties. Aggregation, endotoxin levels, and stability should be looked at carefully.
2. Dilution of stock ADC solution should be done extemporaneously before animal dosing.
3. During the period of animal treatment, formulation is under magnetic stirring at room temperature (20–25 °C), protected from light.
4. Mouse strain and sex should be the one used in pharmacological model. However, these animals have to be non-bearing tumor in order to characterize linker instability not related to tumor processing.
5. Animals are handled and maintained in accordance with the requirements of EEC guideline (1986) and US Federal Guidelines (1985). The animal room conditions are as follows: room temperature, 20–24 °C; relative humidity, 40–70 %; lighting times, 12-h light/12-h dark cycle; air flow, 15–20 changes/h without recirculation; and acclimatization time, at least 6 days. Animals are housed in polysulfone solid bottom floor cages during acclimatization. The bedding is changed at least once a week. Mice are usually housed in groups of three per cage in ventilated cages containing wooden shavings.
6. Preparation of reagent solutions: anti-cytotoxic free drug: stock solution is serially diluted with coating buffer (PBS) to obtain a final concentration of 100 ng/mL. Ag-biotinylated: stock solution is serially diluted with diluent (PBST/0.5 % BSA) to obtain a final concentration of 100 ng/mL. For HRP-Streptavidin: dilute 30.0 μL of stock solution with 5.97 mL of diluent (PBST/0.5 % BSA). TMB Substrate: Color Reagents A and B should be mixed together in equal volumes within 5 min of use. Protect from light. 50 μL of the resultant mixture is required per well.
7. Two separate weightings of each drug are performed to prepare stock solution for calibrations standards and quality controls.
8. In case of multiple analytes, all independent stock solutions are pooled together to obtain a solution at 50.0 μg/mL of each analyte. Working solutions possible dilution scheme for calibration standard samples and quality controls samples:

Working solutions			Used solution	
Conc. (μg/mL)	Final volume (mL)	Solvent	Conc. (μg/mL)	Volume used (μL)
12.5	4.00	Methanol	50.0	1,000
10.0	5.00		50.0	1,000
2.50	4.00		50.0	200
1.25	12.0		50.0	300
0.500	5.00		1.25	2,000
0.250	5.00		1.25	1,000
0.100	5.00		1.25	400
0.0500	5.00		1.25	200

9. Dose level is highly dependent on cytotoxic potency and is defined according to efficacy study or on background knowledge.
10. Any animal found dead or euthanatized due to poor clinical conditions is submitted to a macroscopic examination. Before treatment, animals are placed 3–5 min under UV lamp to dilate the tail vein.
11. Calibration standards are freshly prepared the day of analysis. Example of preparation for an ADC with stock solution A at 6.00 mg/mL: Solution B at 600 μg/mL: 10.0 μL of the stock solution A are added to 90 μL of plasma. Solution C at 100 μg/mL: 30.0 μL of the solution B are added to 150 μL of plasma. Solution D at 10.0 μg/mL: 20.0 μL of the solution C are added to 180 μL of plasma. Solution E at 1.00 μg/mL: 10.0 μL of the solution D at 10.0 μg/mL are added to 90 μL of plasma:

STD ID	(ng/mL)	Preparation
STD9	2,000	30.0 μL sol D 10.0 μg/mL + 120 μL plasma
STD8	1,250	15.0 μL sol D 10.0 μg/mL + 105 μL plasma
STD7	750	15.0 μL sol D 10.0 μg/mL + 185 μL plasma
STD6	500	10.0 μL sol D 10.0 μg/mL + 190 μL plasma
STD5	300	30.0 μL sol E 1.00 μg/mL + 70 μL plasma
STD4	150	15.0 μL sol E 1.00 μg/mL + 85 μL plasma
STD3	100	10.0 μL sol E 1.00 μg/mL + 90 μL plasma
STD2	50	10.0 μL sol E 1.00 μg/mL + 190 μL plasma
STD1	0	100 μL plasma

12. Quality controls are freshly prepared the day of analysis. Example of preparation of quality controls for an ADC with stock solution A at 6.00 mg/mL: Solution B at 600 μg/mL: 10.0 μL of the stock solution A are added to 90 μL of plasma. Solution C at 100 μg/mL: 30.0 μL of the solution B are added to 150 μL of plasma. Solution D at 10.0 μg/mL: 10.0 μL of the solution C are added to 90 μL of plasma. Solution E at 1.00 μg/mL: 10.0 μL of the solution D are added to 90 μL of plasma. QCs are as follows:

ID	ng/mL	Preparation
QC low	150	15.0 μL solution E 1.00 μg/mL + 85 μL of plasma
QC medium	300	30.0 μL solution D 1.00 μg/mL + 70 μL of plasma
QC high	1,000	solution D 1.00 μg/mL

All samples, standards, and QC samples are assayed in duplicate.

13. Bring all the reagents and samples to room temperature before use. All samples, standards, and QC samples are assayed in duplicate.
14. In case of study samples having concentrations higher than the upper limit of quantification, they could be diluted in PBST with 0.5 % BSA (assay buffer) with the last dilution at 1:100 in assay buffer (PBST solution with 0.5 % BSA and 1 % plasma).
15. Protect from light.
16. If color change does not appear uniform, gently tap the plate to ensure thorough mixing.
17. The application of the dilution factor is performed in Watson. Calculations of concentration data and summary statistics are performed in Watson using rounded concentration data. Samples data are reported as ng/mL with three significant digits after the decimal point.
18. TFC parameters and detector parameters are highly dependent on the free drug to be quantified, are specific to that drug, and should be optimized based on the drug.
19. Dilution scheme for calibration standards and quality controls: Vortex to homogenize. Transfer 150 or 400 μL (Std1 and Std8) aliquots into polypropylene tubes for freezing (−80 °C) as described in tables below.

Calibration Standard Samples

Calibration standards (heparinized human plasma)			Used working solutions	
Reference	Conc. (ng/mL)	Final volume (mL)	Conc. (μg/mL)	Volume used (μL)
Std1	1.00	15.0	0.0500	300
Std2	2.00	5.00	0.100	100
Std3	5.00	5.00	0.250	100
Std4	10.0	5.00	0.500	100
Std5	25.0	5.00	1.25	100
Std6	50.0	5.00	2.50	100
Std7	200	5.00	10.0	100
Std8	250	15.0	12.5	300

Vortex to homogenize and transfer 150 or 400 μL (Std1 or Std8) aliquots into propylene tubes for freezing (−80 °C).

Quality Control Samples

Validation and quality controls (heparinized human plasma)			Used working solutions	
Reference	Conc. (ng/mL)	Final volume (mL)	Conc. (μg/mL)	Volume used (μL)
LLOQ	1.00	5.00	0.0500	100
Low—QC1	3.00	10.00	0.150	200
Mid—QC2	25.0	5.00	1.25	100
High—QC3	200	10.00	10.0	200

Vortex to homogenize and transfer 150 μL aliquots into polypropylene tubes from freezing (−80 °C).

20. Alternate dilution schemes are acceptable, as long as final solvent/matrix ratio is kept below 10.0 % for aqueous solvents and 5.0 % for organic solvents.
21. Two separate weightings of each free drug will be performed to prepare stock solution for calibration standards and validation and quality control samples.
22. The calculation model and weighting factor is highly dependent of the free drug(s) analytical response and mass spectrometer source and detector parameters and should be optimized on drug basis.

Acknowledgements

The authors would like to greatly thank Patrick Verdier, Marie-Hélène Pascual, and Olivier Pasquier for providing their lab protocols, for their constructive input, and careful review of this chapter. The authors are grateful to Ingrid Sassoon and Veronique Blanc for giving high-level background and critical reading of the manuscript. We also thank Delphine Valente, Christine Mauriac, Gerard Sanderink, and John Newton for giving relevant review and their support.

References

1. Wu AM, Senter PD (2005) Arming antibodies: prospects and challenges for immunoconjugates. Nat Biotechnol 23:1137–1146
2. Lambert JM (2005) Drug-conjugated monoclonal antibodies for the treatment of cancer. Curr Opin Pharmacol 5:543–549
3. Kratz F, Müller IA, Ryppa C, Warnecke A (2008) Prodrug strategies in anticancer chemotherapy. ChemMedChem 3:20–53
4. Mould DR, Sweeney KR (2007) The pharmacokinetics and pharmacodynamics of monoclonal antibodies—mechanistic modeling applied to drug development. Curr Opin Drug Discov Dev 10(1):84–96
5. Carter PJ, Senter PD (2008) Antibody–drug conjugates for cancer therapy. Cancer J 14:154–169
6. Stephan JP, Kozak KR, Wong WL (2011) Challenges in developing bioanalytical assays for characterization of antibody–drug conjugates. Bioanalysis 3(6):677–700
7. Hamann PR, Hinman LM, Beyer CF, Lindh D, Upeslacis J, Flowers DA, Bernstein I (2002) An anti-CD33 antibody–calicheamicin conjugate for treatment of acute myeloid leukemia. Choice of linker. Bioconjug Chem 13:40–46
8. Trail PA, Willner D, Lasch SJ, Henderson AJ, Hofstead S, Casazza AM, Firestone RA, Hellström I, Hellström KE (1993) Cure of xenografted human carcinomas by BR96-doxorubicin immunoconjugates. Science 261:212–215
9. Chari RVJ (2008) Targeted cancer therapy: conferring specificity to cytotoxic drugs. Acc Chem Res 41:98–107
10. Lewis Phillips GD, Li G, Dugger DL, Crocker LM, Parsons KL, Mai E, Blattler WA, Lambert JM, Chari RV, Lutz RJ, Wong WL, Jacobson FS, Koeppen H, Schwall RH, Kenkare-Mitra SR, Spencer SD, Sliwkowski MX (2008) Targeting HER2-positive breast cancer with trastuzumab-DM1, an antibody–cytotoxic drug conjugate. Cancer Res 68:9280–9290
11. Meister A, Anderson ME (1983) Glutathione. Annu Rev Biochem 52:711–760
12. Blanc V, Bousseau A, Caron A, Carrez C, Lutz RJ, Lambert JM (2011) SAR3419: an anti-CD19-Maytansinoid immunoconjugate for the treatment of B-cell malignancies. Clin Cancer Res 17(20):6448–6458
13. Ikeda H, Hideshima T, Fulciniti M, Lutz RJ, Yasui H, Okawa Y, Kiziltepe T, Vallet S, Pozzi S, Santo L, Perrone G, Tai YT, Cirstea D, Raje NS, Uherek C, Dälken B, Aigner S, Osterroth F, Munshi N, Richardson P, Anderson KC (2009) The monoclonal antibody nBT062conjugated to cytotoxic maytansinoids has selective cytotoxicity against CD138-positive multiple myeloma cells in vitro and in vivo. Clin Cancer Res 15:4028–4037
14. Erickson HK, Lambert JM (2012) ADME of antibody–maytansinoid conjugates. AAPS J 14 (4):799–805
15. Koblinski JE, Ahram M, Sloane BF (2000) Unravelling the role of proteases in cancer. Clin Chim Acta 291:113–135
16. U.S. Food and Drug Administration (2011) FDA approves adcetris to treat two types of lymphoma, for immediate release: 19 Aug 2011. U.S. Food and Drug Administration, Silver Spring, MD, 20993
17. Doronina SO, Toki BE, Torgov MY, Mendelsohn BA, Cerveny CG, Chace DF, DeBlanc RL, Gearing RP, Bovee TD, Siegall CB, Francisco JA, Wahl AF, Meyer DL, Senter PD (2003) Development of potent monoclonal antibody auristatin conjugates for cancer therapy. Nat Biotechnol 21:778–784
18. Erickson HK, Park PU, Widdison WC, Kovtun YV, Garrett LM, Hoffman K, Lutz RJ, Goldmacher VS, Blattler WA (2006) Antibody-maytansinoid conjugates are activated in

targeted cancer cells by lysosomal degradation and linker-dependent intracellular processing. Cancer Res 66:4426–4433
19. Junutula JR, Flagella KM, Graham RA, Parsons KL, Ha E, Raab H, Bhakta S, Nguyen T, Dugger DL, Li G, Mai E, Lewis Phillips GD, Hiraragi H, Fuji RN, Tibbitts J, Vandlen R, Spencer SD, Scheller RH, Polakis P, Sliwkowski MX (2010) Engineered thio-trastuzumab–DM1 conjugate with an improved therapeutic index to target human epidermal growth factor receptor 2-positive breast cancer. Clin Cancer Res 16(19):4769–4778
20. Junutula JR, Bhakta S, Raab H, Ervin KE, Eigenbrot C, Vandlen R, Scheller RH, Lowman HB (2008) Rapid identification of reactive cysteine residues for site-specific labeling of antibody-Fabs. J Immunol Methods 332:41–52
21. Wang L, Amphlett G, Blattler WA, Lambert JM, Zhang W (2005) Structural characterization of the maytansinoid–monoclonal antibody immunoconjugate, huN901-DM1, by mass spectrometry. Protein Sci 14:2436–2446
22. Junutula JR, Raab H, Clark S, Bhakta S, Leipold DD, Weir S, Chen Y, Simpson M, Tsai SP, Dennis MS, Lu Y, Meng YG, Ng C, Yang J, Lee CC, Duenas E, Gorrell J, Katta V, Kim A, McDorman K, Flagella K, Venook R, Ross S, Spencer SD, Lee Wong W, Lowman HB, Vandlen R, Sliwkowski MX, Scheller RH, Polakis P, Mallet W (2008) Site-specific conjugation of a cytotoxic drug to an antibody improves the therapeutic index. Nat Biotechnol 26 (8):925–932
23. Lin K, Tibbitts J (2012) Pharmacokinetic considerations for antibody drug conjugates. Pharm Res 29(9):2354–2366
24. Shen BQ, Xu K, Liu L, Raab H, Bhakta S, Kenrick M, Parsons- Reponte KL, Tien J, Yu SF, Mai E, Li D, Tibbitts J, Baudys J, Saad OM, Scales SJ, McDonald PJ, Hass PE, Eigenbrot C, Nguyen T, Solis WA, Fuji RN, Flagella KM, Patel D, Spencer SD, Khawli LA, Ebens A, Wong WL, Vandlen R, Kaur S, Sliwkowski MX, Scheller RH, Polakis P, Junutula JR (2012) Conjugation site modulates the in vivo stability and therapeutic activity of antibody drug conjugates. Nat Biotechnol 30:184–189
25. Baker MA, Roncari DAK, Taub RN, Mohanakumar T, Falk JA, Grant S (1982) Characterization of compounds shed from the surface of human leukemic myeloblasts in vitro. Blood 60:412–419
26. Black PH (1980) Shedding from the cell surface of normal and cancer cells. Adv Cancer Res 32:75–199
27. Lu Y, Wong WL, Meng YG (2006) A high throughput electrochemiluminescent cell-binding assay for therapeutic anti-CD20 antibody selection. J Immunol Methods 314:74–79
28. Sanderson RJ, Hering MA, James SF, Sun MM, Doronina SO, Siadak AW, Senter PD, Wahl AF (2005) In vivo drug-linker stability of an anti-CD30 dipeptide-linked auristatin immunoconjugate. Clin Cancer Res 11:843–852
29. Stephan JP, Chan P, Lee C, Nelson C, Elliott JM, Bechtel C, Raab H, Xie D, Akutagawa J, Baudys J, Saad O, Prabhu S, Wong WL, Vandlen R, Jacobson F, Ebens A (2008) Anti-CD22-MCC-DM1 and MC-MMAF conjugates: impact of assay format on pharmacokinetic parameters determination. Bioconjug Chem 19(8):1673–1683
30. Fischer SK, Yang J, Anand B, Cowan K, Hendricks R, Li J, Nakamura G, Song A (2012) The assay design used for measurement of therapeutic antibody concentrations can affect pharmacokinetic parameters: case studies. MAbs 4(5):623–631

Chapter 7

Pharmacokinetics and ADME Characterizations of Antibody–Drug Conjugates

Kedan Lin, Jay Tibbitts, and Ben-Quan Shen

Abstract

Pharmacokinetic and absorption, distribution, metabolism, and excretion (ADME) characterization of antibody–drug conjugates (ADCs) reflects the dynamic interactions between the biological system and ADC, and provides critical assessments in lead selection, optimization, and clinical development. Understanding the pharmacokinetics (PK), ADME properties and consequently the pharmacokinetic-pharmacodynamic properties of ADCs is critical for their successful development. This chapter discusses the PK properties of ADCs, types of PK and ADME studies in supporting different stages of development, general design of PK/ADME studies with a focus on ADC-specific characteristics, and interpretation of PK parameters.

Key words Antibody–drug conjugates (ADCs), Clearance, Volume of distribution, Pharmacokinetics, Drug-to-antibody ratio (DAR), Pharmacodynamics, Optimization, Absorption, distribution, metabolism, and excretion (ADME)

1 Introduction

Antibody–drug conjugates (ADCs) are monoclonal antibodies (mAb) bearing cytotoxic drugs covalently bound via a chemical linker [1, 2]. As "targeted chemotherapy," ADCs are designed to be superior to either antibody therapeutics or chemotherapy alone by overcoming their limitations while preserving the merits from both.

Nearly 50 years since the first description of ADCs [3], the field is experiencing a renaissance of intense activities and successes. Brentuximab vedotin (ADCETRIS®) was recently approved for the treatment of relapsed or refractory Hodgkin lymphoma and relapsed or refractory systemic anaplastic large-cell lymphoma [4], and trastuzumab emtansine (T-DM1) is showing promising efficacy in patients with HER2+ metastatic breast cancer [5].

Optimization of these complex molecules can greatly benefit from quantitative and mechanistic understanding of their behavior. Pharmacokinetics of ADC, "what the body does to the drug,"

Laurent Ducry (ed.), *Antibody-Drug Conjugates*, Methods in Molecular Biology, vol. 1045,
DOI 10.1007/978-1-62703-541-5_7, © Springer Science+Business Media, LLC 2013

reflects the dynamic interactions between the biological system and ADC, and provides critical assessments in lead selection, optimization, and clinical development. Specifically, an integrated understanding of the pharmacokinetic and pharmacodynamic principles and their applications to target selection, antibody design, linker/drug selection, and drug-to-antibody ratio (DAR) optimization can help guide the rational development of ADCs with the best safety and efficacy profiles.

In this chapter, we discuss the PK and absorption, distribution, metabolism, and excretion (ADME) properties of ADCs, types of PK/ADME studies in supporting different stages of development, general design of PK/ADME studies with a focus on ADC-specific characteristics, and interpretation of PK/ADME parameters.

2 Pharmacokinetics of ADCs

ADCs consist of two pharmacologically distinct components, the antibody and the cytotoxic small-molecule drug (SMD) (hereafter referred to as drug); this distinction necessitates the understanding of the behavior and fate of both components in vivo. Structurally, the antibody component of the ADC accounts for the majority of the therapeutic agent (approximately 98 % of total ADC by molecular weight). Biologically, the PK of ADCs is strongly influenced by the underlying antibody backbone conferring properties such as target-specific binding, neonatal Fc receptor (FcRn)-dependent recycling, and Fc (fragment, crystallizable) effector functions. Similarly, the absorption, distribution, metabolism, and excretion (ADME) properties of ADCs possess positive attributes associated with unconjugated antibodies, including slow clearance, long half-life, low volume of distribution, and proteolysis-mediated catabolism. However they also retain less desirable characteristics, including poor oral bioavailability, incomplete absorption following intramuscular or subcutaneous administration, immunogenicity, and nonlinear distribution and elimination [6, 7]. Beyond these similarities, many characteristics of ADC are distinct from those of an unconjugated antibody, which need to be considered during ADC development. The small-molecule component of ADCs, conjugation process, and in vivo biotransformation of ADCs are unique and important aspects that require consideration when developing these molecules. Briefly, ADCs are heterogeneous mixtures of molecular entities or drug species, specifically antibodies with multiple drug molecules conjugated at different locations: characteristics that require consideration when evaluating their pharmacology as well as bioanalytical and PK properties. Table 1 shows the comparison of ADC PK with monoclonal antibody and small molecule. Recent reviews have detailed the specific characteristics of ADC PK [8], and this chapter focuses on the more practical

Table 1
General PK comparisons among ADC, small-molecule drug (SMD), and mAb

Property	SMD	ADC	mAB
MW (Da)	Typically <1,000	~150,000	~150,000
PK assays	SMD and relevant metabolites	Conjugate, total antibody, and unconjugated cytotoxic drug	Total antibody
Immunogenicity	No	Yes	Yes
Distribution	High Vd; wide range; can exceed actual volume of the blood and well-perfused tissues	Vc approximates plasma volume Limited tissue distribution	Vc approximates plasma volume Limited tissue distribution
Metabolism	Phase I and Phase II metabolism; CYP450 for ~75 % of drugs	Combination of catabolism via proteolysis and CYP450 metabolism	Catabolism via proteolysis, endocytosis, phagocytosis
Excretion	Mainly biliary secretion and renal excretion	Combination of both SMD and mAb expected	Short peptides and amino acids reused or eliminated via glomerular filtration
Half-life	Short (hours)	Long $t_{1/2}$ (antibody); sustained delivery of SMD	Long (days and weeks); FcRn binding prolongs half-life
Clearance	Low dose: linear High dose: nonlinear	Low dose: nonlinear High dose: linear	Low dose: nonlinear High dose: linear

Vd volume of distribution, *Vc* volume of distribution in central compartment

aspect of ADC PK and ADME. We address analyte selection, study considerations, and application of PK/ADME in ADC optimization in the following sections.

3 Analyte Selection and Key Parameters in Characterizing ADC PK

As discussed in details elsewhere in this book, ADCs are complex and highly heterogeneous. This heterogeneity comes from several sources, including as a result of the conjugation of the drug to the antibody through amino acid such as cysteine and lysine. This process results in a mixture of ADC species differing not only in the number of drugs attached to the antibody, i.e., DAR, but also in the sites of drug linkage [9, 10]. A second source of ADC heterogeneity results from biological or chemical processes following in vivo administration, the deconjugation and degradation of ADCs.

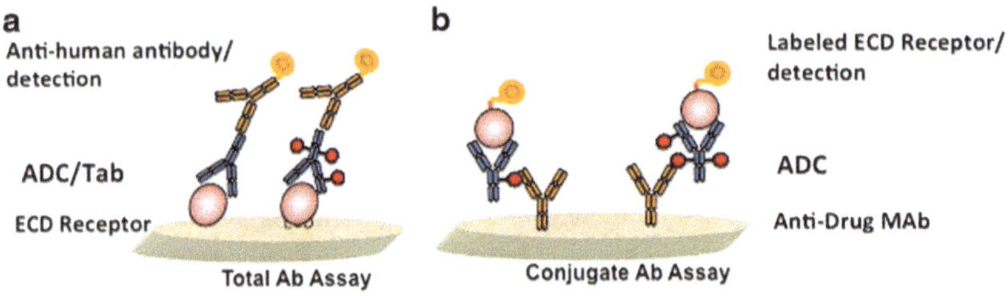

Fig. 1 Typical ELISA formats for ADC analytes. (**a**) Total antibody assay: Capture of ADC antibody using antigen or target extracellular domain (ECD), with detection using labeled antibody to ADC antibody. (**b**) Conjugated antibody assay: Capture of ADC using anti-cytotoxic drug antibody, with detection using labeled antigen or extracellular domain

Table 2
Comparison of analytes, assay format, and their biological significance for characterizing ADC PK

Analytes/assay format	What it measures	Biological significance
Total antibody (Tab) ELISA	Both the conjugated and unconjugated antibody of an antibody of an ADC	Best assessment of antibody-related PK behavior of the ADC
Conjugated antibody ELISA	Antibody with at least one conjugated cytotoxic drug	An estimate of the active ADC concentration, and is the basis for most ADC PK analyses
Conjugated drug LC-MS/MS	Total amount of cytotoxic drug covalently bound to the antibody	An estimate of active drug associated with antibody; reflects both elimination of ADC from systemic circulation and loss of cytotoxic drug from the antibody
Free drug LC-MS or ELISA	Systemic exposure to free drug species released from ADCs	Theoretical assessment of the most prevalent and potent drug species; may reflect the assessment of systemic toxicity

The structural complexity and heterogeneity dictate the need to monitor multiple analytes for ADC PK/disposition for both ADC optimization and development. The commonly monitored analytes may include total antibody (conjugated and unconjugated antibody), conjugated antibody, antibody-conjugated drug, unconjugated antibody, and unconjugated (free) drug. Figure 1 shows the typical ELISA formats for total antibody and conjugated antibody assays. Table 2 summarizes the assay format for each analyte, what is measured, and their biological significance. Multiple analytes help to capture the many facets of the behavior of these complex molecules, such as the rate of drug loss from an ADC (i.e., linker stability), the effect of conjugation on ADC clearance, and ultimately the exposure–response relationship. However, the desire to be comprehensive must be balanced by the practicality, the availability of the technology and reagents, and ultimately the purpose of each study. Two key pharmacokinetic parameters, clearance and volume of distribution, determined from ADC PK studies help elucidate the biological interactions between ADCs and the biological system.

3.1 Clearance

ADC clearance is typically described as the sum of two simultaneous processes: the loss of drug from the ADC (deconjugation), and catabolism of the ADC. Clearance through antibody catabolism is driven primarily by catabolism mediated by specific and saturable antigen-mediated uptake and clearance, and nonspecific high-capacity proteolysis through the interactions between the Fc region of the mAb and Fc receptors. Similar to mAbs, the latter pathway dominates the contribution to clearance for most ADCs at therapeutic doses and leads to linear clearance for ADCs. However, ADCs often exhibit increased clearance and decreased half-lives compared to antibodies [11], presumably owing to the disturbance of tertiary structures from conjugation and altered interactions with clearance pathways.

3.2 Volume of Distribution

The structure of ADCs is dominated by the antibody backbone, and consequently, ADC distribution behavior is usually similar to unconjugated antibodies [12]. Initial distribution is typically limited to the vascular space, with a central compartment volume of distribution similar to plasma volume (~50 mL/kg) [13, 14]. With time, distribution extends to the interstitial space, with a steady-state volume of distribution of approximately 150–200 mL/kg. Similar to unconjugated antibodies, ADC distribution can also be affected by target antigen expression and internalization [15].

The presence of a conjugated cytotoxic drug increases the importance of understanding the distribution of the ADC and, in particular, of the cytotoxic drug. Distribution of unconjugated antibodies to nontarget tissues, via antigen-nonspecific or -specific processes, may have little pharmacologic effect, while distribution and accumulation of an ADC to the same tissues may have profound pharmacologic/toxic effects as a result of the uptake of ADC and subsequent release of the cytotoxic drug or other cytotoxic drug-related catabolites. Interested readers may refer to several recent publications for specific details [15–17].

4 Application of PK in ADC Optimization and Development

The PK studies conducted at different stages of research and development of an ADC serve distinct purposes (Table 3). Early on, the focus of PK studies is to support the selection and optimization of

Table 3
Summary of milestones and studies including PK characterizations at different stages of ADC development

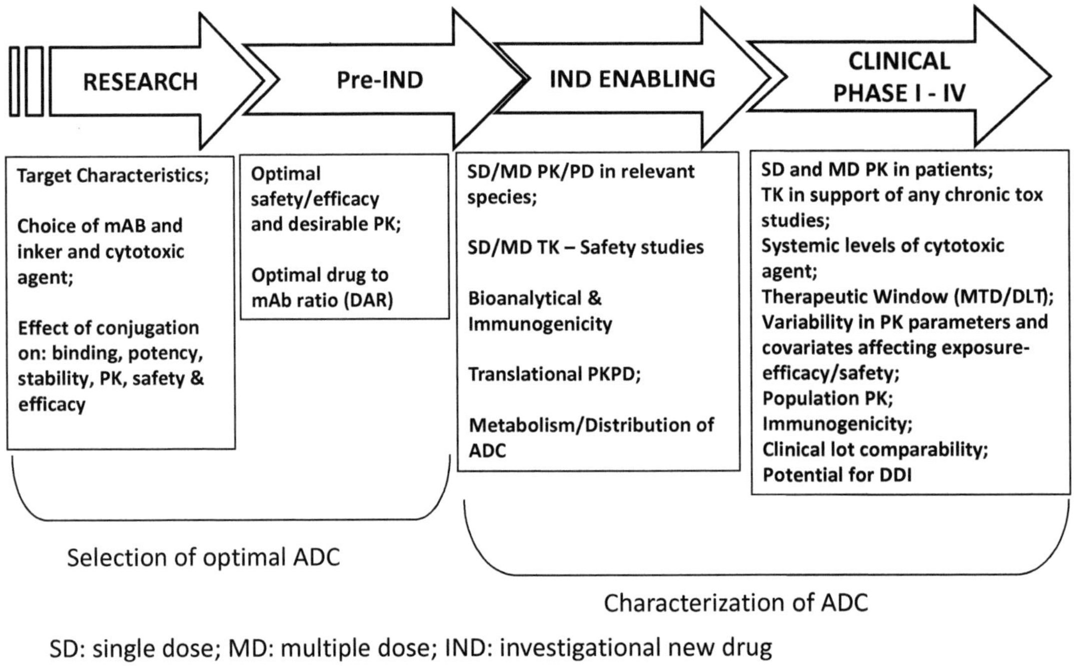

SD single dose, *MD* multiple dose, *IND* investigational new drug, *TK* toxicokinetics

an ADC. During this phase, studies in preclinical species with multiple ADC candidates and unconjugated antibody help provide insights into several aspects of ADC properties, including the interactions between target and ADC (e.g., target-mediated clearance), effect of drug conjugation on antibody pharmacokinetics, linker stability, optimal DAR, and possible pharmacokinetic-pharmacodynamic (PKPD) relationships. For example, comparison of total antibody concentrations of (Tab) PK between an ADC and its unconjugated antibody helps to evaluate the impact of conjugation on the pharmacokinetic behavior of an ADC (Fig. 2) [18, 19].

Once the molecule has been selected, the focus of investigational new drug (IND) enabling studies shifts to full characterization of its pharmacological activities, including PK exposure in efficacy and safety studies, PKPD relationship, and distribution/metabolism. PK evaluation of an ADC continues during clinical development with additional components, such as evaluating drug–drug interaction (DDI) potential (discussed later in the chapter).

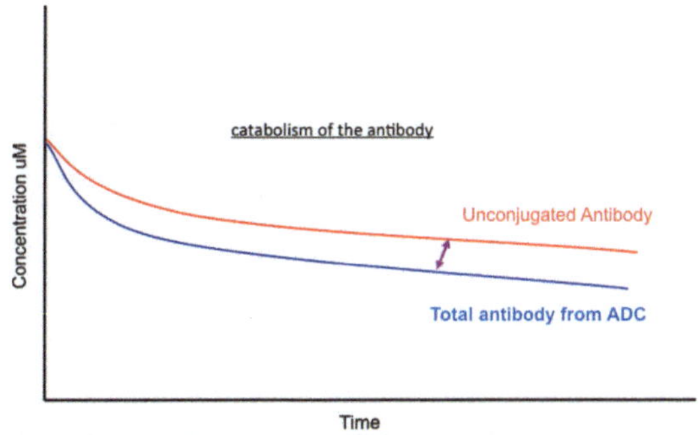

Fig. 2 Comparison of serum or plasma concentration profile of unconjugated antibody (following antibody administration) with total antibody (following ADC administration). Faster decrease in Tab concentrations suggests that ADC pharmacokinetics is affected by conjugation

5 ADC PK Interpretation

Integration of PK information derived from the measurement of multiple ADC analytes can provide critical information during ADC optimization. A critical aspect of ADC behavior is the rate of drug loss from ADC, i.e., linker stability. Qualitative assessment of linker stability can be achieved by comparison of ADC analytes, total antibody, and either conjugated antibody or antibody-conjugated drug. Theoretical plots of this comparison are shown in Fig. 3. For the comparison of total antibody with conjugated antibody, it is typically observed that conjugated antibody concentrations decline more rapidly than Tab concentrations, for reasons explained earlier (decreases in the concentration of ADCs are the result of two processes vs. one process for Tab). The degree of divergence of the curves is indicative of the rate of complete drug loss from the ADC (i.e., DARn-to-DAR zero transition). This is due to the nature of the conjugated antibody assay, which measures all ADC bearing one or more drugs. A greater divergence of the conjugated antibody PK from the Tab PK infers a more rapid loss of drug from the ADC [16, 20–24].

Comparison of Tab and conjugated drug concentrations is best done with concentrations in molar units (Fig. 3). This allows for-clearer visual assessment of the concentration–time profiles of analytes with various molecular weights. Interpretation of the relationship between Tab and antibody-conjugated drug concentrations is, perhaps, less intuitive than for conjugated antibody. Antibody-conjugated drug concentrations decline more rapidly than Tab concentrations because two processes drive the decrease in conjugated drug concentrations: loss of drug from the ADC and elimination of ADC, while Tab concentration changes are driven solely by elimination of ADC and unconjugated antibody. As such,

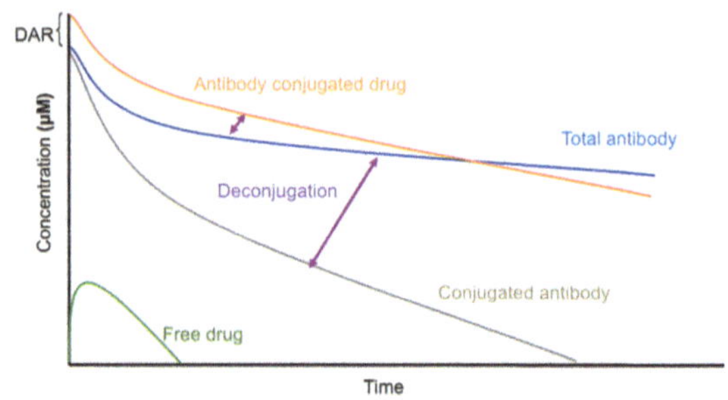

Fig. 3 Comparison of analyte concentration profile following ADC administration. Total antibody (Tab, *blue*) has multi-exponential profile typical of antibody. Conjugated antibody (*gray*) shows more rapid decrease in concentration as a result of antibody elimination and cytotoxic drug deconjugation. Conjugated drug (*orange*) starts at higher concentration than Tab, reflecting its DAR, and then decreases more rapidly than Tab due to antibody elimination and cytotoxic drug deconjugation. Free drug (*green*) concentrations are much lower, increase with time to reflect delay in deconjugation from ADC, and decline over time

the difference in the concentration decrease can be used to infer the rate of drug loss from the ADC [18, 25]. At the time of dosing, the difference in molar concentrations reflects the starting average DAR, and at some time after dosing the two concentrations (total antibody and antibody-conjugated drug) may intersect when the average DAR equals 1.

Overall, comparison of multiple analytes provides quantitative assessment on collective impact of multiple optimization parameters, such as linker stability, conjugation site, and DAR. This information is crucial in guiding the selection and optimization of next generation of ADCs [26–28].

6 ADC ADME Characterization

ADCs contain cytotoxic drugs, and the catabolites of ADCs may hold DDI potential. Therefore, it is of great importance to understand the ADME properties of ADCs and their major elimination pathways, and determine the need for special patient population studies in patients with hepatic or renal impairment. The following questions need to be addressed to understand the ADME properties of ADC and its major catabolites:

- What is linker stability in plasma?
- Which tissue does the ADC distribute to? Any accumulation in any tissue?
- Does conjugation alter distribution? What are the main catabolites in tissue?
- What are the major catabolites and their biological activity?

- What is the major route of elimination and what catabolites are eliminated?
- Is there any DDI potential for the cytotoxic drug/major catabolites?
- Are catabolites translatable across species? Is there a need for conducting clinical DDI or special patient population studies?

In this section, T-DM1 is cited as an example to illustrate how to approach ADC ADME issues. T-DM1 consists of the recombinant anti-epidermal growth factor receptor 2 (HER2) monoclonal antibody trastuzumab conjugated to the maytansinoid DM1 via a non-reducible thioether linkage (MCC). T-DM1 is currently in clinical development for treating HER2-positive metastatic breast cancer and gastric cancer.

6.1 ADC Linker Stability in Plasma

Though ADC linkers are designed to be stable in plasma and to be cleaved only by a few defined release mechanisms such as acidic pH and proteases, drug could be released prematurely in blood, causing systemic toxicity. Previously, Mylotarg®, a chemotherapy agent composed of a humanized IgG4 conjugated with a cytotoxic antitumor antibiotic, calicheamicin, was approved to treat acute myelogenous leukemia. However, Mylotarg was found to have unacceptable toxicity and lack of clinical benefit, which may be in part due to poor linker stability and premature drug release [25, 29]. The current ADCs in clinical development using either valine-citrulline or MCC linker are designed to be stable in plasma and require intracellular lysosomal protease processing to release the drug or active catabolites [30]. In vitro plasma stability studies should be conducted to assess the stability of the linker between antibody and cytotoxic drug, to determine the potential formation of drug-containing products, and to compare stability difference between species. This can be done simply by spiking ADC to plasma at a relevant concentration followed by incubating the mixture at 37 °C in a CO_2 incubator for 0–96 h and analyzing the release of free cytotoxic drug and changes of other analytes (Shen, manuscript in preparation).

6.2 ADC Tissue Distribution

Given the structural properties of ADC, it is expected that the biodistribution of ADCs should be consistent with that described for IgG antibodies [15, 31]. Biodistribution studies of ADC are important to demonstrate that its distribution is similar to unconjugated antibody, i.e., delivery of drug to the specific tumor target without accumulation or persistency in normal tissues. For this purpose, unconjugated antibody and ADC labeled either on antibody (via labeling with [^{125}I]) or drug (via conjugation of antibody with radiolabeled drug) can be administered to tumor-bearing mice or rats and radioactivity in plasma and tissues measured. Comparison of data from these studies would allow the assessment of conjugation on antibody distribution [15, 32–34].

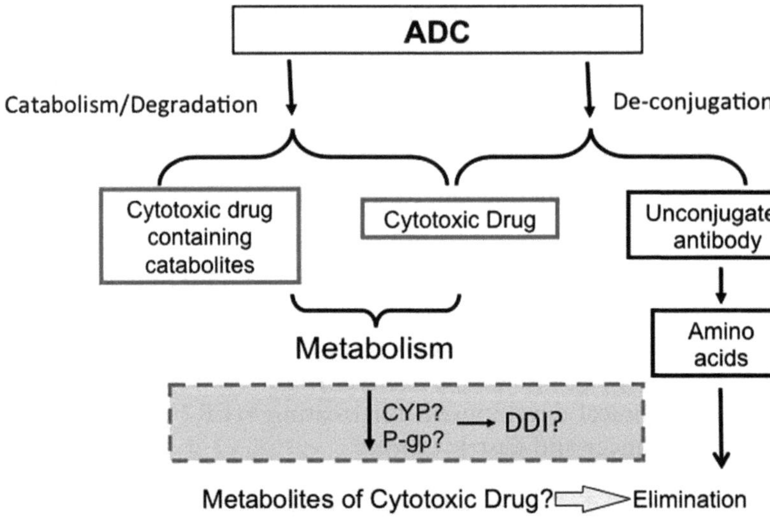

Fig. 4 Diagram of theoretical ADC catabolism. The formation of cytotoxic drug-containing products from ADCs may occur by two concurrent processes: deconjugation and catabolism. The deconjugation process includes release of cytotoxic drug-containing products from the ADC via enzymatic or chemical processes and unconjugated antibody, with preservation of the antibody backbone. The catabolism process includes proteolytic catabolism of the antibody and formation of cytotoxic drug-containing catabolites (free drug or drug–amino acid conjugates)

It is also of great importance to understand the tissue distribution of the cytotoxic drug, whether it is conjugated to the antibody or unconjugated. There are examples in literatures illustrating that ADC and cytotoxic drug distribution could differ between normal tissues and tumor [33]. In some cases, low level of target antigen expression in normal tissues may lead to decreased ADC delivery to tumor and/or increased delivery of cytotoxic drug to normal tissues [35, 36].

6.3 ADC Catabolism/Metabolism and Elimination

The antibody component of ADCs is subject to similar catabolism and elimination processes as that of mAbs. Catabolism and elimination of antibodies have been well studied and are known to be mediated mainly by either receptor-mediated endocytosis or fluid-phase pinocytosis with subsequent trafficking to the lysosome, followed by enzymatic degradation [6, 37, 38]. This occurs mainly in the liver, spleen, lymph nodes, gut, and kidney [39], resulting in degradation to amino acids or peptides with no biologic activity. As expected, ADCs have been shown to undergo similar catabolic processes as mAbs (Fig. 4) [31, 33, 40–42]. Elimination of ADCs warrants additional scrutiny due to their conjugated cytotoxic drugs; proteolytic degradation of ADCs can generate catabolic products that may retain high cytotoxic potency. Cytotoxic drug-containing catabolites are produced either by cleavage of the linker (deconjugation) or by catabolism of the antibody through further intracellular processing [43]. Formation of catabolic products may be linker specific. ADCs with cleavable linkers such as mAb-SPP-DM1 (disulfide) or mAb-vc-MMAE release cytotoxic drug upon linker cleavage [31, 40], and ADCs with noncleavable linkers such as mAb-MCC-DM1 and mAb-mc-MMAF often produce catabolic products that contain the linker–drug conjugated to the amino acid (e.g., lys-MCC-DM1 or cys-mc-MMAF) [32].

In addition to deconjugation through linker cleavage, direct transfer of linker–drug to plasma protein has also been observed [33]. ADCs with linker–drug combination of mc-MMAF were shown to release cytotoxic drug via transfer of linker–drug (mc-MMAF) to thiol-containing albumin in plasma [33]. It is conceivable that similar exchange could occur between ADCs with similar linker structures and other thiol-containing constituents (e.g., glutathione, cystine) in serum/plasma. This example also illustrates the need to investigate the mechanism and products of ADC catabolism using a multi-pronged approach.

Appropriate in vitro studies including catabolism studies in target-expressing cell lines and plasma stability studies across species help to identify ADC degradation products and establish the relevance of preclinical species. A recent report on the effect of conjugation site on the in vivo stability and therapeutic activity of cysteine-engineered thio-antibody–drug conjugates (TDC) nicely demonstrated the utility of such an integrated approach. Plasma stability data of TDCs along with data from in vivo studies confirmed that the stability and therapeutic activity of the antibody conjugate were affected positively by succinimide ring hydrolysis and negatively by maleimide exchange with thiol-reactive constituents in plasma [28]. In vivo studies, on the other hand, corroborate with in vitro study and further shed light on the identity and fate of drug-containing catabolic products.

In addition to understanding the catabolism and distribution of the ADCs, it is equally important to characterize the major route of excretion for ADC and its catabolites. Knowing the major route of elimination would help to determine whether there is a need to conduct a special population study such as hepatic or renal dysfunction patients. In the case of T-DM1, in vivo studies with radiolabeled T-DM1 and DM1 were conducted in rats to characterize the distribution, route of excretion, and the identity of the metabolic products of both T-DM1 and DM1. For example, to determine the major route of elimination, the radiolabeled T-[^{3}H]DM1 or [^{3}H]DM1 was administered to either bile duct-cannulated rats (for bile collection) or non-cannulated rats (for feces and urine collection). Measuring the radioactivity in the excreta including feces, urine, and bile allowed the determination of the rate and route of excretion [28].

Catabolites identified in rats using multiple methodologies were monitored and assessed in humans, which provides valuable information in ADC disposition across species. Knowledge of the identity and pharmacologic properties of these cytotoxic catabolites can be valuable in several ways. Some catabolic products and released drugs, such as S-methyl-DM4 and MMAE, have been shown to contribute to drug efficacy by causing "bystander effect" [40, 41] and provide an advantage in tumors with heterogeneous target expression. On the other hand, the potent and diffusible cytotoxin-containing products contribute to the overall systemic toxicity and harbor the potential for DDI.

6.4 In Vitro DDI Assessment

Similar to other mAb therapeutics, the antibody moiety of an ADC carries low DDI risk [44, 45]. In contrast, the size and structure of ADC catabolic products are similar to small-molecule therapeutics, as described above. These catabolites may be subject to the metabolism and elimination processes associated with SMDs, including cytochromes (CYPs) and drug transporters, which poses a theoretical possibility of DDI when combining with another SMD. While ADC-specific catabolism guidance has not been developed, a well-established framework for DDI evaluation has been described for assessing metabolites for small-molecule therapeutics [46–49]. It is worth pointing out that given the extremely low concentration of free drug released in systemic circulation [11, 50], the likelihood of cytotoxic component of ADC impacting on CYP and transporter activities at clinically relevant doses is low. In contrast, the exposure level of highly potent components of ADCs may be subject to fluctuation in the presence of other SMDs if they share similar metabolism or elimination pathways. Ultimately, the risk of DDI hinges on the exposure response relationships between released cytotoxic drug and efficacy/safety, which has to be evaluated using aforementioned multipronged approach.

7 Conclusions

The development of "antibody–linker–drug" carries great promise in oncology applications; it is, however, complicated by the need to optimize three different moieties, and synchronize them to generate the most desirable pharmacologic effects. Heterogeneity from production and in vivo processing, the necessity to monitor multiple active ADC analytes, complex PKPD relationships, and less understood catabolic and metabolic species are among the considerations in characterizing their unique PK and ADME properties. The growing interest in ADCs, the evolvement of powerful analytical tools, and generation of crucial mechanistic data indicate a promising future for ADC PKPD.

Acknowledgements

The authors would like to thank PKPD colleagues for their constructive input and careful review of this manuscript.

References

1. Carter PJ, Senter PD (2008) Antibody-drug conjugates for cancer therapy. Cancer J 14 (3):154–169
2. Schrama D, Reisfeld RA, Becker JC (2006) Antibody targeted drugs as cancer therapeutics. Nat Rev 5(2):147–159
3. Decarvalho S, Rand HJ, Lewis A (1964) Coupling of cyclic chemotherapeutic compounds to immune gamma-globulins. Nature 202:255–258
4. de Claro RA, McGinn KM, Kwitkowski VE, Bullock J, Khandelwal A, Habtemariam BA, Ouyang Y, Saber H, Lee K, Koti K, Rothmann MD, Shapiro M, Borrego F, Clouse K, Chen XH, Brown J, Akinsanya L, Kane RC, Kaminskas E, Farrell A, Pazdur R (2012) U.S. Food and Drug Administration approval summary: brentuximab vedotin for the treatment of relapsed Hodgkin lymphoma or relapsed systemic anaplastic large cell lymphoma. Clin Cancer Res 18(21):5845–5849. doi:10.1158/1078-0432.CCR-12-1803
5. Blackwell K (2012) Primary results from EMILIA, a phase III study of trastuzumab emtansine (T-DM1) versus capecitabine (X) and lapatinib (L) in HER2-positive locally advanced or metastatic breast cancer (MBC) previously treated with trastuzumab (T) and a taxane. In: 2012 ASCO annual meeting 2012. J Clin Oncol vol 30, 2012 (suppl; abstr LBA1)
6. Lobo ED, Hansen RJ, Balthasar JP (2004) Antibody pharmacokinetics and pharmacodynamics. J Pharm Sci 93(11):2645–2668. doi:10.1002/jps.20178
7. Deng R, Jin F, Prabhu S, Iyer S (2012) Monoclonal antibodies: what are the pharmacokinetic and pharmacodynamic considerations for drug development? Expert Opin Drug Metab Toxicol 8(2):141–160. doi:10.1517/17425255.2012.643868
8. Lin K, Tibbitts J (2012) Pharmacokinetic considerations for antibody drug conjugates. Pharm Res 29(9):2354–2366. doi:10.1007/s11095-012-0800-y
9. Singh R, Erickson HK (2009) Antibody-cytotoxic agent conjugates: preparation and characterization. Methods Mol Biol 525:445–467, xiv. doi:10.1007/978-1-59745-554-1_23
10. Hamblett KJ, Senter PD, Chace DF, Sun MM, Lenox J, Cerveny CG, Kissler KM, Bernhardt SX, Kopcha AK, Zabinski RF, Meyer DL, Francisco JA (2004) Effects of drug loading on the antitumor activity of a monoclonal antibody drug conjugate. Clin Cancer Res 10 (20):7063–7070
11. Girish S, Gupta M, Wang B, Lu D, Krop IE, Vogel CL, Burris Iii HA, Lorusso PM, Yi JH, Saad O, Tong B, Chu YW, Holden S, Joshi A (2012) Clinical pharmacology of trastuzumab emtansine (T-DM1): an antibody-drug conjugate in development for the treatment of HER2-positive cancer. Cancer Chemother Pharmacol 69(5):1229–1240. doi:10.1007/s00280-011-1817-3
12. Tabrizi M, Bornstein GG, Suria H (2010) Biodistribution mechanisms of therapeutic monoclonal antibodies in health and disease. AAPS J 12(1):33–43. doi:10.1208/s12248-009-9157-5
13. Mould DR, Green B (2010) Pharmacokinetics and pharmacodynamics of monoclonal antibodies: concepts and lessons for drug development. BioDrugs 24(1):23–39. doi:10.2165/11530560-000000000-00000
14. Tabrizi MA, Tseng CM, Roskos LK (2006) Elimination mechanisms of therapeutic monoclonal antibodies. Drug Discov Today 11 (1–2):81–88
15. Boswell CA, Mundo EE, Zhang C, Bumbaca D, Valle NR, Kozak KR, Fourie A, Chuh J, Koppada N, Saad O, Gill H, Shen BQ, Rubinfeld B, Tibbitts J, Kaur S, Theil FP, Fielder PJ, Khawli LA, Lin K (2011) Impact of drug conjugation on pharmacokinetics and tissue distribution of anti-STEAP1 antibody-drug conjugates in rats. Bioconjug Chem 22(10):1994–2004. doi:10.1021/bc200212a
16. Tolcher AW, Ochoa L, Hammond LA, Patnaik A, Edwards T, Takimoto C, Smith L, de Bono J, Schwartz G, Mays T, Jonak ZL, Johnson R, DeWitte M, Martino H, Audette C, Maes K, Chari RV, Lambert JM, Rowinsky EK (2003) Cantuzumab mertansine, a maytansinoid immunoconjugate directed to the CanAg antigen: a phase I, pharmacokinetic, and biologic correlative study. J Clin Oncol 21(2):211–222

17. Pastuskovas CV, Mallet W, Clark S, Kenrick M, Majidy M, Schweiger M, Van Hoy M, Tsai SP, Bennett G, Shen BQ, Ross S, Fielder P, Khawli L, Tibbitts J (2010) Effect of immune complex formation on the distribution of a novel antibody to the ovarian tumor antigen CA125. Drug Metab Dispos 38(12):2309–2319. doi:10.1124/dmd.110.034330
18. Xie H, Audette C, Hoffee M, Lambert JM, Blattler WA (2004) Pharmacokinetics and biodistribution of the antitumor immunoconjugate, cantuzumab mertansine (huC242-DM1), and its two components in mice. J Pharmacol Exp Ther 308(3):1073–1082
19. Sapra P, Stein R, Pickett J, Qu Z, Govindan SV, Cardillo TM, Hansen HJ, Horak ID, Griffiths GL, Goldenberg DM (2005) Anti-CD74 antibody-doxorubicin conjugate, IMMU-110, in a human multiple myeloma xenograft and in monkeys. Clin Cancer Res 11(14):5257–5264. doi:10.1158/1078-0432.CCR-05-0204
20. Henry MD, Wen S, Silva MD, Chandra S, Milton M, Worland PJ (2004) A prostate-specific membrane antigen-targeted monoclonal antibody-chemotherapeutic conjugate designed for the treatment of prostate cancer. Cancer Res 64(21):7995–8001
21. Rupp U, Schoendorf-Holland E, Eichbaum M, Schuetz F, Lauschner I, Schmidt P, Staab A, Hanft G, Huober J, Sinn HP, Sohn C, Schneeweiss A (2007) Safety and pharmacokinetics of bivatuzumab mertansine in patients with CD44v6-positive metastatic breast cancer: final results of a phase I study. Anticancer Drugs 18(4):477–485
22. Tijink BM, Buter J, de Bree R, Giaccone G, Lang MS, Staab A, Leemans CR, van Dongen GA (2006) A phase I dose escalation study with anti-CD44v6 bivatuzumab mertansine in patients with incurable squamous cell carcinoma of the head and neck or esophagus. Clin Cancer Res 12(20 Pt 1):6064–6072
23. Burris HA 3rd, Rugo HS, Vukelja SJ, Vogel CL, Borson RA, Limentani S, Tan-Chiu E, Krop IE, Michaelson RA, Girish S, Amler L, Zheng M, Chu YW, Klencke B, O'Shaughnessy JA (2011) Phase II study of the antibody drug conjugate trastuzumab-DM1 for the treatment of human epidermal growth factor receptor 2 (HER2)-positive breast cancer after prior HER2-directed therapy. J Clin Oncol 29(4):398–405. doi:10.1200/JCO.2010.29.5865
24. Advani A, Coiffier B, Czuczman MS, Dreyling M, Foran J, Gine E, Gisselbrecht C, Ketterer N, Nasta S, Rohatiner A, Schmidt-Wolf IG, Schuler M, Sierra J, Smith MR, Verhoef G, Winter JN, Boni J, Vandendries E, Shapiro M, Fayad L (2010) Safety, pharmacokinetics, and preliminary clinical activity of inotuzumab ozogamicin, a novel immunoconjugate for the treatment of B-cell non-Hodgkin's lymphoma: results of a phase I study. J Clin Oncol 28(12):2085–2093. doi:10.1200/JCO.2009.25.1900
25. Sanderson RJ, Hering MA, James SF, Sun MM, Doronina SO, Siadak AW, Senter PD, Wahl AF (2005) In vivo drug-linker stability of an anti-CD30 dipeptide-linked auristatin immunoconjugate. Clin Cancer Res 11(2 Pt 1):843–852, doi:11/2/843 [pii]
26. Dornan D, Bennett F, Chen Y, Dennis M, Eaton D, Elkins K, French D, Go MA, Jack A, Junutula JR, Koeppen H, Lau J, McBride J, Rawstron A, Shi X, Yu N, Yu SF, Yue P, Zheng B, Ebens A, Polson AG (2009) Therapeutic potential of an anti-CD79b antibody-drug conjugate, anti-CD79b-vc-MMAE, for the treatment of non-Hodgkin lymphoma. Blood 114 (13):2721–2729, doi:blood-2009-02-205500 [pii]10.1182/blood-2009-02-205500
27. Lewis Phillips GD, Li G, Dugger DL, Crocker LM, Parsons KL, Mai E, Blattler WA, Lambert JM, Chari RV, Lutz RJ, Wong WL, Jacobson FS, Koeppen H, Schwall RH, Kenkare-Mitra SR, Spencer SD, Sliwkowski MX (2008) Targeting HER2-positive breast cancer with trastuzumab-DM1, an antibody-cytotoxic drug conjugate. Cancer Res 68(22):9280–9290
28. Shen BQ, Bumbaca D, Saad O, Yue Q, Pastuskovas CV, Khojasteh SC, Tibbitts J, Kaur S, Wang B, Chu YW, Lorusso PM, Girish S (2012) Catabolic fate and pharmacokinetic characterization of trastuzumab emtansine (T-DM1): an emphasis on preclinical and clinical catabolism. Curr Drug Metab 13(7):901–910
29. van Der Velden VH, te Marvelde JG, Hoogeveen PG, Bernstein ID, Houtsmuller AB, Berger MS, van Dongen JJ (2001) Targeting of the CD33-calicheamicin immunoconjugate Mylotarg (CMA-676) in acute myeloid leukemia: in vivo and in vitro saturation and internalization by leukemic and normal myeloid cells. Blood 97 (10):3197–3204
30. Ducry L, Stump B (2010) Antibody-drug conjugates: linking cytotoxic payloads to monoclonal antibodies. Bioconjug Chem 21 (1):5–13. doi:10.1021/bc9002019
31. Erickson HK, Park PU, Widdison WC, Kovtun YV, Garrett LM, Hoffman K, Lutz RJ, Goldmacher VS, Blattler WA (2006) Antibody-maytansinoid conjugates are activated in targeted cancer cells by lysosomal degradation and linker-dependent intracellular processing. Cancer Res 66(8):4426–4433

32. Alley SC, Benjamin DR, Jeffrey SC, Okeley NM, Meyer DL, Sanderson RJ, Senter PD (2008) Contribution of linker stability to the activities of anticancer immunoconjugates. Bioconjug Chem 19(3):759–765
33. Alley SC, Zhang X, Okeley NM, Anderson M, Law CL, Senter PD, Benjamin DR (2009) The pharmacologic basis for antibody-auristatin conjugate activity. J Pharmacol Exp Ther 330 (3):932–938
34. Erickson HK, Lambert JM (2012) ADME of antibody-maytansinoid conjugates. AAPS J. doi:10.1208/s12248-012-9386-x
35. Boswell CA, Mundo EE, Zhang C, Stainton SL, Yu SF, Lacap JA, Mao W, Kozak KR, Fourie A, Polakis P, Khawli LA, Lin K (2012) Differential effects of predosing on tumor and tissue uptake of an 111in-labeled anti-TENB2 antibody-drug conjugate. J Nucl Med. doi:10.2967/jnumed.112.103168
36. Boswell CA, Mundo EE, Firestein R, Zhang C, Mao W, Gill H, Young C, Ljumanovic N, Stainton S, Ulufatu S, Fourie A, Kozak KR, Fuji R, Polakis P, Khawli LA, Lin K (2012) An integrated approach to identify normal tissue expression of targets for antibody drug conjugates: case study of TENB2. Br J Pharmacol. doi:10.1111/j.1476-5381.2012.02138.x
37. Lin YS, Nguyen C, Mendoza JL, Escandon E, Fei D, Meng YG, Modi NB (1999) Preclinical pharmacokinetics, interspecies scaling, and tissue distribution of a humanized monoclonal antibody against vascular endothelial growth factor. J Pharmacol Exp Ther 288(1):371–378
38. Braeckman R (ed) (2000) Pharmacokinetics and pharmacodynamics of protein therapeutics, vol 101. Peptide and Protein Drug Analysis. Marcel Dekker, New York
39. Sands H, Jones PL (1987) Methods for the study of the metabolism of radiolabeled monoclonal antibodies by liver and tumor. J Nucl Med 28(3):390–398
40. Erickson HK, Widdison WC, Mayo MF, Whiteman K, Audette C, Wilhelm SD, Singh R (2010) Tumor delivery and in vivo processing of disulfide-linked and thioether-linked antibody-maytansinoid conjugates. Bioconjug Chem 21(1):84–92
41. Okeley NM, Miyamoto JB, Zhang X, Sanderson RJ, Benjamin DR, Sievers EL, Senter PD, Alley SC (2010) Intracellular activation of SGN-35, a potent anti-CD30 antibody-drug conjugate. Clin Cancer Res 16(3):888–897
42. Sutherland MS, Sanderson RJ, Gordon KA, Andreyka J, Cerveny CG, Yu C, Lewis TS, Meyer DL, Zabinski RF, Doronina SO, Senter PD, Law CL, Wahl AF (2006) Lysosomal trafficking and cysteine protease metabolism confer target-specific cytotoxicity by peptide-linked anti-CD30-auristatin conjugates. J Biol Chem 281(15):10540–10547
43. Austin CD, Wen X, Gazzard L, Nelson C, Scheller RH, Scales SJ (2005) Oxidizing potential of endosomes and lysosomes limits intracellular cleavage of disulfide-based antibody-drug conjugates. Proc Natl Acad Sci USA 102(50):17987–17992. doi:10.1073/pnas.0509035102
44. Girish S, Martin SW, Peterson MC, Zhang LK, Zhao H, Balthasar J, Evers R, Zhou H, Zhu M, Klunk L, Han C, Berglund EG, Huang SM, Joshi A (2011) AAPS workshop report: strategies to address therapeutic protein-drug interactions during clinical development. AAPS J 13(3):405–416. doi:10.1208/s12248-011-9285-6
45. Lu D, Girish S, Theil F, Joshi A (2012) Pharmacokinetic and pharmacodynamic-based drug interactions for therapeutic proteins. In: Zhou H, Meibohm B (eds) Drug-drug interaction for therapeutic biologics
46. Baillie TA, Cayen MN, Fouda H, Gerson RJ, Green JD, Grossman SJ, Klunk LJ, LeBlanc B, Perkins DG, Shipley LA (2002) Drug metabolites in safety testing. Toxicol Appl Pharmacol 182(3):188–196
47. Smith DA, Obach RS (2009) Metabolites in safety testing (MIST): considerations of mechanisms of toxicity with dose, abundance, and duration of treatment. Chem Res Toxicol 22(2):267–279. doi:10.1021/tx800415j
48. Bjornsson TD, Callaghan JT, Einolf HJ, Fischer V, Gan L, Grimm S, Kao J, King SP, Miwa G, Ni L, Kumar G, McLeod J, Obach RS, Roberts S, Roe A, Shah A, Snikeris F, Sullivan JT, Tweedie D, Vega JM, Walsh J, Wrighton SA (2003) The conduct of in vitro and in vivo drug-drug interaction studies: a Pharmaceutical Research and Manufacturers of America (PhRMA) perspective. Drug Metab Dispos 31(7):815–832. doi:10.1124/dmd.31.7.815
49. Drug interaction studies—study design, data analysis, implications for dosing, and labeling recommendations (Draft guidance) (2012) http://www.fda.gov/downloads/Drugs/GuidanceComplianceRegulatoryInformation/Guidances/UCM292362.pdf
50. Younes A, Bartlett NL, Leonard JP, Kennedy DA, Lynch CM, Sievers EL, Forero-Torres A (2010) Brentuximab vedotin (SGN-35) for relapsed CD30-positive lymphomas. N Eng J Med 363(19):1812–1821. doi:10.1056/NEJMoa1002965

Chapter 8

Safe Handling of Cytotoxic Compounds in a Biopharmaceutical Environment

Miriam I. Hensgen and Bernhard Stump

Abstract

Handling cytotoxic drugs such as antibody–drug conjugates (ADCs) in a biopharmaceutical environment represents a challenge based on the potency of the compounds. These derivatives are dangerous to humans if they accidentally get in contact with the skin, are inhaled, or are ingested, either as pure compounds in their solid state or as a solution dissolved in a co-solvent. Any contamination of people involved in the manufacturing process has to be avoided. On the other hand, biopharmaceuticals need to be protected simultaneously against any contamination from the manufacturing personnel. Therefore, a tailor-made work environment is mandatory in order to manufacture ADCs. This asks for appropriate technical equipment to keep potential hazardous substances contained. In addition, clearly defined working procedures based on risk assessments as well as proper training for all personnel involved in the manufacturing process are needed to safely handle these highly potent pharmaceuticals.

Key words Cytotoxic compounds, Handling, Occupational exposure, Antibody–drug conjugates

1 Introduction

Many modern medicines are effective with only small doses to achieve a therapeutic effect and therefore have to be highly potent. This is specifically true for cancer therapy, where the drug needs to efficiently kill cancer cells and therefore—to a certain degree—need to be cytotoxic [1]. Antibody–drug conjugates (ADCs) allow to use even more potent cytotoxic drugs in comparison to conventional chemotherapies, as the attachment of the highly active pharmaceutical ingredient (HAPI) to an antibody carrier allows for a targeted therapy with generally less side effects than the use of the HAPI itself [2].

While the possibility to use more potent cytotoxic drugs as a payload of an ADC cancer therapy provokes a lot of optimism in the pharmaceutical industry, it simultaneously poses a challenge for the manufacturers of these novel drugs [3–5]. Cytotoxic small molecule drugs approved as cancer treatment can already reveal severe

Laurent Ducry (ed.), *Antibody-Drug Conjugates*, Methods in Molecular Biology, vol. 1045,
DOI 10.1007/978-1-62703-541-5_8, © Springer Science+Business Media, LLC 2013

Steps	antibody modification	conjugation	formulation
Process	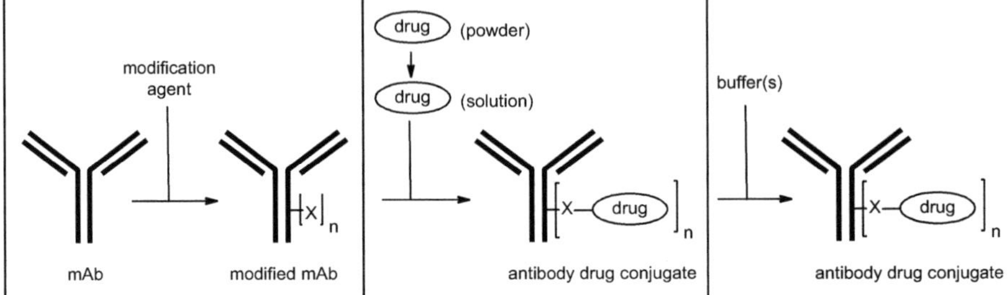		
Safety requirements R&D	Standard hoods, labs	Isolator for solid handling Special hoods, labs for liquid handling	Special hoods, labs
Safety requirements Manufacturing	Standard manufacturing suites	Isolator for solid handling HAPI manufacturing suites	HAPI manufacturing suites

Fig. 1 Typical ADC process based on antibody modification, conjugation and formulation and the safety equipment needed for the safe execution of these steps

side effects with patients when used in therapeutic dosages. The amounts used in the clinic are typically at low mg-scale range for the complete ADC, resulting in a microgram quantity of payload injected in patients. In the manufacturing of an ADC, much larger quantities of the cytotoxic component of the ADC is handled, nourishing concerns for the safety of those who manufacture these drugs or dispose of their waste products. Manufacturing these active compounds calls for safe standard operating procedures (SOPs), containment strategies, and an appropriate, rigorous training to minimize the occupational risks for workers that could come into contact with the cytotoxic payload, the ADC, or related waste.

2 ADC Processes

A typical ADC manufacturing process where a cytotoxic molecule is conjugated to an antibody can be divided in three parts, whereas these parts might differ in their occupational hygiene demand (*see* Fig. 1).

Not all steps in a typical ADC process need the same safety precautions. Usually, the manufacturing of an ADC involves a modification reaction of the monoclonal antibody (mAb) prior to the actual conjugation with the cytotoxic drug. For instance, this can be the partial reduction of the interchain disulfide bridges or the attachment of linker molecules which later will serve as connection points for the payload molecules. Initial steps characteristically involve the use of starting materials such as mAbs and chemicals which do not need a high contamination level as their potency and/or toxicity is quite low. The specific safety challenges of ADC processes are linked to the subsequent conjugation step. The highly potent cytotoxic drug is often brought into the process stream as a stock solution in an organic solvent. The preparation of such a reagent solution involves the handling of the highly potent derivative in powder form. If used in an excess, the cytotoxic compound will partially remain in its unconjugated form in the process solution until appropriate purification steps guarantee the clearance of the surplus free drug species. Thereafter, only the conjugated form of the cytotoxic drug will be present during the following formulation steps, altering the safety requirements further.

In an ADC process, the safety concerns are therefore mainly based on the cytotoxic drug used.

3 Cytotoxic Drugs as ADC Payloads

Predominantly, cytotoxic drugs are therapeutically used for treating cancer. Along with that, a few other medical conditions are being treated with this class of medicines, such as multiple sclerosis, psoriasis, and systemic lupus erythematosus [6].

Cytotoxics include any drug that has a toxic effect on cells, typically by preventing the division (mitosis) of rapidly reproducing cells. As chemotherapeutics, they are commonly used to inhibit the proliferation of cancerous cells. Such substances can be quite powerful, but very often also exhibit severe side effects as they also disturb the growth of healthy quickly dividing cells in the body such as embryonic stem cells, epidermal cells, or hair follicles. Cytotoxic drugs are often known to be:

- Genotoxic—a substance that interacts with DNA, which renders them potentially mutagenic or cancerogenic.
- Carcinogenetic—a substance that may damage the genome or is interfering with cellular metabolic processes leading to the development of tumors in otherwise healthy cells.
- Mutagenic—a substance that alters the DNA of a living being, resulting in mutations that may cause cancer.
- Teratogenic—a substance that is able to disturb the growth and development of an embryo or fetus [7].

The cytotoxins used as warheads in antibody–drug conjugates belong to the most potent drugs used so far. Among others, two classes of natural product-derived compounds proved successful as ADC payload throughout different clinical phases: maytansinoids [8] and auristatins [9] (*see* Fig. 2).

Maytansinoids are based on the structure of the maytansine, originally isolated from maytenus plants. They are inhibiting the assembly of microtubules by binding to tubulin in the cell [10]. Maytansinoids were tested as stand-alone chemotherapeutic agents in different clinical phases but were not approved due to their high

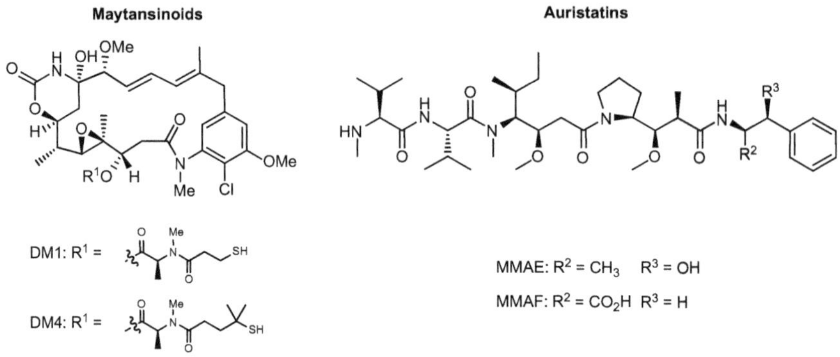

Fig. 2 Structures of the maytansinoids DM1 and DM4 (*left*) and the auristatin derivatives MMAE and MMAF (*right*)

systemic toxicity [8]. In contrast to the attempt to use this class of compounds as classical chemotherapeutic drug, the use of DM1 or DM4 as ADC payloads demonstrated to be successful. The second class of highly potent cytotoxic payloads that proved effective in clinics over the last decade are auristatins, antimitotic drugs that are blocking the polymerization of tubulin. As maytansinoids, auristatin derivatives could not be developed as conventional small molecule drugs due to their high toxicity. When bound to a targeting antibody, e.g., monomethyl auristatin E (MMAE) was successfully tested as ADC payload, with brentuximab vedotin as the pioneering ADC getting approval from the FDA in 2011 [11].

Maytansinoids as well as auristatins are drugs that typically have OELs (occupational exposure limits) in the lower ng/m^3 range, thereby setting the hurdles for ADC manufacturers working with these substances quite high.

4 Occupational Exposure Risks for Co-workers

As mentioned above, the potency of cytotoxic drugs renders them as challenging substances to work with [12]. Even though a drug offers a noteworthy benefit for patients, its handling possesses significant risks for workers if no appropriate manufacturing environment is guaranteed. The main difference between therapeutic benefit and occupational risk is based on the amount of the cytotoxic compound that is used in manufacturing, which is far above the therapeutic dosages used in the clinics with cancer patients. Furthermore, with ADCs the compounds used as payloads are typically not even suitable in their unconjugated form for the use as cancer treatment, based on their high systemic toxicity.

The goal of employers developing and/or manufacturing ADCs is to avoid health effects for their employees or contract workers. Health issues can become apparent either immediately

Table 1
Summary on OEL determination (according to SafeBridge Consultants Inc. [19])

	Category 1	Category 2	Category 3	Category 4
OEL [$\mu g/m^3$]	>500	10–500	0.1–10	<0.1
Toxicity and potency	Low	Moderate	Potent	Highly potent
Typical dosages [mg/kg]	>10	1–10	0.01–1	<0.01
Other characteristics	• Irritant • Low acute or chronic effects	• Moderate to high acute effects • Reversible systemic toxicity	• Mutagens • Carcinogens • Irreversible effects	• Mutagens • Carcinogens • Irreversible effects

while the worker is exposed to questionable substance or in longer terms—weeks, months, or even years after the exposure. Immediate, acute effects of toxic chemicals can include skin, eyes, and mucous membrane irritations, as well as symptoms including nausea, headaches, and dizziness. But particularly risky are those chemicals that have no warning signs such as odor, irritancy, or other rapidly occurring effects, which alert a worker to their presence. The latter might apply to cytotoxic drugs. Cancerogens act of longer duration, rendering an unintended exposure less noticeable for those handling these drugs [13]. But exposure can drastically increase the health risk for employees who work routinely in manufacturing of ADCs, especially if the exposure happens repeatedly.

Therefore, handling strikingly active substances of ADC processes requires a well-defined containment strategy and precisely defined safe handling practices [14].

In order to categorize the toxic potential of chemicals (*see* Table 1), companies have set occupational exposure limits (OELs)—the acceptable amount of a compound allowed in the air of a working area for these drugs as an 8-h time-weighted average. These OELs allow a classification of drugs—the lower the OEL, the greater the potency of the chemical and the more rigorous containment strategy has to be applied for its handling. A four-tier system discussed initially by pharmaceutical companies was evolved over time to form the basis of the SafeBridge system [15, 16]. This system is now well-established and widely accepted among manufacturers of highly potent compounds. SafeBridge's system involves ranking a compound on a scale of 1–4, based on their OELs and mode of action. Category 1, covering low-irritant drugs, with an OEL of 500 $\mu g/m^3$ or higher while Category 2, currently the largest, includes drugs that already exhibit systemic toxicity. Category 3 is the first tier of potent drugs that cause genetic effects, plus organ

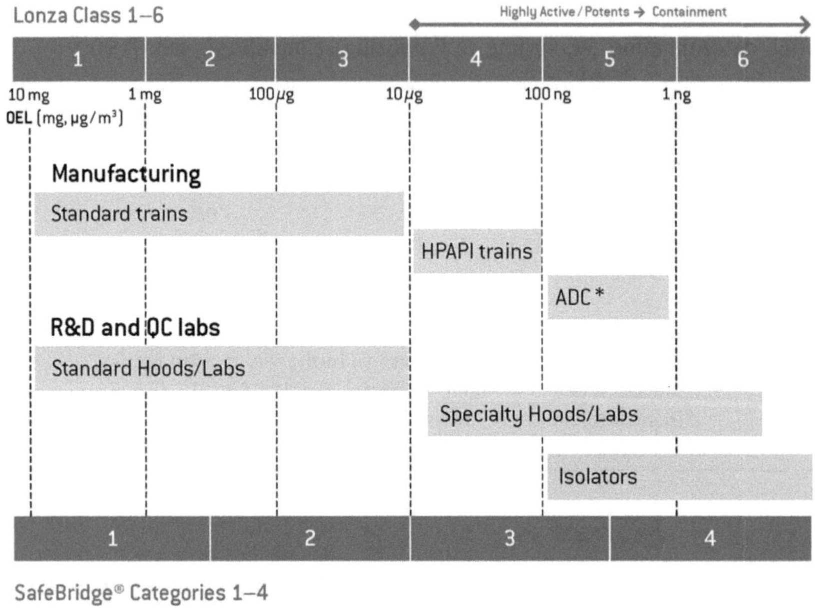

Fig. 3 Lonza classification system compared to SafeBridge categories

toxicity and covers the OEL range between 0.03 and 10 μg/m^3, and finally a tier Category 4 of the most potent compounds limits the exposure to less than 0.03 μg/m^3. In addition, compounds of Category 4 reveal severe acute and/or chronic toxicity.

Some companies have established alternative banding systems. For example, Lonza has defined six classes for compounds, allowing a detailed definition of handling practices based on toxicological properties of the drugs in question (*see* Fig. 3).

For the handling of compounds, some general rules can be considered based on the category. Usually for SafeBridge's Category 1, where the compound has low potency, higher dosage levels and the absorption is slow, it is sufficient to use good lab practices or standard manufacturing practices. In contrast, for the highly potent compounds of Category 4, special procedures are required to handle powders and solutions, access to working areas is restricted and special containment equipment is required to manufacture [3, 14].

5 Risk Mitigation Strategies

5.1 Control of Exposure

In ADC processes, the modification of the antibody typically involves chemicals of the SafeBridge Category 1 or 2 (*see* Chapter 2). In this case, the main focus is clearly on the protection of the process solution from workers. The manufacturing is executed in an aseptic biological manufacturing environment.

The main occupational risk concerns are around the manipulation of the cytotoxic molecules in their solid state as well as solutions thereof. These drugs are typically in SafeBridge Category 4 [17], and the most strict safety precautions have to be taken here. Once conjugated with the antibody, the resulting ADC is still handled under high-containment conditions.

The level of containment is determined by the OELs for the HAPI and the ADC as well as the physical state in which they are handled [18]. Generally, measures to control exposure for Category 3 and 4 materials should be applied in the following order:

- Use totally enclosed systems as the first choice for controlling exposure to carcinogens, unless this is not reasonably practicable.
- Control exposure at source, including, for example, avoiding the generation of dust or aerosols and use of adequate ventilation systems.
- Define appropriate cleaning practices that allow to degrade the cytotoxic compound to nontoxic products or that allow the efficient removal of the active compound.

Furthermore, appropriate organizational measures help reduce the contamination risk:

- Plan work ahead in order to reduce the quantities of drugs used, the number of employees potentially exposed, and their duration of exposure, to the minimum.
- Arrange for the safe handling, storage, and transport of cytotoxic drugs and solutions as well as waste material containing or contaminated by them. Use good hygiene practices as prohibiting eating, drinking, and smoking in areas where drugs are handled and provide washing amenities.
- Train all staff involved in handling cytotoxic drugs or cleaning in the risk, precautions, and accident measures to take.

5.2 Monitoring of the Working Environment

Despite the use of rigorous contained environments, monitoring of the cytotoxic compound level in the working environment is necessary. This can include any periodic test or measurement, which helps to confirm the ongoing effectiveness of the exposure control strategies. On the other hand, accidental spillage of cytotoxic compounds can occur during the manufacturing process, despite all preventive measures taken. For both purposes, analytical methods have to be developed that are able to detect the cytotoxic HAPIs or derivatives thereof in trace amounts. The more potent the compound in question is, the lower the limit of detection and quantification has to be. Monitoring is ideally done by quantifying residual drug amounts in solutions, as swab analysis to detect compounds on surfaces, and through industrial hygiene air monitoring studies.

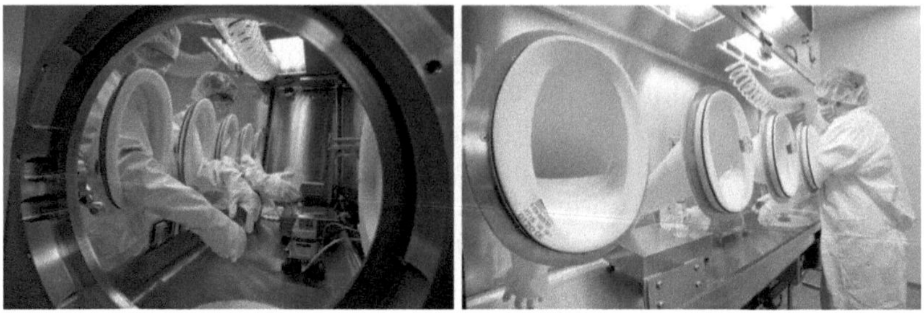

Fig. 4 Isolator in the ADC GMP large scale production plant at Lonza Ltd, Visp, Switzerland

5.3 Personal Protective Equipment

If health and safety risks cannot be properly controlled, personal protective equipment (PPE) has to be used as a good working standard. This also helps mitigating the risk associated with equipment failure or inappropriate handling. The selection of PPE should be based on the performed risk assessment, specific for the properties of the ADC or HAPI in question. It is important to ensure that PPE offers adequate protection for its intended use. Employers need to ensure that employees are trained in the use of PPE and that the equipment is adequately maintained and stored. Effective protection will only be obtained if the PPE chosen is suitable for the task, suited to the wearer and environment, compatible with other PPE in use, in good condition, and worn correctly. The following PPE, among others, are relevant for manufacturers handling ADCs:

Gloves—Where contact with cytotoxic drugs is possible and methods of control other than protective gloves are not reasonably practicable, protective gloves must be provided for employees. The glove material has to be chosen based on the resistance against the cytotoxic drugs and all solvents used in the process.

Eye and face protection—Eye and face protection is relevant, particularly where cytotoxic drugs or drug-containing solutions are being handled outside an enclosed system and there is a risk of splashing or fine powder in the air. A number of options are available including a face shield or visor, goggles, and safety spectacles.

Respiratory protection—The preparation of cytotoxic drug solutions or weighing out of these compounds should be carried out in a suitable safety cabinet or pharmaceutical isolator, avoiding the emission of airborne HAPI powder. At Lonza, cytotoxic drugs in solid form are handled in an isolator at all times (*see* Fig. 4). In ADC processes, this applies to the preparation of stock solutions of these drugs.

Liquids, such as ADC solutions, are handled in Safetech® laminar flow cabinets (*see* Fig. 5). The special design ensures that possible aerosol formation is contained [19]. However, if it is not reasonably practicable to control exposure using enclosure or local

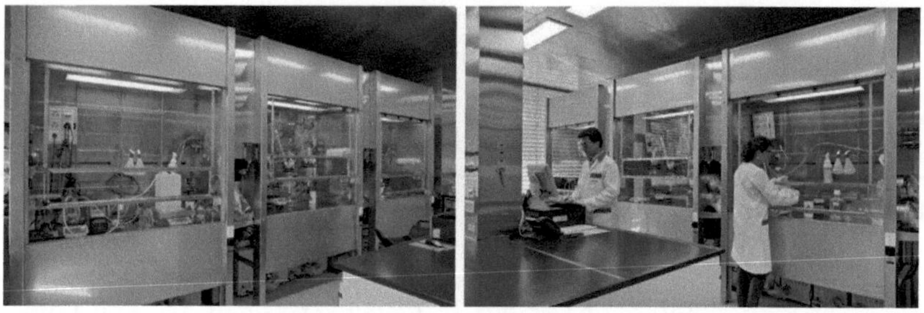

Fig. 5 Safetech laminar flows in the R&D antibody–drug conjugates laboratory at Lonza Ltd, Visp

exhaust ventilation, respiratory protective equipment can be considered to control exposure to powders or aerosols.

Protective clothing—Protective clothing such as gowns, lab coats, or Tyvek® can help prevent contamination of clothes and, subsequently, the skin. The choice of material is important as their absorptive properties may vary.

5.4 Spillages

In case of spillages involving HAPI or ADC derivatives, clear procedures for dealing with such a situation are needed and employees have to be trained accordingly. At Lonza, Visp, the use of spill kits has been established, which must be physically available wherever ADCs or other cytotoxic containing solutions are prepared or being handled. At Lonza, a spill kit contains the following items: Tyvek® overalls, dusk masks, extra arm coverage, shoe covers, gloves, cut-proof gloves, puncture and leak resistant container with absorbent for chemicals, scoop and broom, large plastic disposal bag and cable tie, and waterproof pen and warning tape.

Spillages can be outside of the containment foreseen for the respective ADC or HAPI. Therefore, it is even more crucial to know how to use the proper PPE. Spills should solely be cleaned by staff members that have received the appropriate training. For preventing the contamination of uninvolved and unaware people, spills have to be clearly marked with a warning sign or band. Untrained individuals and any non-staff should vacate the area as soon as it is safe to do so until the spill is cleaned. If feasible, the cleanup should be limited to few people, but there should be at least two people involved as a safety measure.

5.5 Waste Management

The disposal of cytotoxic drug waste and trace contaminated materials (e.g., gloves, gowns, needles, syringes, vials, bottles) presents a possible source of exposure to employees. Bags or containers that are physically robust and also exhibit resistance against chemicals that can be present can be used to collect gloves, gowns, alcohol wipes, and all other potentially contaminated materials. As an example, all waste from R&D or the production plant containing any cytotoxic drug residues as well as liquids up to 25 L which may have traces of these drugs, is collected in color coded polypropylene or polyethylene drums to distinguish them from regular rubbish, labeled with a cytotoxic warning label, and incinerated on site at Lonza Ltd, Visp.

6 Conclusion

ADCs are a class of promising cancer therapeutics that unites the specificity of monoclonal antibodies with the cell-killing properties of cytotoxic drugs. For the manufacturers, ADC processes pose occupational hygiene challenges as the cytotoxins are highly potent. The preparation of stock solutions of the cytotoxin, the conjugation reaction, and following process steps dealing with the ADC are sensitive based on the contamination risk of material and personnel. Strict containment strategies paired with organizational measures allow for the safe manufacturing of these novel therapeutics and finally produce them at commercial scale, for the benefit of the patients.

Acknowledgements

We thank Dr. Jorge Almodovar (Whitaker Post-Doctoral Scholar at Grenoble INP, France) for helpful discussions and inputs regarding the Safe Handling of Cytotoxic Compounds in a Biopharmaceutical Environment.

References

1. Harris CC (1976) The carcinogenicity of anticancer drugs: a hazard in man. Cancer 37:1014–1023
2. Hughes B (2010) Antibody–drug conjugates for cancer: poised to deliver? Nat Rev Drug Discov 9:665–667
3. Axon MW, Farris JP, Mason J (2008) Handling highly potent active pharmaceutical ingredients. Chem Today 26:57–61
4. Thayer AM (2008) Contained chemistry. Synthesizing highly potent compounds is a lucrative and growing niche for custom chemical manufacturers. Chem Eng News 86:17–27
5. Rohrer T (2010) Challenges in the manufacturing of antibody drug conjugates. Innovat Pharmaceut Tech 10–12 http://www.iptonline.com/articles/public/p10-12%20non-print.pdf
6. The State of Queensland (Department of Industrial Relations) (2005) Queensland workplace health and safety strategy: guide for handling cytotoxic drugs and related waste. See http://www.deir.qld.gov.au/workplace/resources/pdfs/cytotoxicdrugs_guide2006.pdf
7. Canadian Association of University Teachers (2011) Cytotoxic drugs fact sheet. 25:1–4 http://cupe.ca/health-andsafety/cytotoxic-drugs
8. Widdison WC, Wilhelm SD, Cavanagh EE, Whiteman KR, Leece BA, Kovtun Y, Goldmacher VS, Xie H, Steeves RM, Lutz RJ, Zhao R, Wang L, Bla WA, Chari RVJ (2006) Semisynthetic maytansine analogues for the targeted treatment of cancer. J Med Chem 49:4392–4408
9. Alley SC, Zhang X, Okeley NM, Anderson M, Law C-L, Senter PT, Benjamin DR (2009) The pharmacologic basis for antibody-auristatin conjugate activity. J Pharmacol Exp Ther 330:932–938
10. Yu T-W, Bai L, Clade D, Hoffmann D, Toelzer S, Trinh KQ, Xu J, Moss SJ et al (2002) The biosynthetic gene cluster of the maytansinoid antitumor agent ansamitocin from

Actinosynnema pretiosum. Proc Natl Acad Sci USA 99:7968–7973

11. Younes A, Yasothan U, Kirkpatrick P (2012) Brentuximab vedotin. Nat Rev Drug Discov 11:19–20
12. Colls BM (1985) Safety of handling cytotoxic agents: a cause for concern by pharmaceutical companies? Br Med J 291:1318–1319
13. Connor TH, McDiarmid MA (2006) Preventing occupational exposures to antineoplastic drugs in health care settings. Cancer J Clin 56:354–365
14. Bormett D (2009) Antibody drug conjugate: a new set of handling and quality control measures. Chem Today 27:23–25
15. Farris JP, Ader AW, Ku RH (2006) History, implementation and evolution of the pharmaceutical hazard categorization and control system. Chem Today 24:5–10
16. Ader AW, Kimmel TA, Sussman RG (2009) Applying health-based risk assessments to worker and product safety for potent pharmaceuticals in contract manufacturing operations. Pharm Outsourcing 10:48–53
17. Watkins KJ (2001) Handle with care—contract pharmaceutical manufacturers find a niche in handling high-potency active ingredients. Chem Eng News 79:31–34
18. Allwood M, Stanley A, Wright P (2002) The cytotoxics handbook, 4th edn. Radcliffe Medical Press, Oxford
19. A1 SafeTech containment strategies, Expositionsschutz durch offene Containments, see http://www.a1-safetech.ch/assets/files/a1safetech_containment_technologies_2012.pdf

Chapter 9

Micro- and Mid-Scale Maleimide-Based Conjugation of Cytotoxic Drugs to Antibody Hinge Region Thiols for Tumor Targeting

James E. Stefano, Michelle Busch, Lihui Hou, Anna Park, and Diego A. Gianolio

Abstract

Currently, the principal chemistries for the preparation of antibody–drug conjugates (ADC) target either lysines or cysteines for coupling cytotoxic drugs for delivery to target cells expressing tumor-specific antigens. All of these chemistries generate populations of molecules which differ in critical properties which are known to affect efficacy, pharmacokinetics, and the therapeutic window. Of key interest are methods to minimize this heterogeneity to achieve reproducible product profiles and efficacy. A current trend in the development of ADC is the evaluation of suitable targets, antibodies, and payloads, occurring well before process development to produce conjugates of clinical quality. This creates a need for an ability to generate comparably high-quality products early in development and at sufficient scale for evaluating in vitro potency and in vivo efficacy, as well as the early identification of any deficiencies in critical quality attributes including solubility and stability. Here we elaborate detailed protocols using maleimide-based chemistry for the conjugation to reduce hinge disulfides in antibodies by several cytotoxic drugs. We present a method for the initial characterization of the reduction/alkylation reaction using polyethylene-glycol (PEG) as a drug surrogate, a 5 mg scale drug conjugation to provide material for initial characterization including cell proliferation assays and a 150 mg scale process for performing efficacy studies in small animals. These methods yield well-defined predictable product profiles at high yield and with low impurities. These procedures include details relevant to the execution of these methods in a safe and contained manner within a typical laboratory environment.

Key words Antibody–drug conjugates, Hinge region disulfides, Maleimide, Reduction, Alkylation, Parallel gel-filtration chromatography, Handling of toxic materials in a laboratory setting, LC-MS analysis

1 Introduction

Conjugation of cytotoxic drugs to antibodies for oncological applications has been accomplished by employing a number of chemistries targeting different functional groups of the protein backbone. Lysine residues and cysteines, generated by the partial reduction of

Laurent Ducry (ed.), *Antibody-Drug Conjugates*, Methods in Molecular Biology, vol. 1045,
DOI 10.1007/978-1-62703-541-5_9, © Springer Science+Business Media, LLC 2013

hinge region disulfides, currently are the most commonly used sites of attachment [1, 2]. One such conjugate, brentuximab vedotin, produced by conjugation of a tubulin inhibitor, monomethyl auristatin E, to an anti-CD30 antibody, has been approved by the US Food and Drug Administration (FDA) in 2011 for use in patients suffering Hodgkin's lymphoma [3, 4]. Because of the multiplicity of both surface lysines (at least 30 per IgG) and hinge disulfides (4 per IgG), such conjugates represent not single entities but a distribution of products which differ with respect to pharmacokinetics, drug loading, and ultimately efficacy [5, 6]. This heterogeneity presents a fundamental challenge in early development in reproducibly obtaining compositional profiles comparable to that of subsequent clinical lots. Although site-directed conjugation to introduced cysteines or unnatural amino acids substantially simplifies this issue, these newer conjugates have not yet been tested in the clinic. Moreover, the site of conjugation has been found to affect in vivo stability, efficacy, and in vitro behavior, and the best sites may depend on the cytotoxic drugs [7–9]. Thus, while perhaps not optimal, ADCs with limited heterogeneity produced by simpler chemistries, for conjugating to targeting antibody candidates, can provide a reasonable platform for evaluating suitable combinations of drug and antibody prior to development or the pursuit of site-specific conjugates.

Many of the cytotoxic drugs used in the context of ADCs are hydrophobic in nature, likely due to a need for efficient escape of the catabolite active drug from the lysosomes after internalization and degradation of the conjugates. The hydrophobicity of the catabolite in the case of cleavable conjugated prodrugs likely plays a significant role in achieving bystander effects which may have bearing on efficacy in some tumor types [10, 11]. This desired property also has an impact on the overall hydrophobicity of the ADC. As a result, the desire to load the antibody with as many drug entities as possible to enhance potency must be balanced against the effect those agents have on the physical properties of the conjugates, significantly affecting the transition toward clinical grade material. Thus, careful control of the processes is essential to obtaining conjugates with both maximum capacity to kill tumor cells and maximum physical stability. Some details of conjugation and purification methods have been published [6] but provide only limited guidance with respect to a strategy for targeting desired average drug/antibody ratio (DAR) values or maintaining a controlled product profile and solubility in a simple manner. This is especially true when lower DAR values are targeted as often appropriate for highly hydrophobic drugs or to limit the abundance of high-DAR species which can have less desirable therapeutic profiles. In the case of conjugation to reduced hinge disulfides, the means to control the process in a manner to minimize the potential for reoxidation and to ensure efficient drug-linker coupling without ultimately resorting to the purification of individual DAR species have not been elaborated. The need to maintain drug-linker solubility during conjugation typically achieved by the use of organic cosolvents also challenges the stability of the protein toward aggregation. Further, specific means to reduce levels of free unconjugated drug have not been disclosed, and the described specifications (typically 0.5 mol%) [12] may not be suitable for the functional characterization of highly cytotoxic agents. In practice, we have found that conditions in the literature [6] using a small excess of drug-linker during conjugations do not ensure complete alkylation by all compounds, leaving product ADCs with significant free thiol contents seen as odd-numbered DAR species by hydrophobic interaction chromatography (HIC) analysis. Increasing the levels of drug-linker to ensure completion of the coupling step challenges the efficiency of subsequent purification steps. Ultimately, the scalability of these processes becomes an important factor in being able to achieve similar profiles at early stages of drug evaluation as well as the scale required for animal studies. Development of a robust process provides additional assurance that both the antibody and loaded drug are compatible and the combination will be appropriate for further development.

A major issue which impacts such efforts is safety. Useful ADC payloads are intrinsically highly toxic but may not be easily inactivated. Passive control by the use of a dedicated laboratory for the process is unlikely to be sufficient to prevent spread of contamination and poses additional burdens and cost of decommissioning or certification of contaminated equipment. The potential exposure of personnel to compounds of uncertain toxicity further poses a legal burden upon the investigating entity to provide a means to actively mitigate risk. Furthermore, personnel involved in product analysis needs to be minimized through steps to reduce the level of free drug which typically shows a nonspecific and higher toxicity profile than the conjugates. The need to maintain an aseptic working environment while maintaining product sterility and low-endotoxin levels adds an additional level of complexity. Providing appropriate means for achieving all of these goals within the context of a scalable process is a significant challenge.

In this chapter we describe detailed procedures for conjugation of maleimide-functionalized drug-linkers to partially reduced antibody hinge region disulfides which is in part based on a published method using tris(2-carboxyethyl)phosphine hydrochloride (TCEP) as reductant [6]. A procedure is provided to pilot reduction conditions using polyethylene-glycol (PEG) as a drug surrogate prior to initiating work with toxic compounds. The conjugation methods subsequently presented in this chapter for both 5 mg pilot and 150 mg preparative scales are performed in a conventional biological safety cabinet (BSC) for the drug coupling and purification steps and yield highly predictable product profiles.

A systematic approach to target a desired product DAR at large scale based on pilot conjugations is delineated. A highly efficient purification process including scavenging of free drug and drug-linker followed by buffer exchange which can be accomplished in a few hours with minimal operator exposure and using fully disposable equipment is described. Both scales yield materials suitable for in vitro cytotoxicity assays and free drug levels routinely below 0.1 mol% with the use of a scavenger and low endotoxin (<0.1 EU/mL). The larger scale provides material for dosing in animal studies.

2 Materials

2.1 Laboratory Supplies and Equipment

1. Conical bottom tube racks, blue (VWR; *see* **Note 1**).
2. Support stand for holding multiple PD-10 columns (*see* **Note 1**).
3. Disposable PD-10 gel-filtration chromatography (GFC) columns (no. 17-0851-01, G.E. Healthcare, Piscataway, NJ).
4. Decapped and autoclaved 5 mL microcentrifuge tubes (no. T2076, Argos Technologies, Elgin, IL), *referred in the text as "Argos 5 mL tubes"*.
5. Column washing reservoir, sanitized with 70 % ethanol (*see* **Note 13**).
6. Hexagonal 7well tube rack for simultaneous stirring of multiple reactions on an electronic stir plate, fashioned from conical bottom tube racks (*for 5 mg scale conjugations—see* **Note 2**).
7. Small animal toenail scissors (no. 1718SS, Integra Miltex, York, PA; *see* **Note 3**), autoclaved.
8. Eppendorf Repeater Plus pipettor (no. 022260201, Eppendorf North America, Hauppauge, NY; *see* **Note 3**).
9. Amicon 30 kDa molecular weight cutoff (MWCO) centrifugal ultrafilters (Ultra 15, no. UFC903024, EMD Millipore Corp., Billerica, MA) or equivalent.
10. Acrodisc 25 mm PF syringe filters, 0.8/0.2 μm Supor membrane (no. 4612, Pall Corporation, Ann Arbor, MI).
11. Steriflip filters, 0.22 μm (no. SE1M179M6, Millipore Corp, Billerica, MA).
12. 5 mM samarium cobalt (SmCo) tumble stir discs (no. VP 779-5, V&P Scientific, San Diego, CA).
13. 13 mm SmCo tumble stir discs (no. VP 779-13, V&P Scientific, San Diego, CA).
14. Endosafe PTS reader (no. PTS100, Charles River Corp., Wilmington, MA), 0.005 EU/mL sensitivity cartridges (no. PTS20005F).

15. Sterile pads (SterileWipe HSII; Cat. no. TX3210, ITW, Kernersville, NC).
16. Lab disc electronic stir plates, three each (no. 3907500, IKA, Wilmington, NC; *see* **Note 3**).
17. Aluminum chilling blocks, 5 × 50 mL (2 ea) (no. 246314, Research Products International, Mount Prospect, IL; *see* **Note 3**).
18. Labquake mixer (Thermo 400110Q; *see* **Note 3**).
19. In-hood dry waste container: 2 gallon (VWR no. 19001-006), discard the lid and line with an 18 × 20 in. reclosable bag (no. S-12319, Uline, Pleasant Prairie, WI; *see* **Note 4**).
20. In-hood sharps disposal container (no. 305543, Becton Dickinson, Franklin Lakes, NJ).
21. UVette disposable plastic cuvettes (no. 952010051, Eppendorf North America, Hauppauge, NY).
22. P200, P500, and P5000 pipettors (Rainin Instrument LLC, Oakland, CA).
23. P5000 filter pipet tips (no. 1050-0810, USA Scientific, Ocala, FL); aseptically loaded into individual 15 mL conical tubes (Falcon no. 352059, BD, Franklin Lakes, NJ), work using aseptic technique over a sterile pad (SterileWipe HSII (*see* above)) to maintain sterility.
24. Combitips Plus, 50 mL, BioPur® (no. 022496140, Eppendorf North America, Hauppauge, NY).
25. CaviWipes (13-1100, Metrex Research Corp., Romulus, MI).
26. Biosafety cabinet (BSC) type I for use with DMSO cosolvent. A type B2 cabinet must be used for volatile toxic cosolvents (e.g., acetonitrile).
27. Chemo Prep Mat, 11 × 19 in., (CST400, Healthcare Safety Systems, Elkhart, IN).
28. Water for injection (WFI).
29. Bio-Rad 10 % polyacrylamide Criterion Stain-Free gels (no. 345-1012, Bio-Rad Laboratories, Hercules, CA).
30. Gel Doc™ System for visualizing Stain-Free gels (such as no. 170-8270, Bio-Rad Laboratories, Hercules, CA, or equivalent) and sample tray (no. 170-8274).
31. Invitrogen NuPAGE 10 % Bis-Tris gels (no. NP0302BOX, Invitrogen Life Technologies, Grand Island, NY).
32. Palm-sized 3.4 × 4 in. aluminized pouch, bottom seal (no. 034MFBOZE04FTN, black) and molecular sieve packets (no. 41MS43, Sorbent Systems, Los Angeles, CA).

33. SpeedVac centrifugal vacuum concentrator (Thermo Savant, Asheville, NC).
34. SDS-PAGE gel scanner with quantitative capabilities. For Stain-Free gels, a Gel Doc™ System (Bio-Rad Laboratories, Hercules, CA) or equivalent. For Coomassie blue-stained gels, an Odyssey Fc (Li-Cor Biotechnology, Lincoln, NE) or equivalent capable of detecting Coomassie infrared fluorescence.
35. TSK Butyl-NPR column (2.5 μm × 4.6 mm × 3.5 cm), Tosoh Bioscience LLC, King of Prussia, PA.
36. TSK G3000SWXL column (7.8 mm ID × 30 cm, Tosoh Bioscience, Tokyo, Japan).

2.2 Reagents

1. Borate buffer: 25 mM sodium borate, 25 mM NaCl, 1 mM diethylenetriaminepentaacetic acid (DTPA) pH 8 (sodium borate titrated with NaOH 0.2 N), prepared in WFI.
2. His/Tween buffer: 20 mM histidine, 0.005 % polysorbate 80 HX2 (NOF Corp., White Plains, NY, USA), pH 6.0 prepared in WFI under aseptic conditions.
3. 0.5 M TCEP (Bond Breaker™, Pierce, Rockford, IL, USA). Store in 100 μL aliquots at −80 °C.
4. 10 % polysorbate 80 HX2 (NOF Corp., White Plains, NY, USA) prepared WFI, sterile filtered, aliquoted, and stored at −80 °C. Referred to as "Tween" in the text.
5. m-dPEG24-MAL (no. 10319, Quanta Biodesign, Powell, OH).
6. Anhydrous dimethylsulfoxide (DMSO) (no. 276855, Sigma). Discard after 6 months of storage at room temperature.
7. 75 % (v/v) DMSO:H_2O (*see* **Note 16**).
8. Maleimide drug-linker. Prepare appropriate-sized single-use powder aliquots for each scale synthesis (e.g., for 6 × 5 mg conjugations, 2.5 μmol; for 150 mg conjugations, 12.5 μmol) in a potent compound facility using an appropriate powder-weighing hood. The disposables described in this procedure were designed to hold 4 mL screw-cap square-bottom vials (e.g., no. C4015-21, National Scientific, Rockwood, TN). Do not exceed 70 % of the vial capacity after dissolution (e.g., 14 μmol at 5 mM). Check to be sure that the pipet tips to be utilized for drug-linker aliquoting will fit into the bottom of the vials. For the vials above, 1,250 μL filter tips (no. 8045, Thermo Scientific, Hudson, NH) are suitable.

9. Falcon 14 mL round-bottom tubes (no. 352059, Becton Dickinson, Franklin Lakes, NJ).
10. PNGase F (N-Glycanase-PLUS®, 10 mU/μL, no. GKE-5010, ProZyme Corporation, Hayward, CA, USA).

3 Methods

3.1 Pilot Conjugations Using Maleimide PEG as a Drug Surrogate

This procedure has proved useful to pilot conditions prior to the introduction of toxins into the process. This method confirms the stability of the antibody toward reduction/alkylation with a non-hydrophobic alkylating agent (discrete-length maleimide PEG) and an initial evaluation of the efficiency of the reduction step which can identify reagent issues or competing thiol reoxidation during conjugation. This is more suitable than 5,5′-dithiobis(2-nitrobenzoic acid) (DTNB) analysis of free thiols since the latter requires a desalting step prior to reaction since DTNB is also susceptible to reduction by any residual unreacted TCEP. Quantitative SDS-PAGE provides data very comparable to LC-MS analysis in a fraction of the time.

1. Buffer exchange the antibody into borate buffer by centrifugal ultrafiltration using 30 kDa MWCO centrifugal ultrafilters and concentrate the final product to obtain no less than 5 mg/mL by A_{280}. Degas briefly in a centrifugal vacuum concentrator (e.g., SpeedVac) or by filtration using a 0.22 μm filter and holding under vacuum for 1–2 min with swirling. Adjust the concentration to 5 mg/mL and prepare 100 μL (0.5 mg) aliquots in 1 mL screw-cap vials.
2. Add an appropriate volume of 1 mM aq. TCEP solution (1:500 dilution) assuming 2 mole thiol generated per mole TCEP and mix gently by tapping. Preferably cover with argon or nitrogen. Incubate for 2 h, first in a water bath to bring to temperature and then in a 37 °C incubator for the remainder of the time. Remove the reactions and allow cooling to room temperature.
3. Prepare a 41.3 mg/mL (33 mM) aq. solution of MAL-mPEG24 (MW = 1,239), assuming a partial specific volume of 1 mL/g for the PEG (i.e., 23.2 μL H_2O per mg PEG). Add 10 μL to each reaction and incubate overnight at room temperature or preferably in a 25 °C incubator.
4. Run aliquots on 10 % Bio-Rad Criterion Stain-Free Tris–HCl gels (4 μg per lane) for direct visualization or Invitrogen 4–12 % Bis-Tris gels (1 μg per lane) for visualization by Coomassie IR

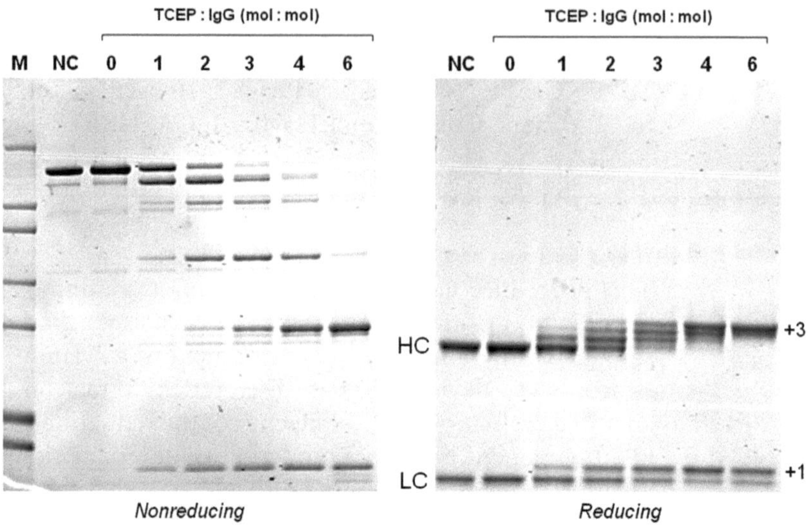

Fig. 1 Partial reduction of an IgG1 with TCEP and alkylation with MAL-dPEG24. Antibody (100 μg IgG in 20 μL borate buffer pH 8) was treated with increasing molar ratios of TCEP for 2 h at 37 °C. Intermediates were immediately alkylated, without further purification, by addition of a tenfold excess MAL-dPEG24. Aliquots (1 μg) were resolved by SDS-PAGE 4–12 % Bis-Tris gels, stained for 5 min with Coomassie blue, and imaged on an Odyssey IR imager. *Left*: nonreduced samples. Fragments represent products of partial reduction/alkylation of interchain disulfides. *Right*: Samples reduced for 10 min at 70 °C with reducing reagent. Note that bands corresponding to up to 3 PEG chains per antibody heavy chain and 1 PEG per light chain are observed without side products, suggesting the process results in conjugation to only the interchain disulfides (NC: negative control—untreated mAb)

fluorescence. For best resolution, perform this step with the gel boxes cooled on ice.

5. For Stain-Free gels, visualize using the appropriate instrumentation (*see* Equipment, Subheading 2.1). For visualizing gels with Coomassie blue, stain and visualize on infrared (IR) fluorescence scanner as described [13]. *See* Fig. 1 for a profile of one analysis obtained with an Odyssey IR scanner. For typical IgG1, there should be maximally one PEGylated product for the light chain and three PEGylated products for the heavy chain. Band assignments made using the ladder pattern produced by intermediate TCEP:IgG ratios gave DAR values identical to LC-MS.

6. Using instrument integration methods provided, determine areas under the peaks, splitting at the peak minima. Calculate PEG/antibody ratio (PAR) by multiplying the percentage area of each peak in the heavy chains by its assigned PEG number and again separately for the light chains and multiplying the sum of those values by two. Figure 2 shows the PAR values obtained by reducing SDS-PAGE and LC-MS. The initial thiol titer was also determined by DTNB assay of the desalted intermediate.

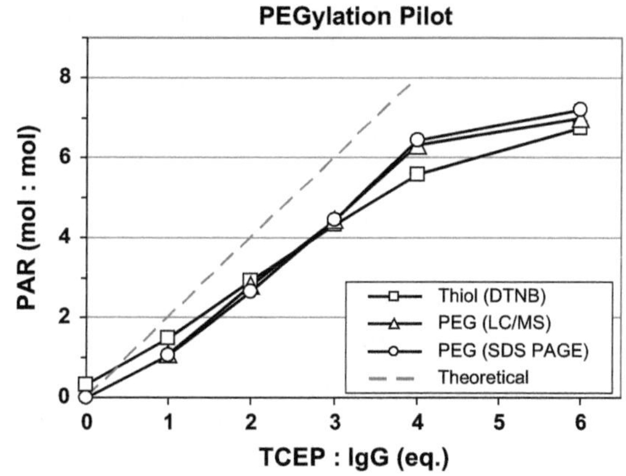

Fig. 2 MAL-dPEG24 as surrogate for drug-linker and to determine conjugatable thiols after reduction. Note the nonzero initial DTNB value and shallower slope, suggesting some nonspecific thiol-like component in the IgG as well as reoxidation of the antibody during the desalting step and prior to reaction with DTNB. A slight lag in the PEG conjugation at low TCEP ratios suggesting the possibility of a slower rate of reduction near TCEP exhaustion is not consistently observed

3.2 ADC Preparation at Pilot (5 mg) Scale

3.2.1 Introduction

The methodology below is based on the preparation of six conjugates (i.e., two antibodies at three TCEP ratios each). We suggest performing these procedures during 2 consecutive days.

Day 1

1. Buffer exchange the antibody into borate buffer by centrifugal ultrafiltration using 30 kDa MWCO centrifugal ultrafilters and concentrate the final product to obtain no less than 5 mg/mL by A_{280}. Weigh to determine the volume, adjust to 5 mg/mL based on $\varepsilon_{280} = 1.37$ mL/mg cm, and store at 4–8 °C. Check endotoxin of a 1:5 dilution.
2. Prepare His/Tween buffer. Check endotoxin level (1:5 dilution in water) prior to use.
3. Assemble column support rack flow-through tube assembly (*see* **Note 1**). The caps are left on the Argos 5 mL tubes in the collection tube rack which are used for storing the conjugates.
4. Assemble a hexagonal reaction tube rack (hex-rack) with tubes (*see* **Note 2**). As described, this rack places the tubes on a Lab Disc electronic stir plate in appropriate positions which permit the simultaneous stirring of up to seven reactions using samarium cobalt (SmCo) magnetic tumble stir discs (*see* **Note 2**). Label the inside and outside of the lids of Argos 5 mL tubes so they will be readable while open and introduce a 5 mm SmCo stir disc to each. Set in a hex-rack (*see* **Note 2**) with the caps open, wrap in aluminum foil, and autoclave. Close the caps after autoclaving.

5. Prepare a column eluate collection rack. Label the caps on 6 Argos 5 mL tubes inside and out (*see* **step 4**), place in a VWR 15 mL conical tube rack in the positions corresponding to where the columns will be placed, wrap in aluminum foil, and autoclave. Close the caps after autoclaving.
6. Prepare the PD-10 GFC columns. One column will be used for each reaction. Provide an additional column as a backup. If low endotoxin is desired, follow this procedure beginning from **step a** below; otherwise proceed to **step e**.
   (a) Spray outside of seven PD-10 columns with 70 % ethanol, transfer to a BSC, uncap, and drain the shipping buffer. Cut the outlet using sterilized small animal toenail clippers and load the columns into the autoclaved column support rack at the same position as the eluate tubes. Align the tops so that the outlets are within the collection tubes without touching their rims and the column bodies are 1–2 mm above the lip of the tubes (Fig. 6). Place the rack into the wash collection reservoir.
   (b) Wash with 25 mL 0.2 N NaOH in 5 mL aliquots applied with a 50 mL Combitip (5.0 mL exactly fills the headspace to the lip of the columns). Cover with a 150 mm sterile culture dish and shroud with the autoclaved foil. Let stand 2 h at room temperature or at 4 °C overnight.
   (c) After incubation, transfer the columns to the wash collection reservoir and wash with another 25 mL 0.2 N NaOH in 5 mL aliquots as before.
   (d) Equilibrate columns with 25 mL His/Tween buffer pH 6 in five 5 mL aliquots. Check the pH, using litmus paper, of the last drop of buffer drawn off with a pipette.
   (e) Store columns in the BSC if using the same day or at 4 °C covered with a culture plate lid and shroud in aluminum foil if to be used the following day.

Day 2

7. Degas the antibody by filtration through a 0.22 μm Steriflip filter and swirl under vacuum for 1 min.
8. Remove and discard the filter membrane assembly. Aliquot the degassed product with reverse pipetting into the autoclaved Argos 5 mL reaction tubes with 5 mm stir discs in the hex-rack. Center on a VWR Lab Disc stirrer at room temperature preset to a speed pre-calibrated to provide efficient but stable stirring.
9. Add 50 mM aq. TCEP solution (1:10 dilution Pierce Bond Breaker) with continuous stirring. Continue stirring for 1 min after the last addition to achieve a uniform solution. The

TCEP:IgG ratios can be adjusted based on PEG titration to center the expected DAR values (twice the TCEP:IgG ratios) around the desired value (typically DAR 4 for thiol-based conjugates).

10. Overlay with N_2 or argon and incubate for 2 h in a 37 °C incubator.
11. Prepare ice-cold 75 % v/v DMSO/water by adding 1.75 mL WFI to 4.5 mL DMSO and chill on ice.
12. Prepare two 1 mL aliquots of dry DMSO for dissolving drug-linker (one for reserve). Keep at room temperature.
13. Chill the TCEP-reduced IgG reactions on wet ice.
14. Prepare a 5 mM drug-linker solution in dry DMSO (*see* **Note 5**).
    (a) Obtain a pre-weighed aliquot (2.5 μmol) of drug-linker powder in a 4 mL vial, preferably in a secondary foil-lined pouch with a drying agent packet, aliquoted in a certified potent compound facility (*see* **Note 5**). Warm the pouch to room temperature on an absorbent pad in the BSC designated for conjugation work.
    (b) Place a disposable vial stand (*see* **Note 6**) on the Chemi prep pad. Remove the vial of drug-linker from its secondary container, tap it down gently to displace powder adhering to the cap, open, and place in the stand. Change gloves and discard into a dry waste container in the hood lined with a reclosable polyethylene bag.
    (c) Dissolve the reagent with dry DMSO to achieve a 5 mM solution, running the solvent around the inner rim of the vial to dissolve all traces of powder. Discard the tip, recap the vial, and swirl until a solution is attained. Avoid inverting the vial and contaminating the cap and threads with liquid (*see also* **Note 7**). Place the vial back on the stand and change gloves and sleeves, discarding in a dry waste container in the hood.
15. Retrieve the chilled IgG solutions in the hex-rack and center over a Lab Disc stir plate in the hood and turn the stir plate on. Adjust the speed if necessary to minimize disc tumbling (*see* **Note 8**).
16. Slowly add 0.167 v/v ice cold 75 % v/v DMSO with continuous stirring. Continue stirring for 1 min to ensure a uniform solution.
17. Add 12 eq. of 5 mM drug-linker in DMSO steadily while stirring, to each reaction (caution—*see* **Note 9**). Discard the tips into the sharps waste container in the hood (*see* **Note 7b**).

18. Overlay the solutions with N_2 or argon and recap. Recap the drug-linker reagent vial and change gloves.
19. Center the reaction rack and tubes on a Lab Disc at 4 °C and stir for 1 h.
20. (Optional). Store the unused portion of drug-linker at −20 °C (*see* **Note 10**).
21. Together, collect the drug-linker vial, the support, and the underlayment pad and place in the dry waste container in the hood. Seal and discard.
22. In some cases, the level of unconjugated hydrophobic drug-linkers in the final product will need to be reduced further (scavenging) by selective binding to a hydrophobic support (*see* **Note 26**) either in suspension [14] or in column format. A cosolvent may also be necessary during this step to suppress antibody binding, but conditions need to be determined empirically. In the event scavenging is required, a suspension format provides a significant safety factor.
23. Transfer the reactions to Argos 5 mL tubes containing pre-washed scavenger resin and 5 mm SmCo stir discs using a P1000 and 1,250 μL filter tip. Cap and place the rack on the Lab Disc stir plate in the hood and stir for 2 h. Set the speed such that the resin reaches a height of at least 70 % of the solution (*see* **Note 11**). The final scavenged product may need to be filtered prior to GFC in the case of a fine resin or if fines are generated in the process, as they may be carried over into the GFC eluate (*see* **Note 12**).
24. Prepare the GFC setup. Unwrap the racked PD-10 column and flow-through tube rack and the collection rack-and-tube assembly and place in the hood. Discard the 150 mm dish covering the columns.
25. Pipet 1 mL of each reaction mixture and scavenged supernatant or filtrate onto a PD-10 column using a P1000 and a 1,250 μL filter tip. Run in, collecting the flow-through. Apply 2 mL His/Tween buffer to all columns with a 50 mL Combitip and run in. Lift the column and collection tube racks together and tap down gently to dislodge any drops hanging from the column outlets. Transfer the columns to the eluate rack and tubes. Apply 3 mL His/Tween buffer to each column and collect. Lift and tap down the racks as before and place the column rack back on the flow-through tube rack before proceeding.
26. Cap and store the pooled eluates at 4 °C. Verify conjugation and obtain preliminary DAR via HIC or UV spectrum in the case of a chromophore in the drug-linker with a λ_{max} other than 280 nm. Determine the concentration by A_{280} (*see* **Note 14**).
27. Aspirate the flow-through fractions and traces of uncollected eluate into toxic waste (*see* **Note 21**). Discard the columns

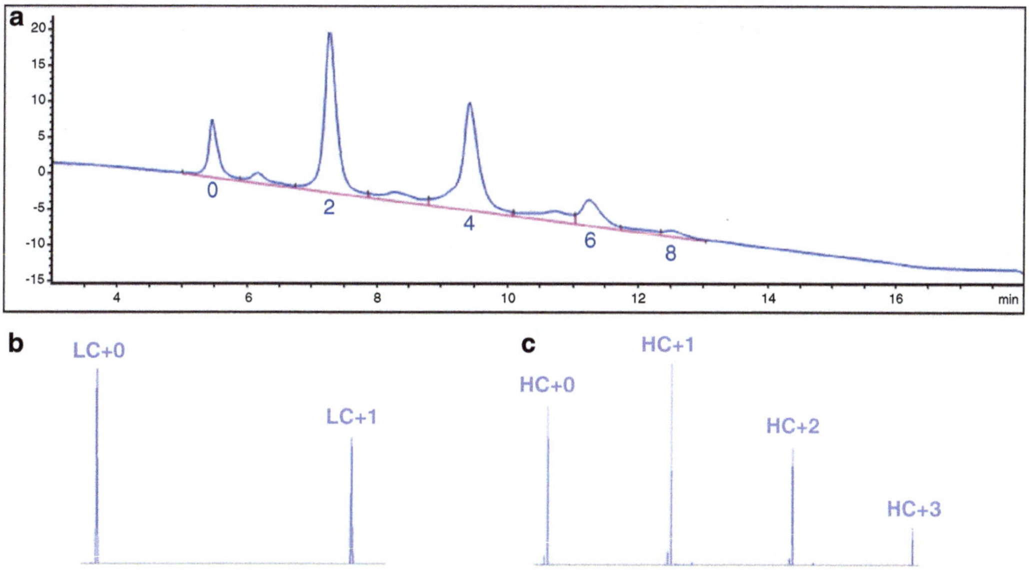

Fig. 3 (**a**) HIC profile obtained for one specific TCEP ratio (1.9 mol:mol TCEP:IgG) conjugation procedure. (**b**) Deconvoluted light-chain LC-MS and (**c**) deconvoluted heavy-chain LC-MS

and their support rack (leaving the columns in place), the flow-through and collection tube racks and tubes, and underlayments into the contaminated dry waste container in the hood. Wipe the hood carefully with CaviWipes, and collect into dry waste in the hood. Seal and transfer the dry waste container liner and transfer to a secondary container in the laboratory for disposal.

28. Determine DAR by HIC and/or LC-MS as described below. Figure 3 shows a typical HIC profile for a conjugation performed at 1.9 mol:mol TCEP:IgG. Figure 4 shows a plot of DAR values versus TCEP:IgG ratio obtained by HIC and LC-MS for the conjugation of two antibodies and two drugs (performed on two occasions) using this procedure. The slope of DAR versus TCEP ratio extrapolated to a zero intercept provides an estimate of the combined efficiency of the combination of reduction and alkylation steps. As shown for two antibodies and two drug-linkers (Table 1), this conjugation efficiency (DAR/(2 × TCEP:IgG ratio)) was around 90 % using DAR values obtained by LC-MS. This suggests that under conditions of excess drug-linker used here, the TCEP: IgG ratio is the principal factor in determining drug loading and that exposed free thiols are largely coupled to drug. This is consistent with the low level of odd-numbered DAR species observed by HIC (Fig. 5b, c).
29. Verify that free drug level is < 0.1 % by LC-MS. Specific conditions and procedures will vary with each drug.

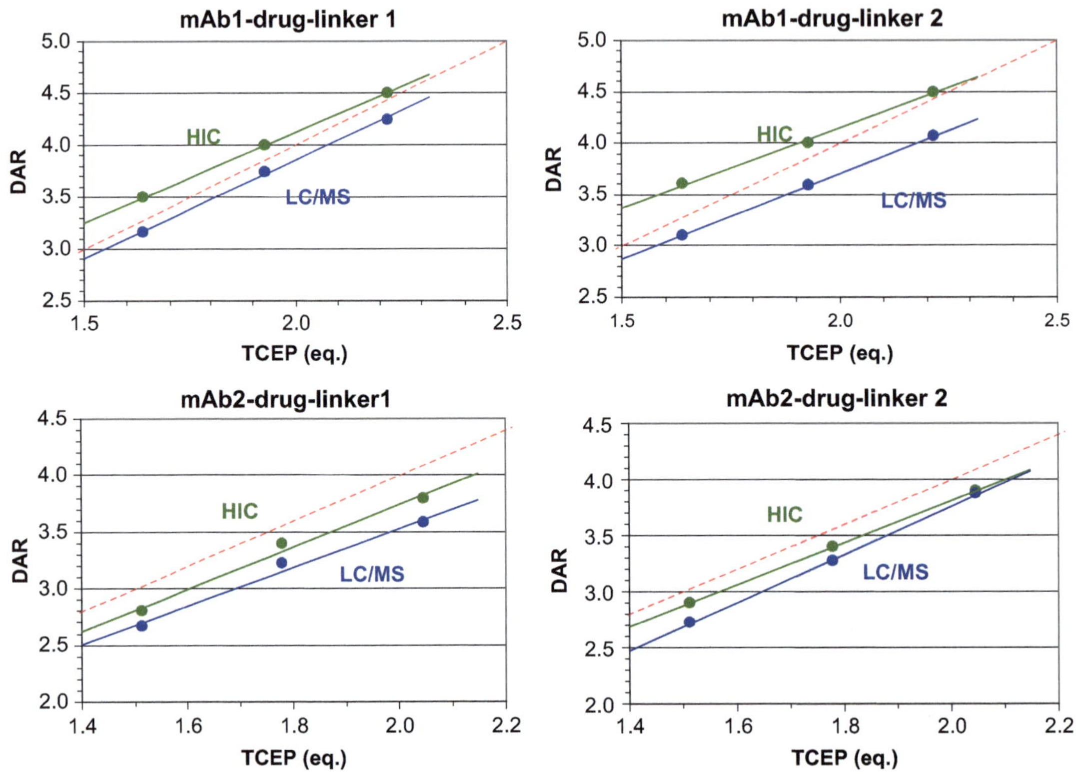

Fig. 4 DAR determined by HIC and LC-MS from pilot-scale conjugations. In some cases, DAR values by HIC exceeded theoretically achievable values (*red dotted line*), possibly reflecting a difference between the actual and theoretical (1.37 mL/mg cm) extinction coefficients. The results of such pilot conjugations are used to establish the proper TCEP ratio for synthesis at larger scale(s)

Table 1
Conjugation efficiency based on DAR values obtained by LC-MS for the experiments described under Subheading 3.2

Conjugation efficiency		
	Drug-linker 1	Drug-linker 2
mAb 1	96 ± 1 %	93 ± 1 %
mAb 2	89 ± 2 %	92 ± 2 %

Two different monoclonal antibodies and two maleimide-functionalized drug-linkers were used. The conjugation efficiency is calculated by the equation Eff (%) = DAR/2 × TCEP (mol : mol IgG) × 100

30. Test selected conjugates for toxicity against appropriate antigen-expressing and non-expressing cell lines. A lack of toxicity against a non-expressing cell line is reasonable evidence of a lack of free drug and/or drug-linker, although cell lines differ in their sensitivity to these compounds.

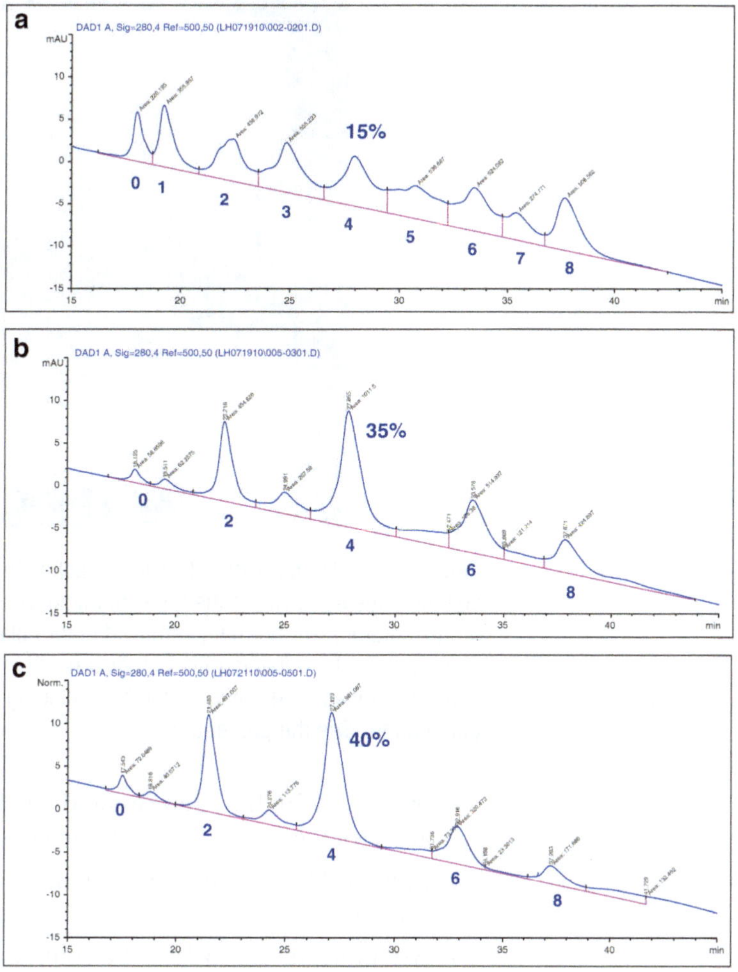

	a	b	c
exp. scale	180 mg	5 mg	135 mg
TCEP	3.7 eq	2.8 eq	2.8 eq
drug-linker	6 eq	12.0 eq.	12.0 eq.

Fig. 5 HIC profiles of conjugations performed at (**a**) TCEP excess, (**b**) drug-linker excess, and (**c**) drug-linker excess. The final DAR values were 4.0, 4.0, and 3.9, respectively

3.3 ADC Preparation at 150 mg Scale

The following protocol is similar to the small-scale protocol but with additional steps for reaction temperature control.

3.3.1 Introduction

Day 1

1. Buffer exchange the antibody into borate buffer by centrifugal ultrafiltration using 30 kDa MWCO centrifugal ultrafilters and concentrate the final product to obtain no less than 5 mg/mL

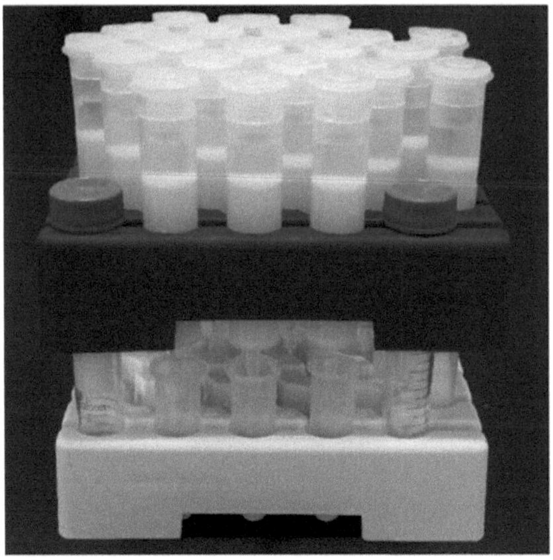

Fig. 6 Assembled parallel GFC column rack with columns in place. Note that the column outlets are within the tubes to minimize potential static effects. The caps on the columns are normally removed before placing in the rack (not as shown). The upper rack containing the columns nests in the bottom rack containing the collection tubes. The entire assembly including columns is discarded following purification. *See* the procedure

by A_{280}. Weigh to determine the volume, adjust to 5 mg/mL, and store at 4–8 °C. Check the endotoxin of a 1:5 dilution.

2. Prepare His/Tween buffer. Check endotoxin (1:5 dilution in water).
3. Assemble and autoclave the column support and flow-through and collection racks as described previously, except filling each of the 21 available wells with decapped 5 mL tubes. Sterilize three 13 mm SmCo tumble stir discs by autoclaving in round-bottom 14 mL Falcon tubes with the caps replaced with 3 in. squares of aluminum foil. Autoclave a pair of small animal toenail scissors.
4. Assemble and sanitize PD-10 columns as described above. Each column will accommodate 2 mL of the scavenged reaction mixture. Provide one additional column as a backup (21 columns for 150 mg scale). Clean, drain, and load the columns in the rack as described above (*see* Fig. 6). Align the column tops using a 150 mm tissue culture dish as a guide (*see* also **step 6(b)** in the small-scale protocol above). Transfer the rack onto a wash collection reservoir and sanitize and equilibrate with His/Tween buffer as described in the 5 mg scale procedure. Store columns in the BSC during NaOH treatment covered with a culture plate lid if to be used the same day or covered and shrouded in aluminum foil at 4 °C if to be used the following day.

5. Calibrate the Lab Disc stirrers at 4 °C and in the BSC using another aluminum block and tube with 35 mL water. It is useful to check the proper suspension of an equivalent amount of Bio-Beads to be used in the procedure (*see* **step 23**).

Day 2

6. Degas the antibody by filtration as described above.
7. Remove the filter assembly; add an autoclaved 13 mm stir disc, cap, and place on a stand over a Lab Disc stirrer which has been preset to a speed providing efficient stable stirring.
8. Slowly add an appropriate amount of 50 mM aq. TCEP solution (1:10 dilution) based on the 5 mg scale titration experiment with continuous stirring. Continue stirring for 1 min after addition to ensure a uniform solution.
9. Overlay with N_2 or argon and cap. Bring the solution to 37 °C in a water bath and incubate for 2 h.
10. Prepare 75 % v/v DMSO/water by adding 1.75 mL WFI to 4.5 mL DMSO and chill on ice.
11. Prepare two 3 mL aliquots of dry DMSO for dissolving drug-linker. Place in the hood and keep at room temperature.
12. Chill the TCEP-reduced IgG solution in the center well of an ice-cold 5 × 50 mL aluminum block (Research Products International) with 1.8 mL water as a heat conductor in the well and place on a Lab Disc stirrer at 4 °C (*see* **Note 15**). Stir for 20 min to bring the solution temperature to <10 °C.
13. While chilling the reduced antibody, prepare a 5 mM drug-linker solution in dry DMSO. Use the precautions outlined in the small-scale protocol (*see* **Notes 5–7**).
    (a) Obtain a pre-weighed aliquot (≥12.5 μmol) of drug-linker powder in a 4 mL vial in a pouch with drying agent packet. Warm to room temperature on a pad in the dedicated BSC.
    (b) Remove the vial from its secondary container, tap it down, open, and place in a disposable vial stand over an absorbent pad (*see* **Note 6**). Change gloves.
    (c) Slowly pipet the appropriate amount of DMSO to obtain a 5 mM solution using a P5000 filter tip and run the solvent around the inside rim of the vial. Recap the vial and swirl (do not invert) until a solution is attained (*see* **Note 7a**). Change gloves.
14. Retrieve the chilled IgG and block, place it on a Lab Disc in the hood, and turn it on at a preset calibrated speed.

15. Add 0.167 volumes ice-cold 75 % v/v DMSO to the IgG in four to five aliquots (e.g., 5 mL in 1 mL aliquots for 30 mL IgG) over a period of 1–2 min allowing for a uniform solution to be attained after each addition. Eppendorf Repeater Plus or motorized repeat pipettors are appropriate. After the last addition, continue stirring for an additional min to draw some of the heat of solution into the block.
16. Add 12 eq. of 5 mM drug-linker in four to six equal aliquots at about 30 s intervals with continuous stirring (e.g., for 150 mg IgG, add 2.4 mL 5 mM drug-linker in six 0.4 mL aliquots). An Eppendorf Combitip may be used for this operation (*see* **Notes 9** and **18**). Recap the vial and change gloves.
17. Overlay the solution with N_2 or argon and cap. Place the reaction block on the Lab Disc at 4 °C for 1 h (*see* **Notes 15** and **17**).
18. (Optional). The unused portion of the drug-linker solution, if significant, can be stored frozen in a secondary container (pouch) with a molecular sieve packet at −20 °C (*see* **Note 10**).
19. Collect the vial support and underpads and discard the dry waste container in the hood.
20. If the reaction product is cloudy, filter the reaction through a Steriflip filter prior to the GFC step. If using a scavenger resin, collect the filter eluate directly onto a bed of washed scavenger in a 50 mL tube (*see* **Note 20**) containing a 13 mm SmCo stir disc. Cap, reweigh to estimate filter recovery, and place the tube on a stand over the Lab Disc stirrer in the BSC and stir for the period required to achieve the desired final free drug limit based on pilot experiments. The resin should rise to at least 70 % of the solution height to ensure efficient scavenging. The stir rate should be predetermined using a practice tube containing buffer and resin only.
21. Unwrap the PD-10 column support and flow-through tube assembly and the collection tube rack-and-tube assemblies and place in the hood. Discard the 150 mm dish covering the columns.
22. Add 2 mL of the filtrate or resin supernatant onto each column using a P5000 pipettor and a 5 mL filter tip. Run in, collecting the flow-through. Then apply 1 mL His/Tween buffer to all columns using a 50 mL Combitip and run in. Lift the column rack and collection tube rack together and tap down gently to dislodge any drops hanging from the column outlets. Transfer the column rack onto the eluate tube rack. Apply 3 mL His/Tween buffer to each column and collect the

eluates. Lift and tap down the rack to dislodge drops and set aside on the flow-through tube rack before proceeding.

23. Collect and pool the eluates using a P5000 and filter tip into a pre-tared 100 mL sterile polycarbonate bottle. Caution: Inserting a P5000 pipet tip to the bottom of the 5 mL tubes will displace and cause loss of a portion of the eluate as well as a contamination event. Draw the solution while lowering the tip and perform this step over a waterproof absorbent pad. Sterile filter the product (e.g., two Steriflip filtration steps). Weigh (*see* **Note 19**) and store the pooled eluate at 4 °C until conjugation is confirmed by HIC or UV spectrum. Determine the concentration by A_{280} (*see* **Note 14**).
24. Aspirate the flow-through fractions and any residual eluate into a toxic liquid waste container in the hood (*see* **Note 21**). Discard the columns and support and both the flow-through and collection tube racks and tubes into the lined dry waste container in the hood. Wipe the hood using CaviWipes. Pull up the reclosable polyethylene bag dry waste container liner, seal, and transfer to contaminated dry waste for disposal.
25. Upon confirmation of conjugation and endotoxin check, aliquot and store the product at −80 °C.

Figure 5 shows the comparison by HIC analysis of conjugations performed under conditions similar to a published procedure [6] with a 3.7-fold molar excess of TCEP and a sixfold excess of drug-linker over mAb (0.8-fold over expected free thiol assuming 100 % efficiency of reduction) (a) or 12-fold molar drug-linker excess over mAb (2.1-fold over expected thiol assuming 100 % efficiency) as used here at 5 mg (b) or 135 mg (c) scale. The drug-linker excess as described here results in mostly even-numbered DAR species lacking free thiols, tighter product profiles, and minimum unconjugated mAb.

3.4 HIC Determination of Drug/Antibody Ratio (DAR)

The procedure is a modification of a published HIC test method [9].

1. Prepare mobile phases: A: 1.5 M ammonium sulfate in 50 mM potassium phosphate pH 7 and B: 20 % isopropanol, 80 % 50 mM potassium phosphate pH 7.0. Mount a TSK gel Butyl-NPR column (2.5 μm, 4.6 mm × 3.5 cm, Tosoh Bioscience) on an HPLC preferably equipped with a diode-array UV detector (DAD, e.g., Agilent 1200) and equilibrate with mobile phase A.
2. Dilute samples to obtain 15–30 μg in 75 μL of 50 mM potassium phosphate pH 7 with sufficient $(NH_4)_2SO_4$ for efficient capture, which may vary with antibody and conjugated drug. It is useful to test a series to establish the optimum $(NH_4)_2SO_4$

concentration for highest absorbance recovery and minimum variation in the average DAR. For most but not all conjugates, a 1:1 mixture with mobile phase B is suitable.

3. Inject 50 μL sample at 0 % B at a flow rate of 1 mL/min at room temperature and hold at 0 % B for 1 min, followed by a gradient of 0–100 % B over 14 min (1 mL/min), holding at 100 % mobile phase B for 2 min, followed by a gradient of 100–0 % B over 1 min before re-equilibrating with 0 % B for 2 min. Follow the absorbance at 280 nm (reference wavelength 500 nm). For drug-linkers with chromophores, their peak wavelength absorbance may be monitored to provide relative peak DAR values [5]. Integrate the A_{280} profiles using manual baselines and splitting at inter-peak minima. The baseline absorbance will typically decline with increasing % B, and baseline subtraction using a suitable blank run checked for reproducibility may be used. The fraction of area under the curve for each peak is multiplied by its assigned DAR and the values summed to obtain the overall DAR. Note that not all drugs are sufficiently hydrophobic to be separated and permit DAR determination by this method. In that case, LC-MS should be used to establish DAR values (Subheading 3.6).

3.5 SE-HPLC Analysis for Aggregation

1. Set up a TSK gel G3000SWXL analytical column (7.8 mm ID × 30 cm, Tosoh Bioscience) with matching guard column on a HPLC (e.g., Agilent 1200) preferably equipped with a diode-array detector (DAD).
2. Equilibrate the column with 0.22 μm filtered 40 mM sodium phosphate and 150 mM sodium chloride pH 7, freshly prepared for each analysis at a flow rate of 0.5 mL/min at room temperature.
3. Inject samples ($\geq$ 50 μg each) in triplicate and follow the UV absorbance at 280 nm for 35 min. Perform a needle wash after each injection and include blank runs between each analyte.
4. Confirm acceptable mass recovery by area under the curve against an unmodified antibody control. Column interactions which occur with some drug-linkers may be controlled by use of cosolvents or buffer excipients [15–17].

3.6 LC-MS Determination of DAR

1. Deglycosylate the sample using 1 μL PNGase F per 100 μg mAb overnight at 37 °C (*see* **Note 22**).
2. Dialyze for 2 h into 25 mM Tris-pH 8.5 in a Mini Slide-A-Lyzer (20 kDa MWCO, no. 69590, Pierce, Rockford, IL) (*see* **Note 23**).
3. Reduce immediately prior to analysis with 20 mM dithiothreitol (DTT) and incubation for 30 min at 37 °C (*see* **Note 24**).

4. Carry out analysis by high-resolution electrospray ionization mass spectroscopy using an initial capture on a C8 reversed-phase column (*see* **Note 25**).
5. Deconvolute the averaged spectrum for all eluted species over a mass range of 10–75 kDa to cover both light and heavy chains which contain m/z from 800 to 2,500 Da.
6. From the deconvoluted spectrum, identify the free and conjugated (mono, di, tri, etc.) species for both the light and heavy chains, where the mass difference between each peak is the mass of the conjugated drug-linker. Separately for heavy and light chain, integrate the peak areas and obtain a weighted peak ratio per chain based on the number of drugs conjugated from the assignments. For example, the peak area of the mono-conjugated light chain plus twice the di-conjugated light-chain peak area is divided by the total peak area of all light-chain species (including the unconjugated) to give the weighted peak ratio for the light chain.
7. Calculate the average DAR by doubling the sum of the light- and heavy-chain weighted peak ratios.

4 Notes

1. The blue conical tube racks for preparing the multicolumn support rack are available through VWR (US no. 89079-526). Drill out all of the wells with a 41/64 in. drill bit (e.g., no. 8870-A55, McMaster-Carr, Robbinsville, NJ) using a drill press at 500 rpm, a feed rate <2 mm/min, and a mineral oil as cutting fluid. Do not increase the feed rate beyond the point of generating ribbons to avoid either shattering or overheating the piece and melting the plastic. The racks should be held down such as with a clear plate during machining to avoid the piece from jumping and gouging the plastic. Machine shops can also be contracted for their fabrication using vertical mills. Debur the racks using mosquito hemostats and machine wash prior to assembling the column support rack. An assembled rack with columns is shown (Fig. 6).
2. To produce the small hexagonal racks for stirring multiple 5 mg conjugation reactions on a Lab Disc stir plate, cut away all but one corner of a VWR conical tube rack (US no. 89079-526) (7 wells total). This can be performed on a radial arm saw with a plastic cutting blade. It is useful to drill the bottom of the center well to also allow visual alignment with the center cross-hairs on the stir plate. Consult a machine shop.

3. The small animal toenail scissors are also available from VWR (US catalog no. 95039-206). The Lab Disc electronic stir plate is also available from VWR (US catalog no. 97056-526). The 50 mL tube aluminum chilling blocks are also available from Fisher (US catalog no. 427901621517421). Labquake tumble stirrers are also available from VWR (US catalog no. 56264-302).
4. Place the liner bag into the container and turn the top half of the bag inside out and pull down around the outside of the container to cover the sides and block any contamination of the container surface. After use, pull the top half of the bag up over the container, turning inside out and zip seal prior to disposal.
5. All of the compounds should be treated as highly toxic. The drug-linkers, although less potent than the free drugs, still pose health risks, especially in conjunction with the use of DMSO which can mediate transport through the skin. Preparation of the drug-linker solution should be performed in a BSC over adsorbent pads using disposable sleeves and double-gloving. Pre-aliquoting of the powder into glass vials within a potent compound facility minimizes the risk of personnel exposure as well as degradation of the maleimide function through exposure to humidity. Compounds in glass vials stored in small metalized foil pouches with molecular sieve packets appear to be stable for many months at −20 °C. These pouches are commercially available (Sorbent Systems, Los Angeles, CA). In choosing the vials for powder aliquots, check to be sure that pipet tips to be used can reach to the corner of the vial bottoms without occluding the orifice and potentially producing aerosols upon solvent addition. The dissolved volume should not exceed 2/3 of the vial capacity.
6. Single-use stands for 4 mL drug-linker vials can be fashioned from sawed 1 in. sections of plastic 25 mL pipets solvent welded with dichloromethane to squares (2 ×2 in.) of 1/16 in. thick acrylic sheet. These provide an unimpeded view of the vial contents and a stable support during the procedure. This is particularly important when working over uneven surfaces typical of most absorbent pads which pose a risk of an unsupported vial tipping over. Dispose of the stands after each use in the contaminated dry waste container in the BSC.
7. *Caution*: (a) Particulate aerosols generated by vigorous addition of DMSO or by brushing of any external powder contamination on the vial during tapping will contaminate the underlayment pad at a position directly beneath the point of handling. If the procedure is performed forward of the centerline in the BSC, contamination will be carried toward the front plenum toward the operator. This was observed by release of fluorescent tracer particles at working height near the

centerline of a standard A1 BSC. Treat the area in front of and behind the working area as a contaminated zone and carefully replace the pad after setting up the conjugation. Decontaminate any exposed metal in this area using CaviWipes immediately after this step and dispose in the solid waste container in the BSC. (b) Tips ejected at a shallow angle into Becton Dickinson swinging-lid sharps containers (which can accommodate aspiration pipets) can ricochet off the rear of the lid and contaminate the hood workspace. Half of the back side of the lids may be cut away before use to prevent this occurrence while retaining the ability to lock the lids closed. Consult a machine shop.

8. Some tumbling of the discs is normal. Setting the stirring speed is best done prior to undertaking the procedures. (VWR Lab Disc stirrers remember the last setting used prior to being turned off).
9. *Caution*: DMSO freezes at about 18 °C. If the addition is too slow, the drug-linker solution will form a frozen plug in the pipet tip. If this occurs, remove the tip from the solution and hold it over the reaction tube until the plug melts (can be up to 1 min).
10. (Optional). The unused portion of the drug-linker solution in DMSO may be returned to the foil pouch secondary container with a molecular sieve packet and stored at −20 °C. Reagents stored in this manner have produced high-quality conjugates after months of storage when used at a several-fold molar excess such as described here. Gloves that have come in contact with the vial should be removed prior to touching the external surfaces of any secondary container or other laboratory surfaces. Ensure that the vial and pouch are supported in a vertical position during freezing to avoid liquid contaminating the cap and external threads.
11. Avoid excessive tumbling of the stir disc during scavenging to prevent fragmentation of the resin. Note that any liquid which splatters on the side of the tubes will not be scavenged and can contaminate the final product and lower the overall efficiency of this process. (Note that the level of free drug after scavenging the conjugate shown in Fig. 6 would correspond to contamination of the final product (30 mL) with only 10 μL of the starting material).
12. If resin fines are generated, the scavenged product slurry may require filtration prior to GFC. This is best performed using an Acrodisc filter with a 0.8 μm prefilter element. Assemble the filters and 5 mL syringes before undertaking this step. On Becton Dickinson syringes, clip the side fins off the plunger assembly using straight-blade toenail scissors (available at any drugstore). This allows easy removal of the plunger and

recovery of remaining slurry in case the filter fouls with the resin, stopping the flow. Pipet the slurry onto the bottom of the syringe barrel-filter assembly, insert the plunger, and drive the solution through using gentle pressure. Do not disassemble the syringe/filter assembly prior to disposal. An appropriate stand to hold the syringes should be fashioned if multiple reactions are filtered.

13. A column washing reservoir can be fashioned from a 150 cm^2 T-flask with the top panel cut with a jigsaw and removed. A section of a 1 mL pipet can be held in place with a rubber stopper to aspirate the liquid. Collect the aspirate into a large side-arm vacuum flask for disposal.

14. A_{280} determination is most safely performed using disposable cuvettes. High-quality UV-transparent cuvettes are available (e.g., Eppendorf UVette) which give accurate UV absorbance values and can be discarded after each use. Read UVettes in the 2 mm path orientation which avoids the need for sample dilution. The use of pedestal-type instruments (e.g., NanoDrop®) should be avoided to minimize the possible spread of toxin in the laboratory. In estimating an average DAR value by spectroscopy, the absorbance of the linker at 280 nm needs to be accounted for [5].

15. The aluminum reaction blocks in the large-scale process may be used for multiple conjugations but can become contaminated, which is not easy to monitor. The block can be kept in a reclosable bag which should be changed after each step where its contamination could occur (such as drug-linker addition). Preferably, the block is stored at 4 °C to facilitate chilling on ice prior to use. Chilling on ice should be performed with the block in the bag.

16. Pre-dilution of DMSO to 75 % (v/v) with water eliminates 50 % of the heat of further dilution and lowers the melting point sufficiently to allow chilling of this reagent to 0 °C, thus minimizing the generation of heat and deleterious effects on the mAb upon addition.

17. The initial block temperature will be about 13 °C and will subsequently drop and stabilize between 9 and 11 °C. The block temperature can be conveniently monitored by a self-adhesive LCD thermometer attached to the block.

18. This procedure was qualified for the use of DMSO as the cosolvent. With the use of more volatile cosolvents or those with low surface tension such as acetonitrile, standard pipet tips introduce a major risk of contamination by dripping. This can be avoided by the use of positive displacement devices such as Combitips. Any air should first be displaced by repeated withdrawal and expulsion of liquid prior to dispensing. Larger

quantities of drug-linker also need to be provided to allow for the dead volume of such devices (the equivalent of two aliquots with a Combitip).

19. A small inexpensive electronic scale of reasonable accuracy (0.1 g) available commercially can be kept in the BSC (away from air flow) and used to determine recovered volumes by weight. If contamination is suspected, it can be discarded.
20. To perform this step in the large-scale procedure, aseptically replace the Steriflip collection tube with the conical tube containing the resin. To ensure sterility, this step can be performed over a sterile pad. Invert the filter and tube assembly containing the scavenged product and resin (which will result in dropping of the resin onto the back of the filter) and screw it onto the top of the uncapped reaction vessel. Attach a vacuum line, invert the assembly, and filter the reaction product onto the resin bed. Tap the assembly down gently; set in a stand with the vacuum line attached and wait an additional min for the last remaining drops to drain. Tap down the assembly again to dislodge any hanging drops. Unscrew the upper tube with filter and discard into contaminated solid waste in the hood.
21. Aspiration of flow-through fractions and uncollected eluates can be performed using a 2 mL tissue culture aspiration pipet and a disposable 250 mL filtration bottle (Corning) with the filter assembly replaced by a one-hole stopper kept in the hood. After each procedure, the pipet is discarded in the sharps container in the hood and the line plugged with a narrow polypropylene tube. Turn off the vacuum and exchange the bottle out, keeping the top, and dispose in accordance with local regulations as toxic liquid waste. Means to support the bottle during aspiration is critical. A polypropylene beaker adhered to the hood surface with double-stick mounting foam tape can be used.
22. Deglycosylation eliminates the mass complexity arising from the heterogeneity of the native heavy-chain glycans.
23. Omit dialysis for more hydrophobic drug-linkers, as it can result in selective loss of higher DAR species and skew the average DAR. Usually, salt concentrations in storage buffers typically used for ADC have little or no effect on the results. Avoid the use of phosphate-containing buffers.
24. Reduction is necessary due to the intrinsically denaturing conditions of mass spectrometry. Without reduction, multiple species are observed, including heavy-heavy, heavy-heavy-light, and heavy-light chains that otherwise highly complicate subsequent analysis.
25. The column is best maintained at an elevated temperature to improve antibody recovery [18, 19].

26. Examples of such resins include LH10 (G.E. Healthcare), Octyl-Sepharose (G.E. Healthcare), or Bio-Beads (Bio-Rad Laboratories) [14]. The suitability for this application must be determined empirically due to differences in drug-linker hydrophobicity.

References

1. Carter PJ, Senter PD (2008) Antibody-drug conjugates for cancer therapy. Cancer J 14:154–169
2. Senter PD (2009) Potent antibody drug conjugates for cancer therapy. Curr Opin Chem Biol 13:235–244
3. Younes A, Yasothan U, Kirkpatrick P (2012) Brentuximab vedotin. Nat Rev Drug Discov 11:19–20
4. Gualberto A (2012) Brentuximab Vedotin (SGN-35), an antibody-drug conjugate for the treatment of CD30-positive malignancies. Expert Opin Investig Drugs 21:205–216
5. Hamblett KJ, Senter PD, Chace DF, Sun MM, Lenox J, Cerveny CG, Kissler KM, Bernhardt SX, Kopcha AK, Zabinski RF, Meyer DL, Francisco JA (2004) Effects of drug loading on the antitumor activity of a monoclonal antibody drug conjugate. Clin Cancer Res 10:7063–7070
6. Sun MM, Beam KS, Cerveny CG, Hamblett KJ, Blackmore RS, Torgov MY, Handley FG, Ihle NC, Senter PD, Alley SC (2005) Reduction-alkylation strategies for the modification of specific monoclonal antibody disulfides. Bioconjug Chem 16:1282–1290
7. Shen BQ, Xu K, Liu L, Raab H, Bhakta S, Kenrick M, Parsons-Reponte KL, Tien J, Yu SF, Mai E, Li D, Tibbitts J, Baudys J, Saad OM, Scales SJ, McDonald PJ, Hass PE, Eigenbrot C, Nguyen T, Solis WA, Fuji RN, Flagella KM, Patel D, Spencer SD, Khawli LA, Ebens A, Wong WL, Vandlen R, Kaur S, Sliwkowski MX, Scheller RH, Polakis P, Junutula JR (2012) Conjugation site modulates the in vivo stability and therapeutic activity of antibody-drug conjugates. Nat Biotechnol 30:184–189
8. Junutula JR, Flagella KM, Graham RA, Parsons KL, Ha E, Raab H, Bhakta S, Nguyen T, Dugger DL, Li G, Mai E, Lewis Phillips GD, Hiraragi H, Fuji RN, Tibbitts J, Vandlen R, Spencer SD, Scheller RH, Polakis P, Sliwkowski MX (2010) Engineered thio-trastuzumab-DM1 conjugate with an improved therapeutic index to target human epidermal growth factor receptor 2-positive breast cancer. Clin Cancer Res 16:4769–4778
9. Junutula JR, Raab H, Clark S, Bhakta S, Leipold DD, Weir S, Chen Y, Simpson M, Tsai SP, Dennis MS, Lu Y, Meng YG, Ng C, Yang J, Lee CC, Duenas E, Gorrell J, Katta V, Kim A, McDorman K, Flagella K, Venook R, Ross S, Spencer SD, Lee Wong W, Lowman HB, Vandlen R, Sliwkowski MX, Scheller RH, Polakis P, Mallet W (2008) Site-specific conjugation of a cytotoxic drug to an antibody improves the therapeutic index. Nat Biotechnol 26:925–932
10. Kovtun YV, Audette CA, Ye Y, Xie H, Ruberti MF, Phinney SJ, Leece BA, Chittenden T, Blattler WA, Goldmacher VS (2006) Antibody-drug conjugates designed to eradicate tumors with homogeneous and heterogeneous expression of the target antigen. Cancer Res 66:3214–3221
11. Okeley NM, Miyamoto JB, Zhang X, Sanderson RJ, Benjamin DR, Sievers EL, Senter PD, Alley SC (2010) Intracellular activation of SGN-35, a potent anti-CD30 antibody-drug conjugate. Clin Cancer Res 16:888–897
12. Pollack VA, Alvarez E, Tse KF, Torgov MY, Xie S, Shenoy SG, MacDougall JR, Arrol S, Zhong H, Gerwien RW, Hahne WF, Senter PD, Jeffers ME, Lichenstein HS, LaRochelle WJ (2007) Treatment parameters modulating regression of human melanoma xenografts by an antibody-drug conjugate (CR011-vcMMAE) targeting GPNMB. Cancer Chemother Pharmacol 60:423–435
13. Luo S, Wehr NB, Levine RL (2006) Quantitation of protein on gels and blots by infrared fluorescence of Coomassie blue and Fast Green. Anal Biochem 350:233–238
14. Spack EG Jr, Packard B, Wier ML, Edidin M (1986) Hydrophobic adsorption chromatography to reduce nonspecific staining by rhodamine-labeled antibodies. Anal Biochem 158:233–237
15. Ejima D, Yumioka R, Arakawa T, Tsumoto K (2005) Arginine as an effective additive in gel permeation chromatography. J Chromatogr A 1094:49–55
16. Ricker RD, Sandoval LA (1996) Fast, reproducible size-exclusion chromatography of biological macromolecules. J Chromatogr A 743:43–50
17. Yumioka R, Sato H, Tomizawa H, Yamasaki Y, Ejima D (2010) Mobile phase containing

arginine provides more reliable SEC condition for aggregation analysis. J Pharm Sci 99:618–620

18. Rehder DS, Dillon TM, Pipes GD, Bondarenko PV (2006) Reversed-phase liquid chromatography/mass spectrometry analysis of reduced monoclonal antibodies in pharmaceutics. J Chromatogr A 1102:164–175
19. Dillon TM, Bondarenko PV, Rehder DS, Pipes GD, Kleemann GR, Ricci MS (2006) Optimization of a reversed-phase high-performance liquid chromatography/mass spectrometry method for characterizing recombinant antibody heterogeneity and stability. J Chromatogr A 1120:112–120

Chapter 10

Protocols for Lysine Conjugation

Marie-Priscille Brun and Laurence Gauzy-Lazo

Abstract

Currently, the most widely used chemical methodology for the conjugation of drugs to monoclonal antibodies involves either lysine or cysteine residues. In this chapter, several methods for the preparation of antibody–drug conjugates (ADCs) through conjugation of drugs to solvent-exposed ε-amino groups of lysine residues are described. These methods apply to various cytotoxic agents, both tubulin binders and DNA-targeting agents and different types of linkers, cleavable or not, peptidic or disulfide-based, for example.

Key words Lysine conjugation, One- and two-step conjugation, Activated ester, Iminothiolane, Maleimido cross-linker, Iodoacetamido cross-linker, Disulfide cross-linker

1 Introduction

Lysine residues exposed at the surface of antibodies (mAbs) are used as sites for drug conjugation as their side-chain amino groups are good nucleophiles. An immunoglobulin (IgG) contains approximately 80–100 lysine residues and most of them are sufficiently exposed or accessible to be reactive.

The main chemistry used for lysine conjugation involves a simple reaction, namely, the formation of a stable amide bond using activated esters of the drug to be conjugated, usually *O*-succinimide reagents like *N*-hydroxysuccinimidyl (NHS) or sulfo-NHS esters. Another approach takes advantage of imido ester compounds like Traut's reagent [1] to form stable amidine bonds which are protonated at physiological pH, thus retaining the native charge of the mAb [2]. Independently of the synthetic strategy, the large number of potential conjugation sites compared to the usually small drug-to-antibody ratio (DAR) results in a stochastic reaction and a heterogeneous product displaying a statistical distribution of loading, sometimes referred to as the "random shotgun loading" of lysine conjugation [3].

Laurent Ducry (ed.), *Antibody-Drug Conjugates*, Methods in Molecular Biology, vol. 1045,
DOI 10.1007/978-1-62703-541-5_10, © Springer Science+Business Media, LLC 2013

Furthermore, it is worth mentioning the possibility to exploit iso(thio)cyanate chemistry that allows the formation of a stable (thio)urea linkage. This methodology has been widely used to fluorescently label antibodies using, for example, fluorescein isothiocyanate [4]. So far, no application to ADC preparation has been disclosed, but such an approach was applied to conjugate camptothecin or doxorubicin to an amine-reactive biopolymer [5] and to prepare radiolabeled antibodies [6].

More recently, site-specific lysine conjugation based on azetidinone chemistry has been described for a particular IgG framework that contains a very reactive lysine on the heavy chain, thus offering two potential sites of conjugation. This lysine displays an unusually low p*K*a around 6 instead of 10–11 that enables the smooth opening of a β-lactam moiety to form a β-alanine peptide bond [7]. So far, no application to ADC preparation has been disclosed, but some detailed procedures have been described for peptide conjugation [8].

2 Materials

All solutions are prepared using analytical grade reagents and ultrapure water, prepared by purifying deionized water to attain a resistivity of 18 MΩ.cm at 25 °C. Antibody and ADC solutions are stored at +4 °C. Ideally drug solutions should be freshly prepared, but if the drug is stable in the organic cosolvent used for conjugation, it can be stored at −20 °C. Drug and ADC solutions have to be carefully handled as they contain highly active cytotoxic compounds. Favor the use of disposable materials, decontaminate the glassware using a drug-destroying solution prior to washing and dispose of waste materials in a septobox to prevent any potential contamination.

1. Pellicon® 3 cassettes and Millex® membranes (Millipore).
2. Sephacryl® S200, Sephadex® G25, SP Sepharose® High Performance, and Superdex® 200 resins (GE Healthcare).
3. Buffer 1: Examples of pH 8 buffers are 50 mM potassium phosphate with or without 50 mM sodium chloride (NaCl), 50 mM 4-(2-hydroxyethyl)-1-piperazineethanesulfonic acid (HEPES) also with or without 50 mM NaCl, or a solution of 50 mM potassium phosphate, 50 mM NaCl, and HEPES 1 N. 2 mM ethylenediaminetetraacetic acid (EDTA) may be added to the buffer.
4. Buffer 2: 10 mM histidine, 130 mM glycine, 5 % w/v sucrose, pH 5.5.
5. Buffer 3: 10 mM phosphate, 140 mM NaCl, pH 6.5.
6. Buffer 4: 10 mM sodium citrate, 135 mM NaCl, pH 5.5.

7. Buffer 5: 50 mM sodium phosphate, 100 mM NaCl, 60 mM sodium caprylate, pH 7.8.
8. Buffer 6: 50 mM phosphate, 100 mM NaCl, pH 7.4.
9. Buffer 7: 50 mM potassium phosphate, 50 mM NaCl, 2 mM EDTA, pH 6.5.
10. Buffer 8: 100 mM HEPES, pH 8.
11. Buffer 9: 50 mM potassium phosphate, 50 mM NaCl, 2 mM EDTA, at a pH between 6.5 and 8.5.
12. Buffer 10: 10 mM phosphate, 140 mM NaCl, pH 6.5 or 7.
13. Buffer 11: 100 mM sodium phosphate, 50 mM NaCl, 2 mM diethylenetriaminepentaacetic acid (DPTA), pH 8.
14. Buffer 12: 50 mM HEPES, 5 mM glycine, 2 mM DPTA, pH 5.5.
15. Buffer 13: 50 mM HEPES, 5 mM glycine, 230 mM NaCl, pH 5.5.
16. Buffer 14: 10 mg/mL glycine, 30 mg/mL sucrose, pH 6.

3 Methods

Conjugating a drug, most often a cytotoxic agent, to an antibody is like combining two different worlds: most highly potent cytotoxic drugs are quite hydrophobic whereas the antibody is hydrophilic. Therefore, the use of an organic cosolvent is often required to increase the poor aqueous solubility of the drug while maintaining both species in solution to perform the covalent linkage. The conjugation of an antibody with a cytotoxic drug can be carried out by either a one- or a two-step process. In the later process, there is an additional modification step of the antibody with a heterobifunctional reagent prior to the addition of the drug. Whatever the process, the final product needs to be purified to remove excess reactants, organic cosolvent, other process additives, as well as reaction by-products. Classical protein purification methods may be used independently or subsequently such as membrane filtration, gel filtration using a desalting resin, size-exclusion chromatography (SEC) to remove aggregates, dialysis in the formulation buffer, or tangential flow filtration (TFF) using a membrane with relevant molecular weight cut-off. In some cases of purification by chromatography, an additional buffer-exchange step may be required to formulate the ADC in the appropriate buffer. Finally, regardless of the conjugation process, determination of the DAR is done by an adequate measurement depending on the drug that has been attached to the antibody. Various techniques may be used, for example, UV-visible, hydrophobic interaction chromatography (HIC) or liquid chromatography coupled to mass spectroscopy (LC-MS), as described in Chapters 16–18.

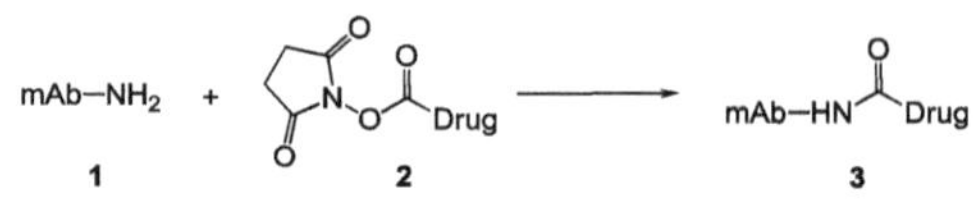

Fig. 1 One-step conjugation

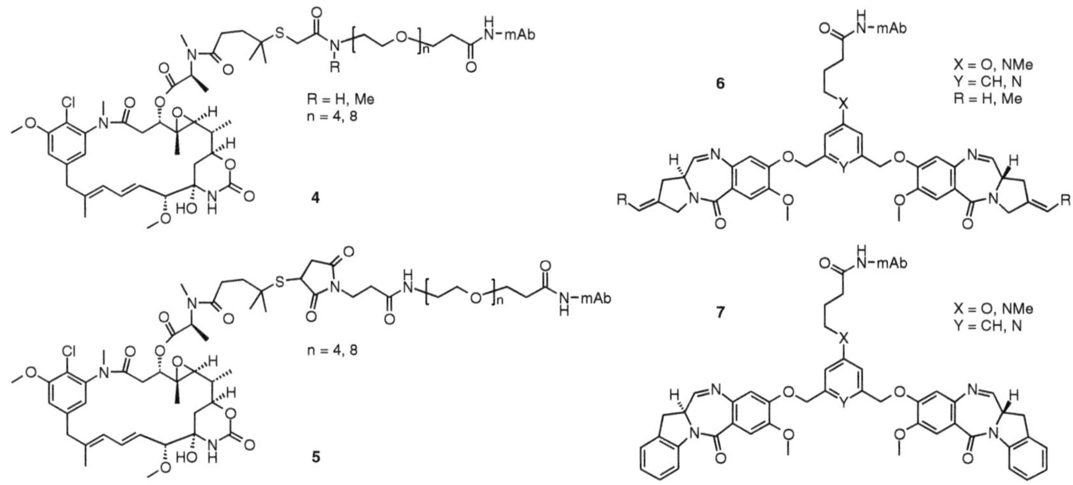

Fig. 2 Structures of some non-cleavable conjugates

3.1 One-Step Conjugation

The one-step conjugation approach consists of directly generating amide bonds by reacting lysine ε-amino groups of the antibody **1** and a drug **2** bearing an amine-reactive group (Fig. 1). NHS esters are often used, but other activated esters can be explored like hydroxybenzotriazole and fluoro- or nitro-phenyl derivatives [9, 10].

This type of conjugation has been widely used for introducing non-cleavable linkers with different cytotoxic agents (Fig. 2), e.g., maytansine derivatives **4** and **5** [11, 12], tomaymycin/pyrrolobenzodiazepine (PBD) dimers **6**, and indolino-benzodiazepine (IBD) dimers **7** [13–15].

The protocols that have been used for these cytotoxic compounds are very similar and a general procedure is described herein:

1. Prepare a solution of the *O*-succinimide-containing cytotoxic drug in *N*,*N*-dimethylacetamide (DMA) at a concentration of approximately 10 mM.
2. The antibody solution is diluted in a pH 8 buffer (buffer 1) and DMA, then treated with a 5- to 20-fold molar excess (depending on the expected DAR and the reactivity of the drug) of the drug solution so that the final concentration of the antibody is around 2.5–5 mg/mL and the final content of DMA does not exceed 20 %. The DMA and drug solution are slowly added to the antibody solution under magnetic stirring.

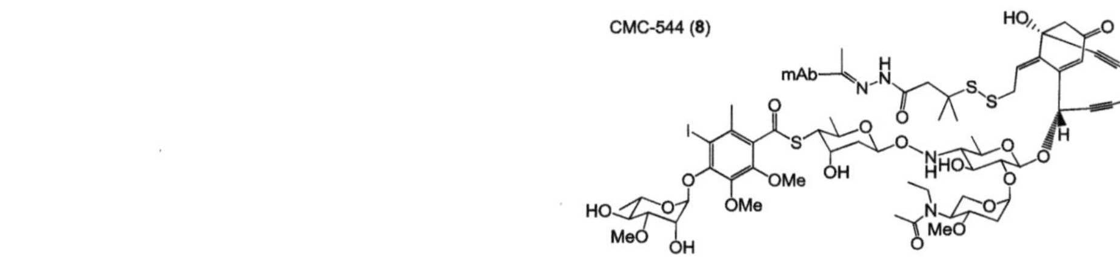

Fig. 3 Inotuzumab ozogamicin, a calicheamicin ADC

3. The solution is stirred for 2–4 h at room temperature. If the expected DAR is not reached, one may add an extra amount of the drug solution and the reaction is continued for two additional hours (*see* **Note 1**).
4. Remove excess of reactant and reaction by-products, and if necessary, exchange the purification buffer to the formulation buffer of the ADC. Some examples are presented hereafter:

   For instance, the maytansinoid conjugates have been purified by TFF on Pellicon® 3 cassettes and diafiltrated against ten sample volumes of buffer 2 or by gel filtration on a Sephadex® G25 desalting resin followed by dialysis in the formulation buffer.

   For PBD conjugates **6**, after clarification on 0.45 or 5 μm membrane, the crude conjugation media was purified by SEC on a Superdex® 200 prep grade column using buffer 3. The monomeric conjugated antibody-containing fractions were pooled and concentrated by centrifugation on a 10 or 50 kDa membrane.

   For IBD conjugates **7**, purification was carried out by gel filtration on a Sephadex® G25 desalting resin followed by dialysis using buffer 4.

A one-step approach may also be used for the preparation of ADCs bearing cleavable linkers, such as for the conjugation of calicheamicin derivatives to provide, for example, inotuzumab ozogamicin or CMC-544 (Fig. 3) [16–18].

A prerequisite for this kind of conjugation is that the drug-linker construct has to be generated prior to conjugation. The available amine-reactive group is again an activated ester, and the following alternative protocol has been used in this particular case:

1. Prepare a solution of the cytotoxic drug in dimethylformamide (DMF) or propylene glycol.
2. Dissolve the mAb in buffer 5.
3. Under stirring, slowly add a 4- to 6-fold molar excess of the drug solution, so that the final mAb concentration is 5 mg/mL, the final drug concentration is 1 mg/mL, and the final content of organic cosolvent is 15 % for DMF or 30 % for propylene glycol.

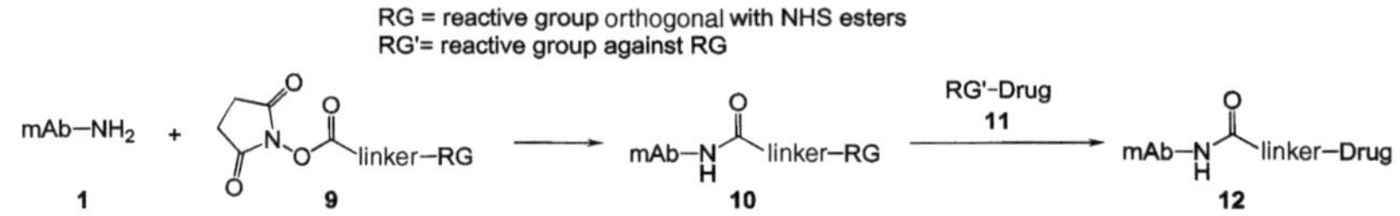

Fig. 4 Two-step conjugation

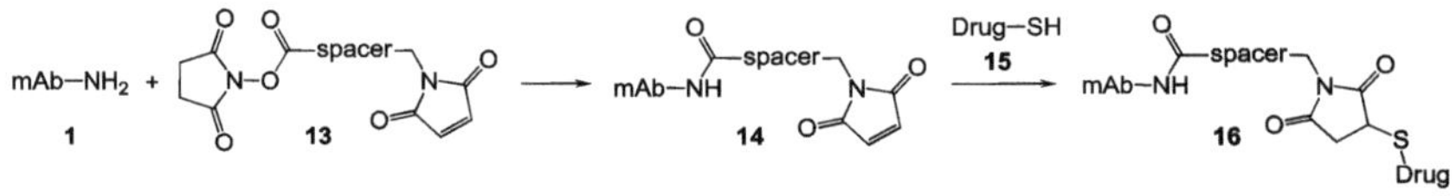

Fig. 5 Maleimido-based conjugation

4. React for 3 h at room temperature.
5. After filtration over a Millex® membrane, purify the crude medium by SEC on Sephacryl® S200 using buffer 6.

3.2 Two-Step Conjugation Using O-Succinimide Reagents

This type of conjugation first proceeds with the modification of the lysine residues of antibody **1** to introduce chemical functionalities that are able to subsequently react with specific reactive groups present on the drug **11** (Fig. 4). The antibody-linker intermediate **10** resulting from this first step is usually called "modified antibody."

Methods will be described with *O*-succinimide reagents for the introduction of maleimido, iodoacetamido, or pyridyldisulfide moieties. The modified antibody may be characterized in terms of an available reactive group in order to calculate the appropriate quantity of drug required for the second step.

Whatever the chemical functionality introduced during the modification step, the conjugation of the drug to the modified antibody is rather similar, since the reactive group carried by the drug is always a sulfhydryl moiety. Each modification step will be described separately and subsequently the conjugation to the drug as a general protocol. Sulfo-NHS derivatives are more soluble than the classical NHS esters and can be used to increase the cross-linker solubility.

3.2.1 Introduction of a Maleimido Group

This kind of modified antibody is usually obtained by reaction with maleimido-containing derivatives such as **13** (Fig. 5). One of the most widely used cross-linkers of this type is succinimidyl 4-(*N*-maleimidomethyl)-cyclohexane-1-carboxylate (SMCC, **19**). For example, it has been successfully used to link the maytansinoid DM1 to Herceptin™ to provide trastuzumab emtansine (T-DM1 **17**, Fig. 6, Kadcyla™ which was approved by the FDA in February 2013) [19], as well as PBD-based ADC **18** [20].

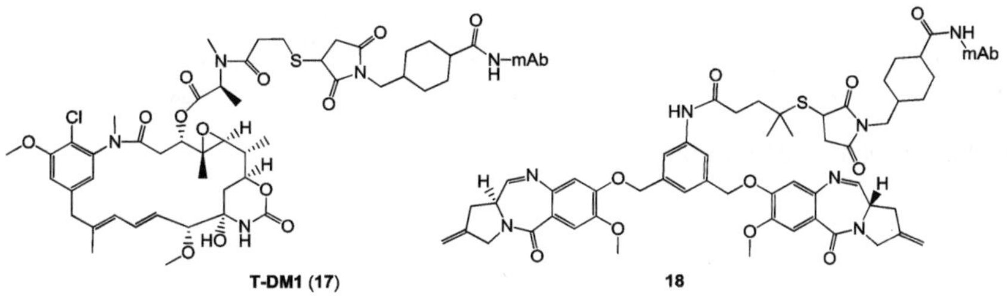

Fig. 6 Structures of some maleimido-based conjugates

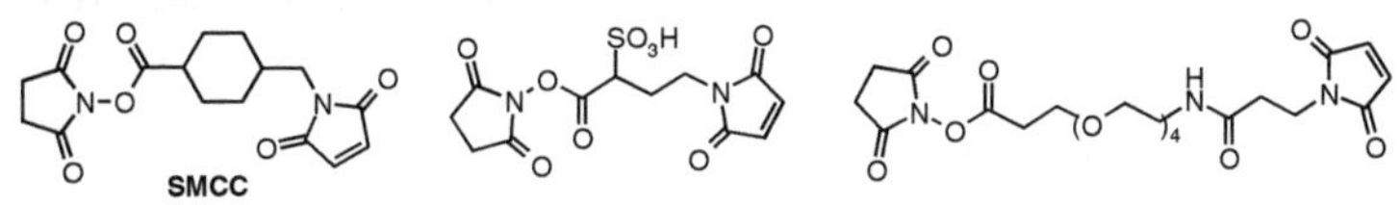

Fig. 7 Representative examples of maleimido cross-linkers

Hydrophilic linkers bearing either a negatively charged sulfonate group such as **20** [21] or a neutral PEG moiety such as **21** [22] have also been used to enable higher loading of hydrophobic drugs without triggering aggregation of the resulting ADC (Fig. 7) [23].

A general procedure that has been used to attach DM1 or DM4 to different antibodies via SMCC **19** or hydrophilic linkers consists of the following steps [21–25]:

1. Prepare a solution of maleimido linker in DMSO for SMCC or DMA for hydrophilic linkers at a concentration around 20 mM.
2. Dilute the mAb at a concentration >8 mg/mL in buffer 7.
3. Under stirring, slowly add DMSO or DMA, followed by a 7.5- to 10-fold molar excess of the SMCC solution or a 5- to 50-fold molar excess of the hydrophilic linker solution, so that the final concentration of the mAb is approximately 8 mg/mL and the final content of organic cosolvent is 5 % (*see* **Note 2**).
4. React for 2 h at room temperature under stirring (*see* **Note 3**).
5. Remove excess reactant and reaction by-products by gel filtration using a Sephadex® G25 desalting resin with buffer 7.

An alternative protocol has been used for conjugation of a pyrrolo-benzodiazepine (PBD) dimer using a similar linker to afford ADC **18** [20]: DMA was used as the cosolvent instead of DMSO and gel filtration performed with buffer 8.

Determination of the number of SMCC linkers per molecule of antibody may be done on a small aliquot of the modified antibody using a subtractive Ellman's assay (UV method) [25]. The sample may be treated with an excess of β-mercaptoethanol followed by 5,5′-dithiobis-2-nitrobenzoic acid (DTNB) to determine the remaining thiol ($\varepsilon_{412\text{nm}} = 14{,}150/\text{M/cm}$ for TNB).

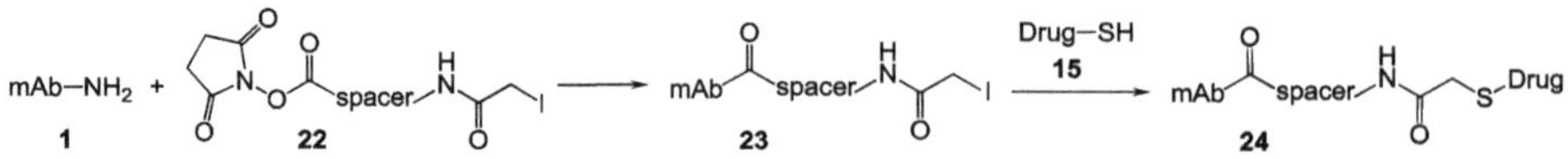

Fig. 8 Iodoacetamido-based conjugation

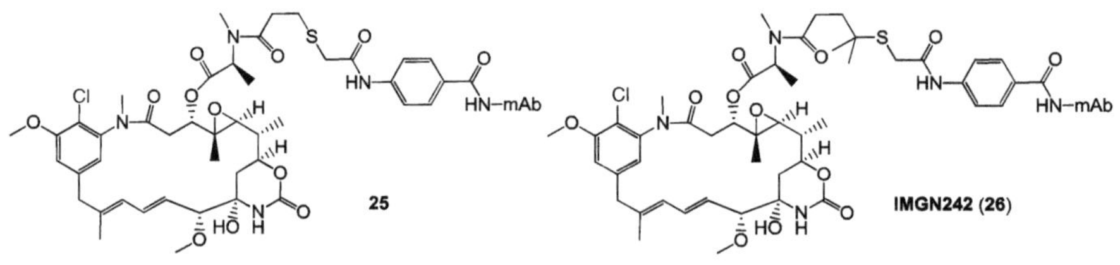

Fig. 9 Maytansinoid–thioacetamido conjugates

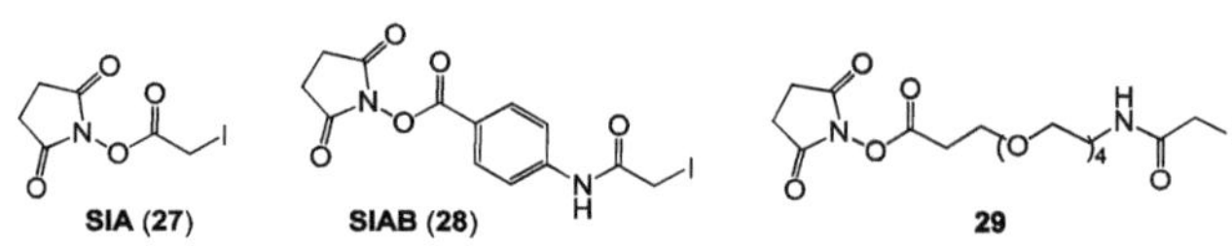

Fig. 10 Representative examples of iodoacetamido cross-linkers

3.2.2 Introduction of an Iodoacetamido Group

Several haloacetyl-based derivatives are available for use as ADC linkers (Fig. 8). Among them, iodoacetyl-based derivatives have been the most commonly used, due to a higher reactivity against sulfhydryl moiety compared to bromoacetyl-based derivatives, for instance. One of the most widely used cross-linkers of this type is *N*-succinimidyl (4-iodoacetyl)aminobenzoate (SIAB **28**, Fig. 10). It has been successfully used to link maytansinoid derivatives DM1 (ADC **25**, Fig. 9) and DM4 (e.g., huC242-DM4 or IMGN242 **26**) to various antibodies [24, 25].

Nevertheless, one can use other derivatives, from the simplest *N*-succinimidyl iodoacetate (SIA, **27**) to a more hydrophilic iodoacetyl-PEG linker **29** (Fig. 10) [11].

A standard protocol for such a modification step may be the following, based on the procedure that has been used to attach DM1 to several antibodies using SIAB **28** [24, 25]:

1. Prepare a solution of SIAB **28** in DMSO at a concentration around 18 mM.
2. Dilute the mAb at a concentration >20 mg/mL in buffer 7.
3. Under stirring, slowly add DMSO, followed by a 7- to 10-fold molar excess of the drug solution, so that the final concentration of the mAb is 20 mg/mL and the final content of DMSO is 5 %.

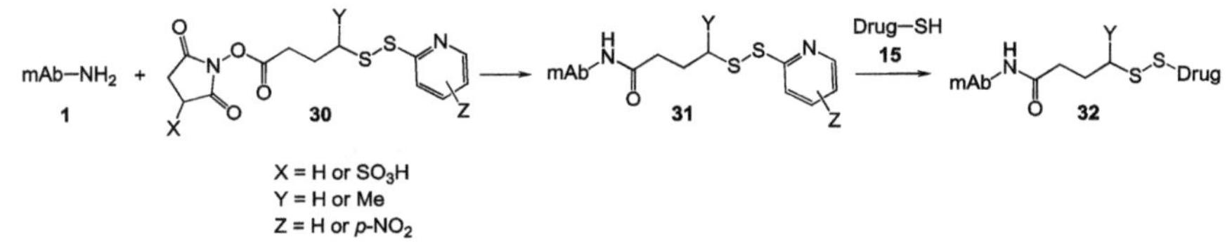

Fig. 11 Pyridyldithio-based conjugation

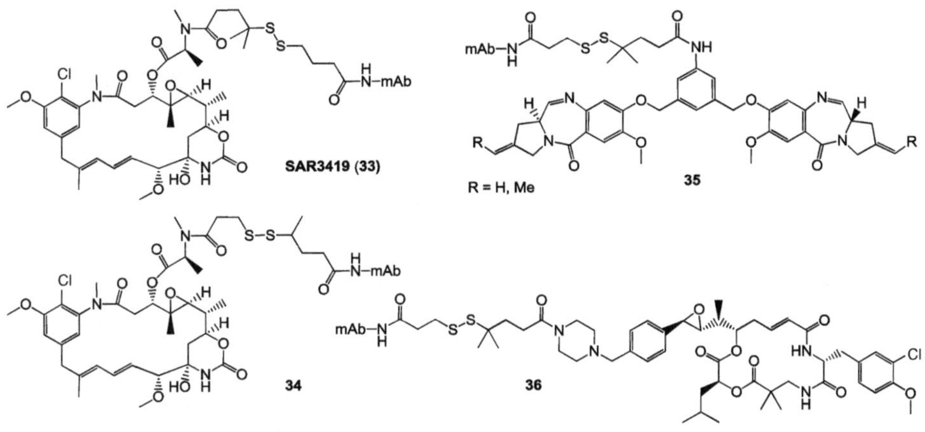

Fig. 12 Structures of some disulfide conjugates

4. Protect the reaction from light and stir for 2 h at room temperature.
5. Remove excess reactant and reaction by-products by gel filtration using a desalting resin with buffer 7 and add 1 N sodium hydroxide until pH 8, the pH required for subsequent conjugation.

The yield of modification of the antibody by SIAB **28** is assumed to be quantitative, based on SIAB stoichiometry.

3.2.3 Introduction of a Pyridyldisulfide Group

The antibody **1** is first activated by the introduction of sulfhydryl-reactive moieties such as (nitro-) pyridyldisulfides **30** that are subsequently displaced by the free sulfhydryl group of the drug **15** (Fig. 11). This method has been developed by ImmunoGen and widely used for the preparation of ADCs bearing a cleavable disulfide linker [26, 27]. It has been successfully used with the maytansinoid DM4 to provide huB4-SPDB-DM4 (SAR3419 **33**, Fig. 12) [28], together with DM1-based ADC **34**, PBD-based ADC **35** [20], and cryptophycin-based ADC **36** [29].

Commonly used pyridyldisulfide linkers (Fig. 13) are the commercially available *N*-succinimidyl-3-(2-pyridyldithio)propionate (SPDP, **37**) or the *N*-succinimidyl-4-(2-pyridyldithio)butanoate (SPDB, **38**) [30]. Sterically hindered disulfide linkers like **39** and **40** have also been developed to modulate the release of the drug [30, 31].

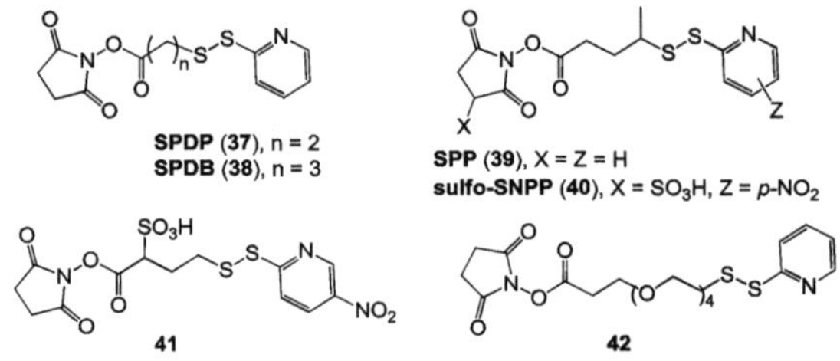

Fig. 13 Representative examples of disulfide cross-linkers

As for maleimido-based conjugation, hydrophilic - sulfonate **41** or PEGylated **42** - linkers have been prepared [21–23]. Nitro-substitution on the pyridine ring renders the pyridyldithio moiety more reactive towards displacement by a sulfhydryl derivative and may be used with poorly reactive drugs.

A general procedure has been used to attach maytansinoid or PBD derivatives to antibodies using disulfide linkers [20, 23, 25, 26, 30]. Here is the most widely used protocol:

1. Prepare a solution of the cross-linker in ethanol or DMA at a concentration near 10 or 20 mM for hydrophilic linkers.
2. Dilute the mAb at a concentration >8 mg/mL in buffer 7.
3. Under stirring, slowly add ethanol or DMA, followed by a 4- to 7-fold molar excess of the SPDB **38** solution (depending on the expected final DAR) or a 5- to 50-fold molar excess of the hydrophilic linker solution, so that the final concentration of the mAb is around 8 mg/mL and the final content of organic cosolvent is 5 %.
4. React for around 2 h at room temperature under stirring (*see* **Note 3**).
5. Remove excess reactant and reaction by-products by gel filtration using a Sephadex® G25 desalting resin with buffer 9.

Determination of the number of linkers per molecule of antibody depends on the nature of the linker. For instance, determination of the number of SPDB **38** per molecule of antibody may be done using a small aliquot of the modified antibody by treating the sample with an excess of 50 mM DTT and determining the release of pyridine-2-thione by UV measurement ($\varepsilon_{343\text{nm}} = 8{,}080/\text{M/cm}$ and $\varepsilon_{280\text{nm}} = 5{,}100/\text{M/cm}$). Determination for sulfo-SNPP **40** linker may be done by direct absorbance measurement at 325 nm knowing that $\varepsilon_{325\text{nm}} = 10{,}964/\text{M/cm}$ for the 4-nitropyridyl-2-dithio group linked to the antibody [30], whereas determination for hydrophilic sulfo-linker **41** may be done by addition of DTT to an aliquot of modified antibody to assay the release of 2-mercapto-4-nitropyridine ($\varepsilon_{394\text{nm}} = 14{,}205/\text{M/cm}$, [21]).

An alternative "one-pot" protocol (without purifying the crude medium of the modification step) has been used for conjugation of cryptophycin derivatives using a SPDB **38** linker [29].

1. Prepare a solution of SPDB **38** linker in DMA at a concentration around 15 mM.
2. Dilute the mAb at a concentration >8 mg/mL in buffer 7 and add 1 N HEPES solution to adjust the pH at 8.
3. Under stirring, slowly add DMA, followed by a 5- to 10-fold molar excess of the linker solution (depending on the final expected DAR), so that the final concentration of the mAb is around 8 mg/mL and the final content of DMA is 5 %.
4. React for 2 h at room temperature under stirring and engage into the second step without prior purification.

The yield of modification is assumed to be quantitative, based on SPDB stoichiometry.

3.2.4 Second Step: Introduction of the Drug

Whatever the specific chemical functionality introduced during the modification step, the second step introducing the sulfhydryl-containing drug **15** is quite standard. A general protocol may be the following:

1. Prepare a solution of drug **15** in DMA at a concentration between 1 and 5 mM.
2. Dilute the modified mAb in the appropriate reaction buffer if necessary.
3. Under stirring, add DMA, followed by a 1.5- to 7-fold molar excess of the drug solution over the linker content, so that the final concentration of the mAb is around 2.5–12.5 mg/mL and the final content of DMA does not exceed 20 %.
4. React for 20 h at room temperature (*see* **Note 4**). Protect from light in the case of SIAB-modified antibody.
5. Remove excess reactant and reaction by-products and formulate. Some examples are described hereafter:

   DM1, DM4, and PBD conjugates have been purified by gel filtration using a Sephadex® G25 desalting resin or dialysis in buffer 10.

   For cryptophycin conjugates, the crude conjugation media were clarified over a 5 μm Millex® membrane and purified by SEC on a Superdex® 200 prep grade column using buffer 3 with 10–20 % by volume of *N*-methylpyrrolidone (NMP). The monomeric conjugated antibody-containing fractions were pooled and concentrated by centrifugation on a 50 kDa membrane. The purification buffer was exchanged by gel filtration on a Sephadex® G25 desalting resin to deliver the ADC in the final buffer, for example, buffer 3.

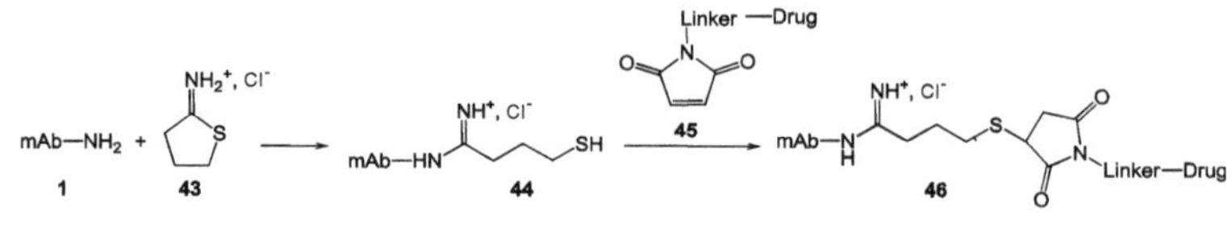

Fig. 14 Iminothiolane-based conjugation

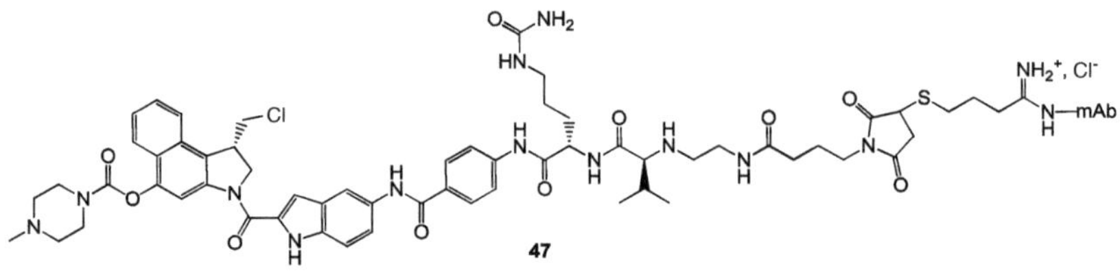

Fig. 15 A duocarmycin ADC bearing an amidine linker

3.3 Two-Step Conjugation Using Iminothiolane Reagents

Iminothiolane reagents are used for the introduction of sulfhydryl groups on lysine residues of antibody **1**; these thiol groups are able to subsequently react with specific reactive groups like the maleimido moiety present on the drug **45** (Fig. 14).

Several substituted iminothiolane hydrohalides have been described [32], but so far, the only iminothiolane successfully applied to the preparation of ADCs is 2-iminothiolane **43** (Fig. 14) also named Traut's reagent [1]. It can react with drugs carrying any sulfhydryl-reactive group, the mostly used so far for ADC being the maleimido group.

The following protocol has been used to attach duocarmycin derivatives bearing a cathepsin B-sensitive linker to antibodies (Fig. 15) [33]:

1. Dilute the mAb at a concentration >5 mg/mL in buffer 11.
2. Under stirring, slowly add a 10-fold molar excess of 2-iminothiolane **43**, so that the final concentration of the mAb is 5 mg/mL.
3. React for 1 h at room temperature under stirring.
4. Remove excess reactant and reaction by-products and exchange buffer to conjugation buffer by diafiltration using a 10 kDa TFF cassette with buffer 12; adjust the concentration of the modified antibody at 2.5 mg/mL and determine the thiol concentration. This determination may be done on a small aliquot of the modified antibody by treating the sample with an excess of 4,4′-dithiodipyridine (DTDP) to assay the release of thiopyridine by UV measurement ($\varepsilon_{324\text{nm}} = 19{,}800/\text{M/cm}$).
5. Prepare a drug solution in DMSO at a concentration of 5 mM.

6. Under stirring, slowly add a 3-fold molar excess of the drug solution per thiol.
7. React for 1.5 h at room temperature under stirring.
8. After filtration through a 0.2 μm membrane, quench the reaction by addition of a 10-fold molar excess per thiol of a 100 mM solution of *N*-ethylmaleimide in DMSO for 1 h at room temperature.
9. Remove aggregates, excess reactant, and reaction by-products by filtration through a 0.2 μm membrane followed by cation-exchange (CEX) chromatography using a SP Sepharose® High Performance CEX column eluted with buffer 13.
10. Formulate the ADC by diafiltration using a 10 kDa TFF cassette with buffer 14, add Dextran 40 to a final concentration of 10 mg/mL, and "sterilize" by filtration through a 0.2 μm membrane.

4 Notes

1. Stirring may be stopped during this step and replaced by slight heating to 30 °C. The DAR can be monitored by an appropriate technique, depending on the drug (see, e.g., methods described in Chapters 16–18).
2. Concentration may reach 20 mg/mL in some cases. The molar excess of linker solution depends on its reactivity and the expected DAR.
3. For less reactive linkers, the reaction can proceed for up to 24 h.
4. Stirring may be stopped during this step and replaced by slight heating to 30 °C.

References

1. Traut RR, Bollen A, Sun T-T, Hershey WB, Sundberg J, Pierce LR (1973) Methyl 4-mercaptobutyrimidate as a cleavable cross-linking reagent and its application to *Escherichia coli* 30S ribosome. Biochemistry 12:3266–3273
2. Wilbur DS (1992) Radiohalogenation of proteins: an overview of radionuclides, labeling methods, and reagents for conjugate labeling. Bioconjugate Chem 3:433–470
3. Wang L, Amphlett G, Blättler WA, Lambert JM, Zhang W (2005) Structural characterization of the maytansinoid-monoclonal antibody conjugate, huN901-DM1, by mass spectroscopy. Protein Sci 14:2436–2446
4. Jobbagy A, Kiraly K (1966) Chemical characterization of fluorescein isothiocyanate–protein conjugates. Biochim Biophys Acta 124:166
5. Chen Q, Sowa D, Gabathuler R (2004) The use of isocyanate linkers to make hydrolyzable active agent biopolymer conjugates. WO2004/008101
6. Wilbur DS, Chyan M-K, Nakamae H, Chen Y, Hamlin DK, Santos EB, Kornblit BT, Sandmaier BM (2012) Reagents for astatination of biomolecules. 6. An intact antibody conjugated with a maleimido-closo-decaborate(2-) reagent via sulfhydryl groups had considerably higher kidney concentrations than the same antibody conjugated with an isothiocyanato-closo-decaborate(2-) reagent via lysine amines. Bioconjugate Chem 23:409–420
7. Gavrilyuk JI, Wuellner U, Barbas CF III (2009) β-Lactam-based approach for the chemical programming of aldolase antibody 38C2. Bioorg Med Chem Lett 19:1421–1424

8. Gavrilyuk JI, Wuellner U, Salahuddin S, Goswami RK, Sinha SC, Barbas CF III (2009) An efficient chemical approach to bispecific antibodies and antibodies of high valency. Bioorg Med Chem Lett 19:3716–3720
9. Tietze LF, Goerlach A, Beller M (1988) Glycosidation, X. Synthesis of glycoconjugates of acetal-glycosides with lysine and tripeptides for selective cancer therapy. Liebigs Ann Chem 565–577
10. Mier W, Hoffend J, Krämer S, Schuhmacher J, Hull WE, Eisenhut M, Haberkorn U (2005) Conjugation of DOTA using isolated phenolic active esters: the labeling and biodistribution of albumin as blood pool marker. Bioconjugate Chem 16:237–240
11. Singh R, Kovtun Y, Wilhelm SD, Chari R (2010) Potent conjugates and hydrophilic linkers. WO2010/126551
12. Bouchard H, Commerçon A, Fromond C, Mikol V, Parker F, Sassoon I, Tavares D (2011) New maytansinoids and the use of said maytansinoids to prepare conjugates with an antibody. WO2011/039721
13. Bouchard H, Chari RVJ, Commerçon A, Deng Y (2009) Cytotoxic agents comprising new tomaymycin derivatives and their therapeutic use. WO2009/016516
14. Li W, Fishkin NE, Zhao RY, Miller ML, Chari RVJ (2010) Novel benzodiazepine derivatives. WO2010/091150
15. Commerçon A, Gauzy-Lazo L (2011) Conjugates of pyrrolo[1,4]benzodiazepine dimers as anticancer agents. WO2011/023883
16. Hinman LM, Hamann PR, Wallace R, Menendez AT, Durr FE, Upeslacis J (1993) Preparation and characterization of monoclonal antibody conjugates of the calicheamicins: a novel and potent family of antitumor antibiotics. Cancer Res 53:3336–3342
17. Hamann PR, Hinman LM, Beyer CF, Lindh D, Upeslacis J, Flowers DA, Bernstein I (2002) An anti-CD33 antibody–calicheamicin conjugate for treatment of acute myeloid leukemia. Choice of linker. Bioconjugate Chem 13:40–46
18. Hamann PR, Hinman LM, Hollander I, Beyer CF, Lindh D, Holcomb R, Hallett W, Tsou H-R, Upeslacis J, Shochat D, Mountain A, Flowers DA, Bernstein I (2002) Gemtuzumab ozogamicin, a potent and selective anti-CD33 antibody–calicheamicin conjugate for treatment of acute myeloid leukemia. Bioconjugate Chem 13:47–58
19. Lewis Phillips GD, Li G, Dugger DL, Crocker LM, Parsons KL, Elaine Mai E, Blättler WA, Lambert JM, Chari RVJ, Lutz RJ, Wong WLT, Jacobson FS, Koeppen H, Schwall RH, Kenkare-Mitra SR, Spencer SD, Sliwkowski MX (2008) Targeting HER2-positive breast cancer with Trastuzumab-DM1, an antibody–cytotoxic drug conjugate. Cancer Res 68:9280–9290
20. Gauzy L, Zhao R, Deng Y, Li W, Bouchard H, Chari RVJ, Commerçon A (2007) Cytotoxic agents comprising new tomaymycin derivatives and their therapeutic use. WO2007/085930
21. Chari RVJ, Zhao RY, Kovtun Y, Singh R, Widdison WC (2009) Cross-linkers and their uses. WO2009/134977
22. Singh R, Kovtun Y, Wilhelm SD, Chari RVJ (2009) Potent conjugates and hydrophilic linkers. WO2009/134976
23. Zhao RY, Wilhelm SD, Audette C, Jones G, Leece BA, Lazar AC, Goldmacher VS, Singh R, Kovtun Y, Widdison WC, Lambert JM, Chari RVJ (2011) Synthesis and evaluation of hydrophilic linkers for antibody maytansinoid conjugates. J Med Chem 54:3606–3623
24. Steeves R, Lutz R, Chari R, Xie H, Kovtun Y (2005) Method of targeting specific cell populations using cell-binding agent maytansinoids conjugates linked via a non-cleavable linker, said conjugates, and methods of making said conjugates. WO2005/037992
25. Chari RVJ, Widdison WC (2004) Cytotoxic agents comprising new maytansinoids. US2004/0235840
26. Widdison WC, Wilhelm SD, Cavanagh EE, Whiteman KR, Leece BA, Kovtun Y, Goldmacher VS, Xie H, Steeves RM, Lutz RJ, Zhao R, Wang L, Blättler WA, Chari RVJ (2006) Semisynthetic maytansine analogues for the targeted treatment of cancer. J Med Chem 49:4392–4408
27. Lambert JM (2010) Antibody-maytansinoid conjugates: a new strategy for the treatment of cancer. Drugs Future 35:471–480
28. Blanc V, Bousseau A, Caron A, Carrez C, Lutz RJ, Lambert JL (2011) SAR3419: an anti-CD19-maytansinoid immunoconjugate for the treatment of B-cell malignancies. Clin Cancer Res 17:6448–6458
29. Bouchard H, Brun M-P, Commerçon A, Zhang J (2011) Novel conjugates, preparation thereof, and therapeutic use thereof. WO2011/001052
30. Widdison WC (2004) Cross-linkers with high reactivity and solubility and their use in the preparation of conjugates for targeted delivery of small molecule drugs. WO2004/016801
31. Kellogg BA, Garrett L, Kovtun Y, Lai KC, Leece B, Miller M, Payne G, Steeves R, Whiteman KR, Widdison W, Xie H, Singh R, Chari

RVJ, Lambert JM, Lutz RJ (2011) Disulfide-linked antibody–maytansinoid conjugates: optimization of in vivo activity by varying the steric hindrance at carbon atoms adjacent to the disulfide linkage. Bioconjugate Chem 22:717–727

32. Carroll SF, Goff DA (1990) Hindered linking agents and methods. WO1990/06774
33. King DJ, Terrett JA, Gangwar S, Cardarelli JM, Raonaik C, Pan C (2009) Conjugates of anti-RG1 antibodies. WO2009/073524

Chapter 11

Engineering THIOMABs for Site-Specific Conjugation of Thiol-Reactive Linkers

Sunil Bhakta, Helga Raab, and Jagath R. Junutula

Abstract

Antibody conjugates are used in many therapeutic and research applications and are generated by chemically linking a cysteine or lysine residue to potent chemotherapeutic drugs or other functional groups through a flexible linker. Recently, we have engineered THIOMABs (antibodies with engineered reactive cysteine residues) for site-specific conjugation and showed that these antibody conjugates display homogeneous labeling with optimal in vitro and in vivo characteristics. Here, we describe protocols for engineering, selection, and site-specific conjugation of THIOMABs with thiol-reactive linkers.

Key words Antibody conjugate, THIOMAB, Site-specific conjugation, Antibody–drug conjugate (ADC), Engineered ADCs

1 Introduction

Antibody-based targeted therapeutics have revolutionized our approach to treating a variety of human diseases as over 30 monoclonal antibodies (mAbs) have so far been approved for use in many indications, including cancer [1]. Several mAbs (rituximab, trastuzumab, cetuximab, and bevacizumab) have shown profound clinical benefit in the treatment of some types of cancers, and many others are currently in clinical development [2]. Antibodies developed against tumor-specific cell-surface antigens often lack or display poor therapeutic activity; hence, alternate strategies have been explored to enhance their activity, including antibody–drug conjugates (ADCs). ADCs specifically deliver a highly potent toxic agent directly to cancer cells, thereby combining antibody tumor targeting specificity with the enhanced antitumor activity of toxic agents [3–5]. Antibodies have been conjugated to a variety of cytotoxic drugs such as auristatins, calicheamicins, duocarmycins, maytansinoids, and other small-molecule chemotherapeutic agents to generate ADCs that display selective killing of target tumor cells in vitro and in mouse-tumor xenograft studies [6–15].

Laurent Ducry (ed.), *Antibody-Drug Conjugates*, Methods in Molecular Biology, vol. 1045,
DOI 10.1007/978-1-62703-541-5_11, © Springer Science+Business Media, LLC 2013

Cytotoxic drugs and other small molecules are generally conjugated to antibodies either through lysine ε-amino groups or through cysteine sulfhydryl groups activated by reducing interchain disulfide bonds. These conventional conjugation methods result in heterogeneous antibody conjugate products with a mixture of different molar ratios of conjugated species to antibody linked at different sites [16–19]. In order to create more homogeneously loaded ADCs better suited to clinical development, we recently created antibodies with engineered cysteines to enable thiol conjugation at these specific sites, named THIOMABs [17, 18]. THIOMAB–drug conjugates are superior to conventional ADCs because these conjugates exhibit uniform distribution of linker-drugs and being equivalently efficacious, they also display superior safety with respect to liver and bone marrow toxicity in rats and monkeys [17, 18]. This chapter describes protocols for engineering, selection, and conjugation of THIOMABs to thiol-reactive linkers. Additionally, we also describe methods associated with analytical (quantitation of linker-drugs attached to antibody) and functional characterization (binding and in vitro potency) that can be applied to both engineered and conventional ADCs. Engineered THIOMABs have been successfully used to conjugate cytotoxic drugs for therapeutic applications and also to conjugate biotin, fluorophore, or radiolabels for antibody-based research and imaging applications [20, 21].

2 Materials

2.1 Site-Directed Mutagenesis

1. IgG1-heavy and light-chain expression plasmids.
2. Forward and reverse primers with desired cysteine substitution (*see* **Note 1**).
3. PfuUltra high-fidelity DNA polymerase and 10× buffer (Agilent) (*see* **Note 2**).
4. 100 mM dNTP mix (Roche).
5. DpnI (New England Biolabs).
6. Subcloning grade *E. coli*-competent cells (*see* **Note 3**).
7. LB-medium.
8. LB-agar plates containing 50 μg/mL carbenicillin/ampicillin or other appropriate selection antibiotics.

2.2 THIOMAB Production

1. IgG1-heavy and light-chain expression plasmids with desired cysteine substitution.
2. HEK293 cells.
3. Fugene® HD transfection reagent (Roche) (*see* **Note 4**).
4. Cell growth medium: Ham's F-12: high glucose DMEM (50:50) supplemented with 10 % heat-inactivated fetal bovine serum and 2 mM L-glutamine (Invitrogen).

5. Opti-MEM medium (Gibco).
6. Gibco 293 freestyle medium (Gibco).
7. Protein A-Sepharose beads (GE Healthcare Life sciences).
8. 1× Phosphate buffered saline (PBS): 8 g NaCl, 0.2 g KCl, 1.13 g Na_2HPO_4, 0.2 g KH_2PO_4, water to 1 L and adjust pH to 7.2 with 6 N HCl.
9. Elution buffer: 0.1 M acetic acid.
10. Neutralization buffer: 1 M Tris–HCl, pH 8.0.

2.3 Conjugation

1. Conjugation buffer: 50 mM Tris–HCl, pH 7.5, 2 mM EDTA.
2. 100 mM DTT.
3. HiTrap SP FF column 1 mL (GE Healthcare Bio-Science AB).
4. Cation-exchange chromatography (CEX) binding buffer: 20 mM succinate, pH 5.0.
5. CEX elution buffer: 50 mM Tris–HCl, pH 7.5, 150 mM NaCl.
6. 100 mM dehydroascorbic acid (DHAA): Dissolved in *N*, *N*-Dimethylacetamide (DMA) (*see* **Note 5**).
7. Biotin-PEO-maleimide (Pierce): Dissolved in water.
8. Maytansine (DM1)-MPEO-maleimide (Genentech): Dissolved in DMA.

2.4 Hydrophobic Interaction Chromatography (HIC) and Mass Spectrometric (LC–MS) Analysis

1. Butyl HIC NPR column, 2.5 μm, 4.6 mm × 3.5 cm (Tosoh Bioscience).
2. HIC buffer A: 50 mM potassium phosphate, pH 7.0, and 1.5 M ammonium sulfate.
3. HIC buffer B: 50 mM potassium phosphate, pH 7.0, 20 % isopropanol.
4. ChemStation software (Agilent Technologies).
5. Deglycosylation enzyme: PNGase F (New England Biolabs).
6. Polymeric reversed phase column (PL 1912-1802, PLRPS 1000 Å, 50 mm × 2.1 mm, 8 μm (Agilent Technologies).
7. Mobile phase A: 0.05 % trifluoroacetic acid in water.
8. Mobile phase B: 0.04 % trifluoroacetic acid in acetonitrile.
9. MassHunter software (Agilent Technologies).
10. THIOMAB–drug conjugates, e.g., Thio-trastuzumab-mpeo-DM1 (HC-A118C and LC-V205C variants) (Genentech).
11. Conventional ADC, e.g., Trastuzumab-mcc-DM1 (Genentech).

2.5 Cell-Surface Binding

1. Cell lines expressing high levels of target antigen (e.g., SK-BR-3, a Her2 expressing cell line for Trastuzumab conjugates).
2. 96-well round-bottom falcon plates (Becton Dickinson).

3. Cell growth medium: Ham's F-12: high-glucose DMEM (50:50) supplemented with10 % heat-inactivated fetal bovine serum and 2 mM L-glutamine (Invitrogen).
4. 1× PBS: 8 g NaCl, 0.2 g KCl, 1.13 g Na_2HPO_4, 0.2 g KH_2PO_4, water to 1 L and adjust pH to 7.2 with 6 N HCl.
5. FACS-binding buffer: PBS buffer, pH 7.2 containing 1 % bovine serum albumin.
6. Trastuzumab (Genentech).
7. Thio-trastuzumab-mpeo-DM1 (Genentech).
8. Phycoerythrin-labeled goat antihuman Fc secondary antibody (Jackson ImmunoResearch).

2.6 In Vitro Potency

1. Antigen-expressing cells.
2. 96-well flat clear-bottom black plates (Corning).
3. Cell growth medium: Ham's F-12: high-glucose DMEM (50:50) supplemented with 10 % heat-inactivated fetal bovine serum and 2 mM L-glutamine (Invitrogen).
4. Unconjugated antibody, e.g., Trastuzumab (Genentech).
5. THIOMAB–drug conjugate, e.g., Thio-trastuzumab-mpeo-DM1 (Genentech).
6. Nonbinding negative control conjugate, e.g., Thio-anti-CD22-mpeo-DM1 (Genentech).
7. CellTiter-Glo® Luminescent Cell Viability Assay kit (Promega) (*see* **Note 6**).

3 Methods

3.1 Site-Directed Mutagenesis

1. Set up 25 μL PCR reaction containing 1× PFU DNA polymerase buffer, 20 mM dNTP mixture, 200 ng of each forward and reverse mutagenic primers, 100 ng double-stranded IgG-heavy chain expression plasmid, and 0.5 μL of HF PFU DNA polymerase (2.5 U/mL).
2. Incubate PCR reactions in a thermal cycler for 2 min of denaturation step at 95 °C, followed by 20 cycles of 30 s denaturation at 95 °C, 30 s annealing at 52 °C, and 10 min of extension at 68 °C (*see* **Note 7**).
3. Add 1 μL of DpnI (10 U/μL) to each PCR sample and incubate at 37 °C for 3 h (*see* **Note 8**).
4. Add 1 μL of above DpnI-treated PCR sample to 50 μL *E. coli*-competent cells and incubate the cells on ice for 30 min.
5. Do the heat-shock treatment for 30 s at 42 °C and transfer reaction tubes back to ice for 2 min.

6. Add 150 μL of LB-medium to the reaction tube and keep at 37 °C incubator shaker for 30 min.
7. Plate *E. coli* cells on LB-agar carbenicillin plates and transfer the plates to 37 °C incubator for 16 h.
8. Inoculate single colonies in 5 ml LB-medium containing 50 μg/mL carbenicillin and grow cultures for 12–14 h.
9. Isolate the plasmid DNA using Qiagen miniprep isolation kit and perform DNA sequencing to verify desired cysteine mutation and also unwanted nonspecific mutations that may have caused due to PCR.

3.2 Small-Scale THIOMAB Production in HEK293 Cells

1. Day 1: Seed 1×10^7 HEK293 cells into T175 flasks with 30 mL of cell growth medium and grow them overnight at 37 °C in CO_2 incubator.
2. Day 2: Dilute 15 μg of IgG-light chain and 15 μg of IgG-heavy chain construct consisting desired cysteine substitution into a total of 1.5 mL of Opti-MEM medium at 0.02 μg/mL (*see* **Note 9**).
3. Place 1.5 ml of diluted DNA into a sterile non-siliconized reaction tube and add 90 μL of Fugene® HD transfection reagent directly into the medium containing diluted DNA (*see* **Note 10**).
4. Vortex DNA:transfection reagent complex for 2 s and incubate at room temperature (20 °C) for 15 min.
5. Carefully add transfection complex dropwise to the cells and mix the medium gently (*see* **Note 11**).
6. Transfer T175 flask to 37 °C CO_2 incubator for 24 h.
7. Day 3: Aspirate growth medium, wash gently with 15 mL PBS, and add 30 mL of Gibco 293 Freestyle medium and incubate the cells at 37 °C for 5 days.
8. Day 8: Collect medium, spin at 1,000 × *g*, and transfer the supernatant to 50 mL Falcon tubes, add 0.5 mL Protein A-sepharose beads and place the tube on a rotator at 4 °C for 3–4 h.
9. Wash the beads with 50 mL of ice-cold PBS buffer four times and elute the bound antibody with 2 mL of elution buffer. Immediately neutralize eluted sample with 0.5 mL of 1 M Tris–HCl, pH 8.0. Repeat the elution step once more and pool the samples (*see* **Note 12**).
10. Concentrate the sample to a final concentration of 5 mg/mL with Amicon ULTRA-15 centrifugal filters and buffer exchange with 50 mM Tris–HCl containing 2 mM EDTA by repeated concentration steps using centrifugation at 4,000 × *g*.

3.3 Conjugation with Thiol-Reactive Linkers

1. Add 14 μL of 100 mM DTT (40-fold molar excess) to the 5 mg (1 mL) of THIOMAB (thio-trastuzumab) in the conjugation buffer and incubate the reaction mixture at room temperature (~20 °C) for 16 h (*see* **Notes 13** and **14**).
2. Use approximately 1/50th reaction volume of 10 % acetic acid to adjust the pH to 5.0 (*see* **Note 15**).
3. Load the sample (~1.035 mL) on HiTrap SP FF cation-exchange chromatography column, then wash the column with 10 column volumes of CEX binding buffer and elute with 3 mL of CEX elution buffer.
4. Add 5 μL of 100 mM DHAA (15-fold molar excess) to the antibody at room temperature for 3 h to reoxidize the native interchain disulfide bonds while leaving the engineered cysteines unpaired (*see* **Note 16**).
5. Add the BMPEO-DM1 or biotin-PEO-maleimide (2.5- to 3-fold molar excess) and incubate at room temperature (~20 °C) for 1 h (*see* **Note 17**).
6. Purify the antibody conjugate or ADC using cation-exchange chromatography as described above in **step 3** of Subheading 3.3.
7. Analyze the antibody conjugate or ADC by LC–MS and HIC to examine percent conjugation. LC–MS profile examples of partially (Fc-V280C THIOMAB) and fully conjugated (Fc V278C THIOMAB) variants are illustrated in Fig. 1. Optimal THIOMABs that result 100 % conjugation can be screened using biotin-PEO-maleimide linker prior to conjugating with desired cytotoxic drug.

3.4 Quantitation of Number of Drugs per Antibody

1. HIC analysis: Inject 50 μg of ADC diluted in an equal volume of 2× HIC buffer A onto a butyl column of HIC.
2. Elute with a linear gradient from 0 to 70 % HIC buffer B at 0.8 mL/min and monitor the protein peak using UV280 absorption.
3. Use, e.g., ChemStation software to resolve and quantify antibody species with different ratios of drug per antibody (*see* **Note 18**). Examples of a HIC profile for Thio-trastuzumab-mpeo-DM1 variants (HC-A114C and LC-V205C) and a conventional ADC (Trastuzumab-mcc-DM1) are illustrated in Fig. 2.
4. In order to deglycosylate the ADC for molecular weight determination by mass spectrometry, add 1 μL of PNGase F enzyme to 100 μg of ADC and incubate at 37 °C for 16 h.
5. LC–MS analysis: Reduce antibody conjugate in 10 mM DTT for 15 min.

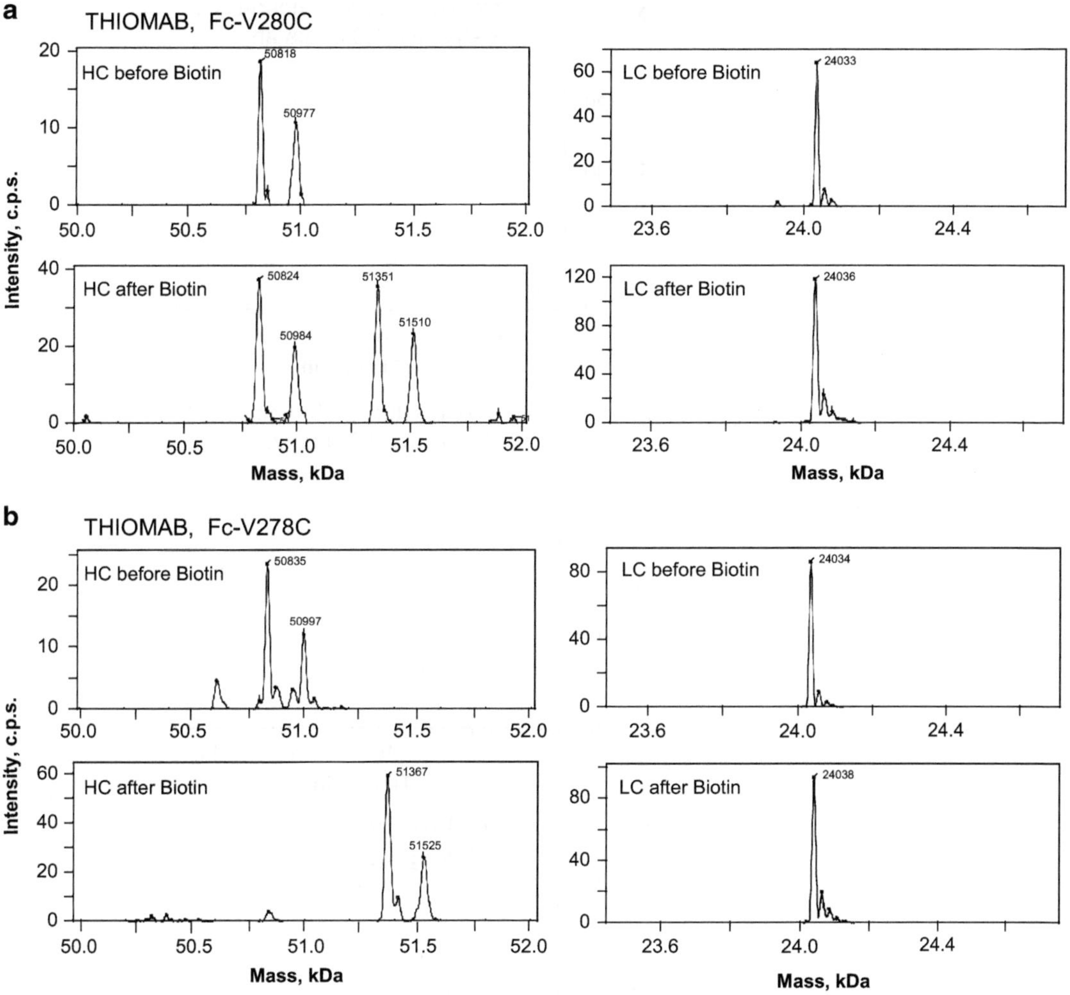

Fig. 1 Conjugation of THIOMABs with reactive cysteines in the Fc region to biotin-PEO-maleimide. LC–MS analysis revealed that conjugation of Fc-V280C (**a**) was partial (<2 biotins/ab) while Fc-V278C THIOMAB (**b**) was fully conjugated (two biotins/ab). As expected, there is no conjugation to the light chain (LC). Kabat numbering is used to define the cysteine substitution in the antibody

6. Inject (2 μg) on a polymeric reversed phase column at 80 °C using a linear gradient from 34 % mobile phase B to 42 % mobile phase B in 10 min at a flow rate of 0.5 mL/min with detection at 280 nm.
7. Mass–spec analysis of the eluted peaks is performed using a LC–MS instrument such as a 9520 ESI Q-TOF Accurate Mass. MassHunter software (Agilent Technologies) is used to deconvolute the spectra and to determine the masses of the eluted peaks.

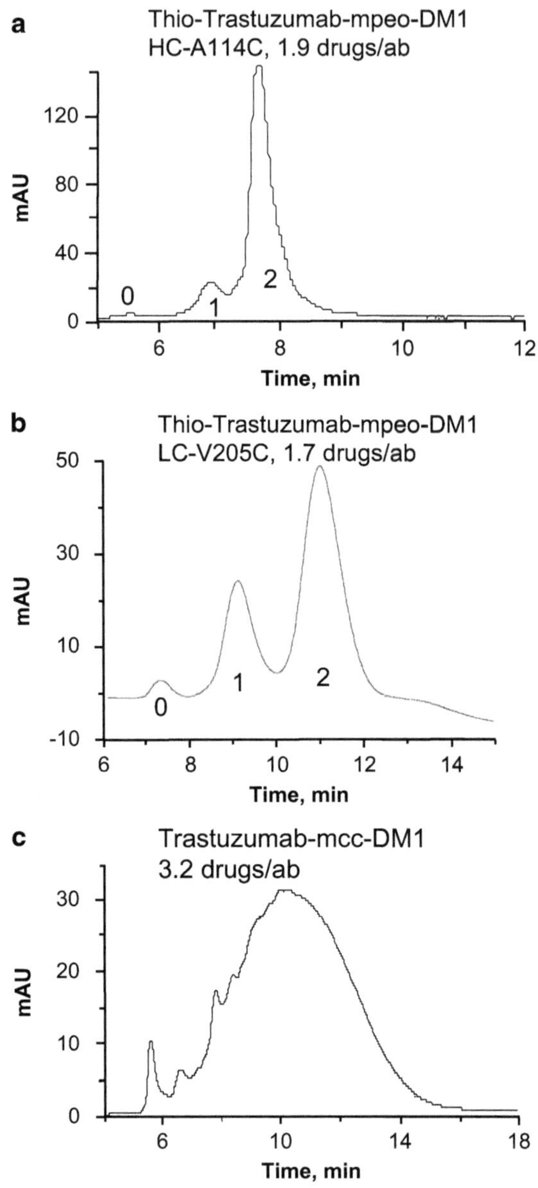

Fig. 2 HIC analysis for engineered ADCs. Number of drugs (DM1) conjugated to antibody was determined by HIC analysis for engineered ADCs (**a**, **b**). In contrast, this procedure cannot be applied for a conventional ADC, where DM1 is conjugated through lysine residues (**c**) because of mixture of ADC species. **a**: HC-A114C ADC; **b**: LC-V205C ADC; **c**: Trastuzumab-mcc-DM1

8. The average DAR (based on the A280 measurement) is determined by using the mole fraction of each of the mass-identified heavy- and light-chain species after chromatographic resolution. Examples of a LC–MS profile for intact, deglycosylated Thio-trastuzumab-mpeo-DM1 variants (HC-A114C and LC-V205C) and a conventional ADC (Trastuzumab-mcc-DM1) are illustrated in Fig. 3.

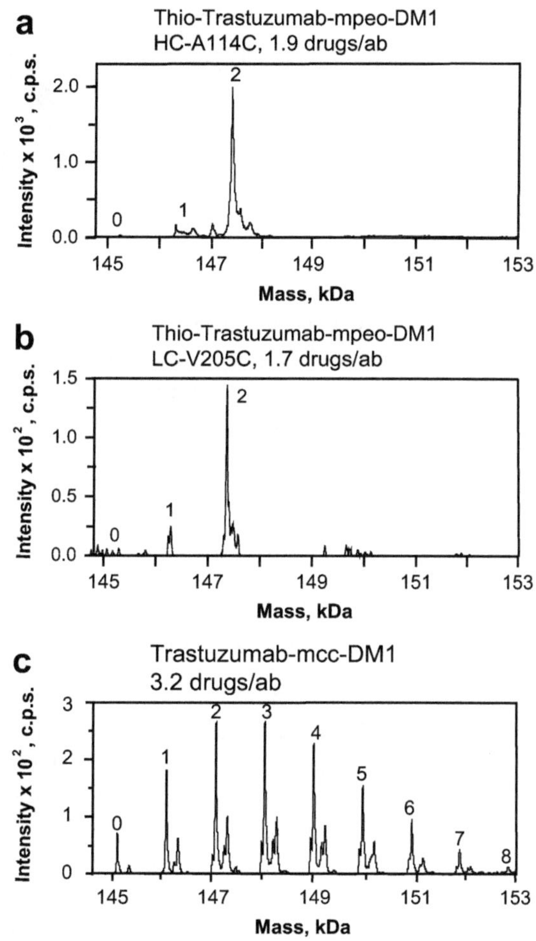

Fig. 3 LC–MS profiles for ADCs. LC–MS analysis of intact, deglycosylated Ab,\ is used to determine both quality (homogeneity of drug load) and quantity (number of drugs per antibody) of conjugated molecules to antibodies. **a**: HC-A114C ADC; **b**: LC-V205C ADC; **c**: conventional Trastuzumab-mcc-DM1 ADC conjugated via lysines

3.5 Cell-Surface Binding of Engineered ADCs

1. Detach SK-BR-3 cells with 1 mM EDTA or other nonenzymatic cell detachment solution and resuspend in FACS buffer at 2×10^6 cells/mL. Dispense 100 μL cells into each well of a round-bottom 96-well plate (*see* **Note 19**).
2. Add Trastuzumab, Thio-trasuzumab-mpeo-DM1, or negative control nonbinding conjugate such as Thio-anti-CD22-mpeo-DM1 at several concentrations ranging from 0 to 5 μg/mL and incubate on ice for 1 h.
3. Spin down 96-well plate at $300 \times g$ for 5 min. Aspirate the buffer and wash the cell pellet by resuspending in 200 μL of FACS buffer. Repeat this step two times.

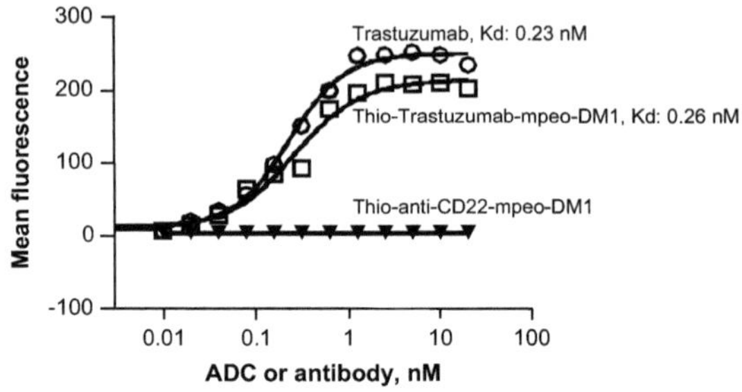

Fig. 4 Functional binding of ADC to target antigen. Engineered thio-trastuzumab-mpeo-DM1 shows similar binding to that of unconjugated Trastuzumab with Her2-expressing SK-BR-3 cells, indicating that conjugation has not disrupted antigen recognition. In contrast, a control Thio-anti-CD22-mpeo-DM1 does not bind to these cells due to lack of CD22 target antigen

4. Add secondary phycoerythrin-labeled goat antihuman Fc secondary antibody at 1:2,500 dilution and incubate on ice for 1 h.
5. Wash three times as in **step 3**.
6. Resuspend cells in 3 % paraformaldehyde and analyze by FACS using a FACS caliber. Cell-surface binding of Thio-trastuzumab-mpeo-DM1, Trastuzumab (positive control), and Thio-anti-CD22-mepo-DM1 (negative control) is illustrated in Fig. 4 (*see* **Note 20**).

3.6 In Vitro Potency of Engineered ADCs

1. Day 1: Seed 5,000 antigen-expressing cells, e.g., SK-BR-3 (75 μL) into each well of a black-walled 96-well plate and incubate cells at 37 °C for overnight (*see* **Note 21**).
2. Day 2: Add 25 μL of unconjugated Trastuzumab or test article ADC (Thio-trastuzumab-mpeo-DM1 or nonbinding negative control Thio-anti-CD22-mpeo-DM1) at varying concentrations ranging from 0 to 10 μg/mL. (*see* **Note 22**).
3. Incubate plates at 37 °C CO_2 incubator for 3 days (*see* **Note 23**).
4. Day 5: Add an equal volume (100 μL) of CellTiter-Glo® Luminescent Cell Viability Assay reagent, mix on a titer plate shaker for 5 min.
7. Measure the luminescence in a luminometer, such as Envision PerkinElmer plate reader. Luminescent values were normalized to 100 % for 0 μg/ml and percent cell killing is plotted against ADC concentration. IC_{50} values can be calculated using appropriate software, such as GraphPad PRISM analysis or

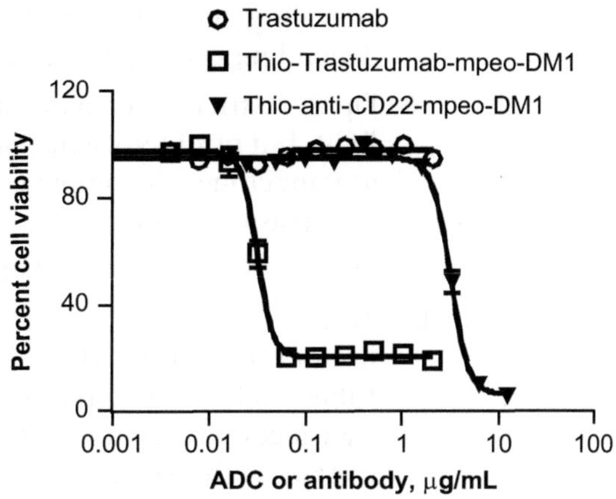

Fig. 5 In vitro cell proliferation assay for functional characterization of ADCs. Engineered Thio-trastuzumab-mpeo-DM1 showed potent (IC_{50}: 30 ng/mL) target-dependent cell killing compared to its unconjugated antibody. A control Thio-anti-CD22-mpeo-DM1 shows nonspecific cell killing (IC_{50}: 3,000 ng/mL) activity at over 100-fold higher concentrations than Thio-trastuzumab-mpeo-DM1

Kaleidagraph. Examples of cell killing with Thio-trastuzumab-mpeo-DM1 (with cytotoxic drug), Trastuzumab (without cytotoxic drug), and Thio-anti-CD22-mpeo-DM1 (negative control ADC) are illustrated in Fig. 5.

4 Notes

1. Design an oligonucleotide primer with minimum of 15 bases to the 3′ side of the desired cysteine mutation and 10–15 bases to the 5′ side.
2. Other high-fidelity PCR-grade DNA polymerases can be substituted. Please note that Taq DNA polymerase may introduce unwanted mutations during PCR.
3. Other subcloning grade *E. coli* chemical competent cells (DH5α, XL1-Blue, or other equivalent competent cells) can be used.
4. Other transfection reagents can be substituted with corresponding changes to the transfection protocol provided by the manufacturer.
5. Keep it at 37 °C for 15 min to dissolve the DHAA and use freshly prepared DHAA stock solution.
6. Prepare CellTiter-Glo Reagent as per manufacturer instructions.
7. In general, using 52 °C as an annealing temperature in the PCR should produce the desired result, but optimization of

annealing temperature in the PCR reaction may be needed depending on GC content.

8. DpnI restriction enzyme digests template DNA used in the PCR, but not DNA synthesized during PCR, thereby enriching mutant clones. Incomplete DpnI digestion could result in wild-type plasmid clones.
9. Do not use medium containing antibiotics during transfection.
10. Need to optimize required transfection reagent to obtain maximum transfection efficiency, and do not use siliconized tips or tubes while setting up DNA:transfection reagent complex. Add transfection reagent directly to DNA solution without allowing contact with plastic surface.
11. Add DNA:transfection reagent to the medium dropwise carefully without disturbing attached cells to the flask/plate. Since 293 cells loosely attach to plastic, one must be more careful adding DNA:transfection reagent.
12. Immediately neutralize the eluted antibody sample to avoid antibody denaturation/mis-folding due to prolonged exposure to acid/low pH.
13. Conditions described for conjugation reaction are scalable to lower or higher amounts (0.1–100 mg scale) of antibody conjugate preparations used for research and preclinical studies.
14. Engineered cysteines on the antibody surface are usually blocked with cysteine or glutathione present in the growth medium (post-transfection incubation period). Therefore, reduction with DTT followed by a purification step and reoxidation of the intra-chain disulfides is important to remove cysteine or glutathione adducts and to reactivate the thiol groups on the engineered cysteines for conjugation with thiol reactive linkers.
15. Conjugation reaction also can be diluted to adjust the pH by adding 5 volumes of 20 mM succinate pH 5.0 if the conjugation reaction is scaled in a small volume.
16. Critical step of conjugation reaction: *Monitor the reoxidation reaction by LC–MS by observing appearance of intact IgG mass peak and disappearance of reduced light- and heavy-chain mass peaks. Over incubation of oxidation step could result in oxidation of engineered cysteines thus resulting in poor conjugation yields.*
17. If it is a hydrophobic cytotoxic drug, then the drug should be diluted into DMA to bring the final DMA concentration in reaction mixture to the minimum of 5 %. To obtain optimal conjugation results, biotin-PEO-maleimide may have to be used at 10- to 50-fold molar excess due to poor quality of the biotin-PEO-maleimide reagent. Maleimide groups are also not

very stable at neutral pH and often undergo hydrolysis upon storage. To avoid this, use freshly prepared biotin-PEO-maleimide stock solution.

18. Chromatographic separation of antibody DAR species by HIC or reverse phase column on LC–MS is possible for cytotoxic drugs that impart a significant increase in hydrophobicity to the antibody. However, HIC analysis method cannot be used for all ADCs. If chromatographic resolution of peaks is not achieved on the reverse phase LC–MS column, then the relative abundance of the deconvoluted masses is used to calculate number of drugs per antibody.
19. Do not use trypsin to detach cells from plate or flask prior to FACS analysis as trypsin would enzymatically digest cell-surface proteins. Instead use 1 mM EDTA to separate cells from plastic surface.
20. It is important to include unconjugated antibody along with its corresponding ADC while setting binding experiments. This helps analyzing whether drug conjugation resulted in the loss of antibody binding to the target antigen.
21. Black with clear-bottom plate can also be used for imaging to monitor the cell death by microscope in addition to measuring luminescence.
22. It is important to use a control ADC that does not to bind the target cells as a negative control in order to quantitate any nonspecific ADC activity that may result either due to target antigen-independent pinocytic uptake of the ADC or linker instability, which can release free drug from the antibody into the growth medium.
23. ADC incubation with cells can vary from 3 to 7 days depending on the cell line's rate of cell proliferation, drug resistance, target copy number, target internalization, and other factors could influence its cell death properties. Therefore, it is important to determine the ADC incubation period to achieve an optimal cell-killing curve for each given ADC and cell line.

References

1. Reichert RM (2012) Marketed therapeutic antibodies compendium. MAbs 4:413–415
2. Reichert JM, Dhimolea E (2012) The future of antibodies as cancer drugs. Drug Discov Today
3. Beck A, Haeuw JF, Wurch T, Goetsch L, Bailly C, Corvaia N (2011) The next generation of antibody–drug conjugates comes of age. Discov Med 10:329–339
4. Carter PJ, Senter PD (2008) Antibody–drug conjugates for cancer therapy. Cancer J 14:154–169
5. Polakis P (2005) Arming antibodies for cancer therapy. Curr Opin Pharmacol 5:382–387
6. Doronina SO, Toki BE, Torgov MY, Mendelsohn BA, Cerveny CG, Chace DF, DeBlanc RL, Gearing RP, Bovee TD, Siegall CB,

Francisco JA, Wahl AF, Meyer DL, Senter PD (2003) Development of potent monoclonal antibody auristatin conjugates for cancer therapy. Nat Biotechnol 21:778–784

7. Fossella F, McCann J, Tolcher A, Xie H, Hwang LL, Carr C, Berg K, Fram R (2005) Phase II trial of BB-10901 (huN901-DM1) given weekly for four consecutive weeks every 6 weeks in patients with relapsed SCLC and CD56-positive small cell carcinoma. J Clin Oncol 23:660S
8. Francisco JA, Cerveny CG, Meyer DL, Mixan BJ, Klussman K, Chace DF, Rejniak SX, Gordon KA, DeBlanc R, Toki BE, Law CL, Doronina SO, Siegall CB, Senter PD, Wahl AF (2003) cAC10-vcMMAE, an anti-CD30-monomethyl auristatin E conjugate with potent and selective antitumor activity. Blood 102:1458–1465
9. Helft PR, Schilsky RL, Hoke FJ, Williams D, Kindler HL, Sprague E, DeWitte M, Martino HK, Erickson J, Pandite L, Russo M, Lambert JM, Howard M, Ratain MJ (2004) A phase I study of cantuzumab mertansine administered as a single intravenous infusion once weekly in patients with advanced solid tumors. Clin Cancer Res 10:4363–4368
10. Henry MD, Wen SH, Silva MD, Chandra S, Milton M, Worland PJ (2004) A prostate-specific membrane antigen-targeted monoclonal antibody-chemotherapeutic conjugate designed for the treatment of prostate cancer. Cancer Res 64:7995–8001
11. Liu CN, Tadayoni BM, Bourret LA, Mattocks KM, Derr SM, Widdison WC, Kedersha NL, Ariniello PD, Goldmacher VS, Lambert JM, Blattler WA, Chari RVJ (1996) Eradication of large colon tumor xenografts by targeted delivery of maytansinoids. Proc Natl Acad Sci U S A 93:8618–8623
12. Naito K, Takeshita A, Shigeno K, Nakamura S, Fujisawa S, Shinjo K, Yoshida H, Ohnishi K, Mori M, Terakawa S, Ohno R (2000) Calicheamicin-conjugated humanized anti-CD33 monoclonal antibody (gemtuzumab zogamicin, CMA-676) shows cytocidal effect on CD33-positive leukemia cell lines, but is inactive on P-glycoprotein-expressing sublines. Leukemia 14:1436–1443
13. Phillips GDL, Li GM, Dugger DL, Crocker LM, Parsons KL, Mai E, Blattler WA, Lambert JM, Chari RVJ, Lutz RJ, Wong WLT, Jacobson FS, Koeppen H, Schwall RH, Kenkare-Mitra SR, Spencer SD, Sliwkowski MX (2008) Targeting HER2-positive breast cancer with trastuzumab–DM1, an antibody–cytotoxic drug conjugate. Cancer Res 68:9280–9290
14. Polson AG, Calemine-Fenaux J, Chan P, Chang W, Christensen E, Clark S, de Sauvage FJ, Eaton D, Elkins K, Elliott JM, Frantz G, Fuji RN, Gray A, Harden K, Ingle GS, Kljavin NM, Koeppen H, Nelson C, Prabhu S, Raab H, Ross S, Stephan JP, Scales SJ, Spencer SD, Vandlen R, Wranik B, Yu SF, Zheng B, Ebens A (2009) Antibody–drug conjugates for the treatment of non-Hodgkin's lymphoma: target and linker-drug selection. Cancer Res 69:2358–2364
15. Tse KF, Jeffers M, Pollack VA, McCabe DA, Shadish ML, Khramtsov NV, Hackett CS, Shenoy SG, Kuang B, Boldog FL, MacDougall JR, Rastelli L, Herrmann J, Gallo M, Gazit-Bornstein G, Senter PD, Meyer DL, Lichenstein HS, LaRochelle WJ (2006) CR011, a fully human monoclonal antibody–auristatin E conjugate, for the treatment of melanoma. Clin Cancer Res 12:1373–1382
16. Hamblett KJ, Senter PD, Chace DF, Sun MM, Lenox J, Cerveny CG, Kissler KM, Bernhardt SX, Kopcha AK, Zabinski RF, Meyer DL, Francisco JA (2004) Effects of drug loading on the antitumor activity of a monoclonal antibody drug conjugate. Clin Cancer Res 10:7063–7070
17. Junutula JR, Flagella KM, Graham RA, Parsons KL, Ha E, Raab H, Bhakta S, Nguyen T, Dugger DL, Li G, Mai E, Lewis Phillips GD, Hiraragi H, Fuji RN, Tibbitts J, Vandlen R, Spencer SD, Scheller RH, Polakis P, Sliwkowski MX (2010) Engineered thio-trastuzumab–DM1 conjugate with an improved therapeutic index to target human epidermal growth factor receptor 2-positive breast cancer. Clin Cancer Res 16:4769–4778
18. Junutula JR, Raab H, Clark S, Bhakta S, Leipold DD, Weir S, Chen Y, Simpson M, Tsai SP, Dennis MS, Lu YM, Meng YG, Ng C, Yang JH, Lee CC, Duenas E, Gorrell J, Katta V, Kim A, McDorman K, Flagella K, Venook R, Ross S, Spencer SD, Wong WL, Lowman HB, Vandlen R, Sliwkowski MX, Scheller RH, Polakis P, Mallet W (2008) Site-specific conjugation of a cytotoxic drug to an antibody improves the therapeutic index. Nat Biotechnol 26:925–932
19. Wang L, Amphlett G, Blattler WA, Lambert JM, Zhang W (2005) Structural characterization of the maytansinoid–monoclonal antibody immunoconjugate, huN901-DM1, by mass spectrometry. Protein Sci 14:2436–2446

20. Junutula JR, Bhakta S, Raab H, Ervin KE, Eigenbrot C, Vandlen R, Scheller RH, Lowman HB (2008) Rapid identification of reactive cysteine residues for site-specific labeling of antibody-Fabs. J Immunol Methods 332:41–52

21. Tinianow JN, Gill HS, Ogasawara A, Flores JE, Vanderbilt AN, Luis E, Vandlen R, Darwish M, Junutula JR, Williams SP, Marik J (2010) Site-specifically 89Zr-labeled monoclonal antibodies for ImmunoPET. Nucl Med Biol 37:289–297

Chapter 12

Enzymatic Antibody Modification by Bacterial Transglutaminase

Patrick Dennler, Roger Schibli, and Eliane Fischer

Abstract

Enzymatic posttranslational modification of proteins permits more precise control over conjugation site than chemical modification of reactive amino acid side chains. Ideally, protein modification by an enzyme yields completely homogeneous conjugates with improved properties for research or therapeutic use. As an example, we here provide a protocol for bacterial transglutaminase (BTGase)-mediated conjugation of cadaverine-derivatized substrates to an IgG1, resulting in stable bond formation between glutamine 295 of the antibody heavy chain and the substrate. This procedure requires enzymatic removal of N-linked glycans from the antibody and yields a defined substrate/antibody ratio of 2:1. Alternatively, a mutant aglycosylated IgG1 variant may be generated by site-directed mutagenesis. The mutation introduces an additional glutamine and yields a substrate/antibody ratio of 4:1 after coupling. Finally, we describe an ESI-TOF mass spectrometry-based method to analyze the uniformity of the resulting conjugates. The presented approach allows the facile generation of homogeneous antibody conjugates and can be applied to any IgG1 and a wide range of cadaverine-derivatized substrates.

Key words Bacterial transglutaminase, BTGase, Site specific, Stoichiometric, Antibody–drug conjugates, Enzymatic conjugation, Mass spectrometry, Antibody conjugation, Antibody modification

1 Introduction

Conventional approaches for coupling small molecules to monoclonal antibodies are based on chemical modification of lysine or cysteine residues, which typically yields heterogeneous products. In contrast, precise control over stoichiometry and conjugation sites gives rise to homogenous preparations with reduced batch-to-batch variation and favorable properties. Notably, optimization of drug load and the exclusive use of conjugation sites which do not impair targeting properties or stability have been shown to improve the therapeutic index of antibody–drug conjugates [1, 2].

An elegant approach to reduce heterogeneity of antibody conjugates is site-specific linkage of substrates by enzymatic conjugation. Enzymes are restrictive in the acceptance of conjugation

Laurent Ducry (ed.), *Antibody-Drug Conjugates*, Methods in Molecular Biology, vol. 1045,
DOI 10.1007/978-1-62703-541-5_12, © Springer Science+Business Media, LLC 2013

sites as they usually require a consensus sequence or are influenced by the tertiary structure of the protein. In addition to site specificity, enzymatic conjugation has the advantage of being performed at physiological pH, temperature, and ionic strength, thus allowing mild reaction conditions. A variety of enzymes can potentially be used to form stable bonds between defined sites on a protein and a drug derivative [3]. In many cases, the specificity of the enzyme requires introduction of a peptidic tag or mutation to the native antibody sequence prior to the conjugation step [4]. While introduction of such tags allows exact control over the conjugation site, it precludes direct modification of native antibodies and requires time-consuming recombinant engineering of the antibody sequence. In some cases, however, antibodies can be directly used for enzymatic conjugation without prior recombinant engineering. For example, glycosyltransferases have been used to modify the N-linked glycans on the Fc part of IgGs with sugar analogs [5, 6] resulting in relatively uniform conjugates.

We recently described an approach for enzymatic modification of antibodies at a defined conjugation site using bacterial transglutaminase (BTGase) from *Streptomyces mobaraensis* [7]. Transglutaminases (TGase) are a large family of enzymes (EC 2.3.2.13) that catalyze the covalent cross-linking of Gln- and Lys-containing peptides or proteins by formation of an isopeptide bond. There are eight different TGases in mammals (e.g., factor XIIIa), but also lower organisms such as algae, fungi, or bacteria express TGases. The advantage of using BTGase instead of mammalian TGases is its robustness, Ca^{2+} independency, and high reaction rate. But most importantly, BTGase has a low substrate specificity and can therefore accept a wide range of lysine-containing substrates [8, 9]. It even accepts 5-aminopentyl groups and can therefore be used to couple cadaverine-derivatized entities to an antibody.

On the other hand, BTGase is much more selective towards the protein-bound Gln residues. Both protein chain flexibility and neighboring amino acids influence if a particular Gln can be modified by TGases [10]. Antibodies generally lack such a site and are not efficiently modifiable by BTGase. However, after removal of the carbohydrate moiety, a unique conjugation site is exposed that allows attaching exactly one substrate to each heavy chain at amino acid Q295 (Fig. 1 top lane). By site-directed mutagenesis, we introduced an additional Gln-residue at position 297 (N297Q) [11], resulting in an aglycosylated variant of the antibody which can then be modified with exactly two substrates per heavy chain (Fig. 1 bottom lane).

In this chapter, the enzymatic conjugation of cadaverine-derivatized molecules, including biotin–cadaverine, to a monoclonal antibody is described [7]. The protocol includes deglycosylation of the antibody heavy chain by the enzyme PNGase F and

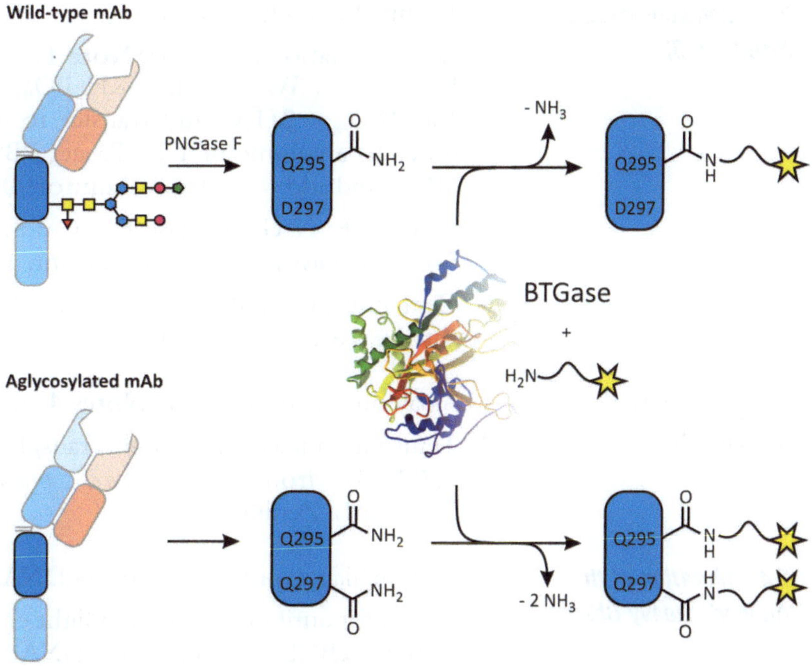

Fig. 1 Conjugation of cadaverine-derivatized substrates to an IgG1 (*top*) and an aglycosylated variant (*bottom*). Data for crystal structure of BTGase from Protein Data Bank, Research Collaboratory for Structural Bioinformatics, Rutgers University, New Brunswick, www.rcsb.org, code 1IU4, processed with Molsoft ICM-Browser

subsequent modification by BTGase. We then outline the generation of a mutant variant (N297Q) of the antibody heavy chain by site-directed mutagenesis that can be used to couple exactly four substrates. In addition, a protocol for mass spectrometric identification of the conjugates is provided.

2 Materials

All buffers and solutions were prepared by using Millipore water unless indicated otherwise.

2.1 Antibodies and Substrates

1. Antibody solution: Antibody in PBS 1× or Tris–HCl, stored at −20 °C in 1.5–3 mg/mL stock solutions (10–20 mM, pH 7.0–7.4).
2. EZ-Link® Pentylamine–Biotin (biotin–cadaverine as white powder, Pierce), 10 mM in PBS 1×, store aliquots at −20 °C (*see* **Note 1**).
3. Cadaverine-derivatized substrates (*see* **Note 2**).

2.2 Deglycosylation (See Note 3)

1. 1.5 mL Eppendorf tubes.
2. Deglycosylation buffer (*see* **Note 4**):
   PBS (10×): Weigh 2.1 g KH_2PO_4, 90 g NaCl, and 4.8 g $Na_2HPO_4 \times 2H_2O$ and transfer to a 1 L glass bottle. Add water to a volume of 1 L. To get PBS 1×, use 100 mL PBS (10×) and add water to a volume of 900 mL. Adjust pH to 7.2.
3. PNGase F: *N*-Glycosidase F (EC 3.5.1.52) from *Flavobacterium meningosepticum*, recombinant, 1,000 U/mL, Roche.
4. Centrifugal ultrafiltration: Vivaspin 500, 50 kDa MWCO PES, Sartorius Stedim Biotech.

2.3 Enzymatic Conjugation

1. Assay buffer: PBS 1× (*see* **Notes 4** and **5**).
2. Transglutaminase: Bacterial Transglutaminase (BTGase, EC 2.3.2.13) from *Streptomyces mobaraensis*, recombinant, 50 U/mL, Zedira.

2.4 Mutation of the Antibody Heavy Chain

1. Mammalian expression vector pcDNA3.1+, Invitrogen.
2. cDNA for antibody heavy and light chains (we used cDNA for chimeric chCE7 antibody in pcDNA3.1+).
3. Restriction enzymes: *Hind*III and *Bam*HI, Fermentas.
4. Pfu DNA polymerase, Fermentas.
5. *E. coli* strain XL1-Blue.
6. Ampicillin (Amp), Sigma-Aldrich.
7. Primers, Microsynth (*see* **Note 6**):

   Primer 1: (5′-GCTGGCTAGCGTTTAAACTTAAGC-3′).

   Primer 2: (5′-CACCCGGTACGTGCTTTGGTACTGCTCCTCCC-3′).

   Primer 3: (5′-GGGAGGAGCAGTACCAAAGCACGTACCGGGTG-3′).

   Primer 4: (5′-GCGGATCCTCATTTACCCGGAGACAGG-GAGAG-3′).

2.5 Analysis by Mass Spectrometry

1. Guan-buffer: 7.5 M Guanidine–HCl, 0.1 M Tris–HCl, and 1 mM EDTA buffer pH 8.5. Weigh 0.3152 g of Tris–HCl (Sigma) and transfer to a glass vial. Add 18.75 mL of 8 M Guanidine–HCl (Pierce) followed by 40 μL of 0.5 M EDTA (Fisher). Adjust the pH to 8.5 by addition of concentrated NH_4OH (28 % aqueous solution). Add water to a final volume of 20 mL (*see* **Note 5**).
2. Reducing agent: 1 M DTT. Weigh 0.1543 g DTT, transfer it to a 1.5 mL Eppendorf vial, and dissolve it in 1 mL of 50 mM NH_4HCO_3.

3. Column: POROS 10 R1 60 mm × 1 mm, Dr. Maisch GmbH, Spherical Polystyrenedivinylbenzene.
4. Mass spectrometer: Waters Micromass LCT Premier (LC-ESI-TOF).
5. LC parameters: Acetonitrile + 0.1 % formic acid (solvent A), water + 0.1 % formic acid (solvent B), and isopropanol (solvent C). Gradient: 0–3 min, 15 % A, 80 % B, 5 % C; 3–20 min, 15 % A to 80 % A, 80 % B to 15 % B, 5 % C; 10 min re-equilibration time. Flow: 0.3 mL/min, column temperature: 25 ± 2 °C.
6. Analyze MS data with MassLynx V4.1. Raw data was deconvoluted with MaxEnt1.

3 Methods

3.1 Deglycosylation of IgG1

1. Incubate the antibody (1 mg) in PBS 1× buffer overnight at 37 °C with 6 U of PNGase F (*see* **Note 7**).
2. Remove the enzyme by ultrafiltration using a Vivaspin column MWCO 50 kDa. Apply the reaction mixture onto the column, and centrifuge at 4,000–6,000 × *g*. Wash three times with buffer (*see* **Note 8**). Resuspend deglycosylated antibody in a suitable volume of buffer for further processing. Analyze deglycosylation by mass spectrometry (*see* **Note 7**).

3.2 Enzymatic Conjugation by BTGase

1. Mix the antibody (final concentration, 1 mg/mL), 60 equivalents of cadaverine-derivatized substrate (biotin–cadaverine), BTGase (final concentration, 1 U/mL), and PBS 1× buffer (*see* **Note 5**). Incubate the reaction mixture at 37 °C overnight (*see* **Note 9**).
2. Remove excess substrate and enzyme by ultrafiltration as described in Subheading 3.1, **step 2**.
3. Under the experimental conditions described here, the coupling reaction was observed to be complete after 4 h.

3.3 Site-Directed Mutagenesis and Preparation of Aglycosylated IgG1

1. The overall cloning procedure is outlined in Fig. 2. Using the cDNA of the antibody heavy chain as template, perform a PCR with the following primer pairs: (a) Primer 1 and Primer 2 and (b) Primer 3 and Primer 4 (1 min 95 °C, 1 min 55 °C, 3 min 68 °C, 20 cycles) (*see* **Note 6**).
2. After gel purification, combine the two primary PCR products and run a second PCR with the flanking primers (Primer 1 and Primer 4) to get the complete, mutated heavy chain including *Bam*HI and *Hind*III restriction sites.
3. Digest the resulting DNA fragment with the restriction enzymes *Bam*HI and *Hind*III (37 °C, 3 h). Gel purify.

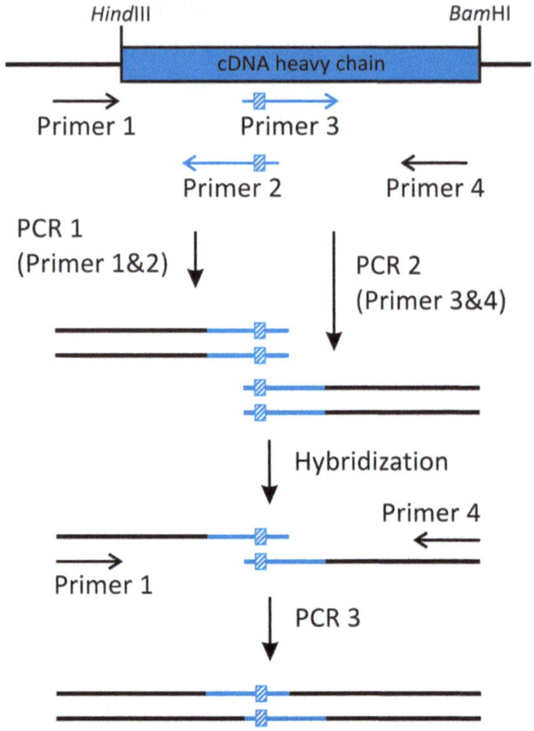

Fig. 2 Introduction of mutation N297Q by site-directed mutagenesis using standard overlapping PCR techniques (*Blue*/*white* stripes, mutation)

4. Clone the mutated cDNA of the heavy chain into the *Hind*III/*Bam*HI site of the pcDNA3.1+ vector (*see* Fig. 3). Transform *E. coli* strain XL1-Blue and select ampicillin-resistant colonies. Purify DNA for transfection of mammalian cells.
5. Express the aglycosylated IgG1 variant in an appropriate mammalian expression system and purify (*see* **Note 10**).

3.4 Quality Control of the Reaction by Mass Spectrometry

1. Mass Spectrometry: Mix 10 μg of antibody and 1M DTT (final concentration, 20 mM) in an MS sample vial. Add Guan-buffer to a volume of 50 μL and incubate the mixture at 70 °C for 30 min. Inject 5 μL (*see* **Note 11**).
2. Process and analyze the data by using appropriate software (e.g., MassLynxV4.1). Usually, two distinct peaks can be detected which correspond to light and heavy chain of the antibody (*see* Fig. 4a). Process the respective raw data (*see* Fig 4 c, d) using MaxEnt1 to get deconvoluted mass spectra of the light (*see* Fig. 4c) and heavy chain (*see* Fig. 4d) (*see* **Note 12**). The expected mass difference between unconjugated and conjugated heavy chain represents the molecular weight of the substrate $MW_{substrate}$ minus 17 Da due to loss of ammonia

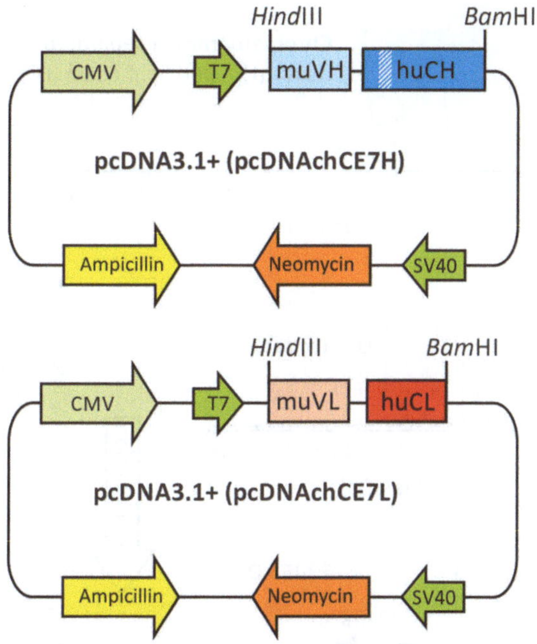

Fig. 3 Expression of an aglycosylated antibody variant (*Blue/white* stripes, mutation). The two vectors are co-transfected into HEK-293 cells

during the conjugation reaction. Accordingly, an increase in mass of 2× ($MW_{substrate}$−17 Da) is expected after conjugation to the mutant aglycosylated heavy chain (*see* **Note 13**).

4 Notes

1. We propose to include biotin–cadaverine as a positive control for the enzymatic reaction conditions. Conjugation with this substrate is usually fast and should result in 100 % modified antibody under the experimental conditions described here. Successful conjugation of biotin–cadaverine results in a mass shift of 311 Da.
2. BTGase accepts a wide range of lysine- or cadaverine-derivatized entities as substrates. For example, we described the synthesis of various cadaverine-derivatized chelators for radiometal labeling [7]. However, not all cadaverine-containing molecules will be conjugated equally well by BTGase. Steric hindrance of bulky molecules and limited solubility may impair the enzymatic reaction. DMSO may be used as a solvent as concentrations up to 5 % in the reaction buffer do not inhibit BTGase catalysis. The active site of the enzyme contains a free cysteine residue, which precludes the coupling of thiol-reactive substrates (e.g., maleimide-functionalized),

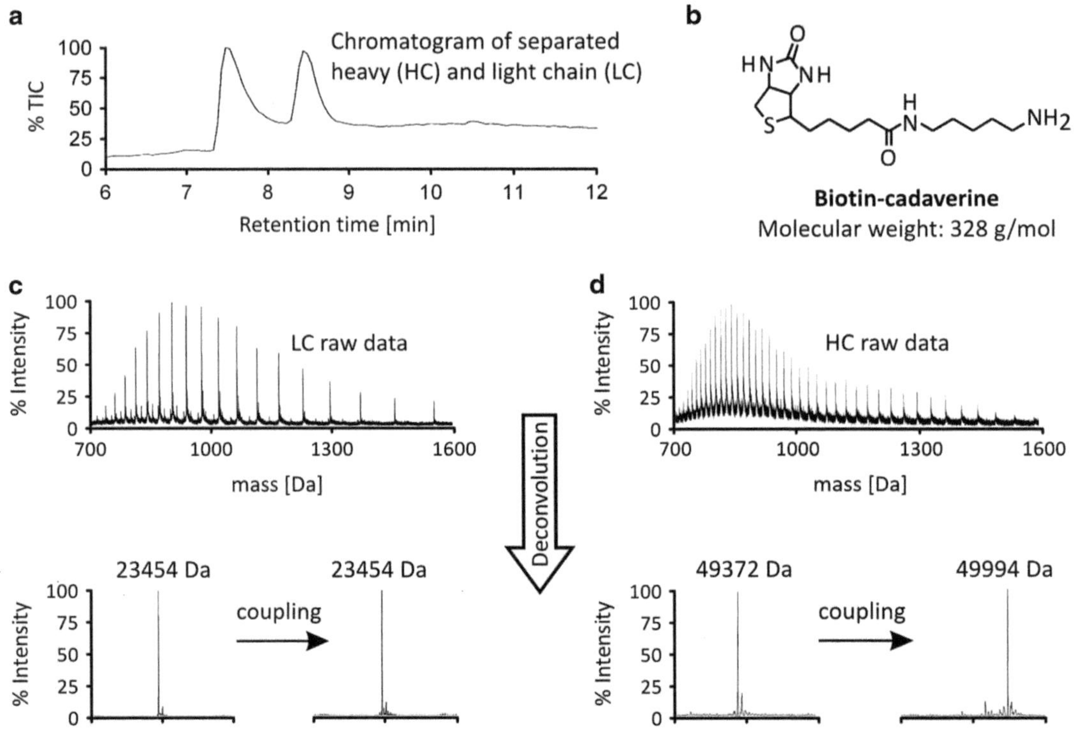

Fig. 4 (**a**) Liquid chromatography of heavy and light chain. (**b**) Chemical structure of biotin–cadaverine. (**c**) Raw data of IgG1 light chain (*top*) and deconvoluted data before (*bottom, left*) and after coupling (*bottom, right*). The light chain remains unaffected. (**d**) Raw data of IgG1 heavy chain (*top*) and deconvoluted data before (*bottom, left*) and after coupling (*bottom, right*). The mass difference between uncoupled and coupled heavy chain is 622 Da which corresponds to two biotin–cadaverine molecules (MW: 328 Da, 2×328 Da $= 656$ Da) attached to the heavy chain by BTGase under the loss of two ammonia molecules (2×17 Da $= 34$ Da) (*see* also Fig. 1)

because they irreversibly inactivate the enzyme. We observed that substrates with two or more terminal amines may result in antibody cross-linking, even at high molar excess of substrates in the reaction mixture.

3. Deglycosylation of antibodies is important if quantitative modification at Q295 is attempted. However, upon recombinant introduction of the mutation Q297N, it is not necessary.
4. Alternatively, 40 mM Tris–HCl pH 7.0 (40 mM Tris–HCl, pH 7.0: Weigh 4.85 g Trizma® base and add water to a volume of 900 mL. Adjust pH with 1 M HCl to 7.0) can be used for storage, deglycosylation, and conjugation with BTGase. The following buffers are not recommended to use with BTGase conjugation:
   (a) 0.2 M Na_2HPO_4/NaH_2PO_4 pH 6 or 7.
   (b) 0.1 M Citric acid/Na_2HPO_4 pH 6 or 7.
   (c) 0.2 M Imidazole–HCl pH 7.

Buffering capacity: Depending on the substrate, pH in the assay may rise/drop. We observed a decline in enzymatic activity at pH below 6 and above 8.

5. Reducing metal contamination to a minimum is essential if transition metal chelators (e.g., DOTA) are being coupled to antibodies. Thus, metal-free tools (e.g., spatula and bottles for storage) for the preparation of required buffers and solutions as well as potassium-free PBS 1× buffer for the conjugation assay are recommended.
6. We describe the expression of recombinant antibody by co-transfection of heavy and light chain on two separate pcDNA3.1 plasmids. If the antibody sequence is cloned into a different vector or if other restriction enzymes are used, the sequences of the flanking primers (Primers 1 and 4) need to be adjusted accordingly. The mutagenic primers (Primers 2 and 3) and the flanking Primer 4 are specific for the human IgG1 sequence. Their sequence needs to be modified if other isotypes are used.
7. The kinetics of deglycosylation may vary for each antibody preparation, depending on isotype, producing cell line, etc. For example, murine isotypes IgG2a and IgG2b need extended reaction time and/or increased PNGase F concentration. The conditions need to be evaluated in case other isotypes are used. Deglycosylation of antibodies may affect their stability and some deglycosylated antibodies are prone to aggregation.
8. This centrifugation step allows a buffer change. The centrifugation time needs to be adjusted individually and depends on the antibody concentration, the speed of the centrifuge, and the volume loaded into the tube.
9. The efficiency and kinetics of the conjugation reaction are strongly influenced by the structure of the substrate, the BTGase concentration, the pH value of the reaction mixture, and the incubation time. To achieve complete conversion, the optimal conditions need to be evaluated for each case.
10. Affinity purification on Protein A or Protein G sepharose columns is usually not impaired by the aglycosylated Fc part.
11. Adjust injection volume to your MS System. Treatment with Guan-buffer and DTT reduces the antibody to heavy and light chains which can then be analyzed separately (e.g., no. of substrates conjugated to light and heavy chain). The isopeptide bond introduced by BTGase is stable under the described conditions (reducing conditions, 70 °C and slightly basic pH). However, the integrity of the coupled molecule needs to be verified after sample treatment, as unstable chemical entities may give rise to additional mass peaks in the spectrum. Mass spectrometry allows the estimation of modified and

unmodified portion of deglycosylated antibody in the reaction mixture, particularly with regard to completeness of the reaction. Due to mass heterogeneity of glycosylated antibodies, other methods should be considered for such cases. Depending on the substrate, the reaction may also be qualitatively assessed by other approaches, including SDS-PAGE, fluorimetry, immunoassays, or radiodetection.

12. The retention times of heavy and light chain depend on the column, the conjugated molecules, and the individual antibody sequence. It is therefore not possible to predict which of the two peaks corresponds to heavy and light chain, and in some cases, they may even co-elute. Nevertheless, heavy and light chain can be identified by looking at the distribution of the charged states (peaks) of the raw data. The mass difference between the individual peaks of the heavy chain is smaller compared to the light chain (*see* Fig. 4b).
13. In principle, the variable regions of an antibody may contain additional conjugation sites that are recognized by BTGase. Modification of such a site may impair the antibodies binding ability. We strongly suggest functional testing of the antibody after conjugation, especially if more than the expected numbers of attached moieties are detected by mass spectrometry.

Acknowledgement

This work was supported by the Swiss National Foundation (SNF, Grant Nr 132611).

References

1. Junutula JR, Flagella KM, Graham RA, Parsons KL, Ha E, Raab H, Bhakta S, Nguyen T, Dugger DL, Li G, Mai E, Lewis Phillips GD, Hiraragi H, Fuji RN, Tibbitts J, Vandlen R, Spencer SD, Scheller RH, Polakis P, Sliwkowski MX (2010) Engineered thio-trastuzumab-DM1 conjugate with an improved therapeutic index to target human epidermal growth factor receptor 2-positive breast cancer. Clin Cancer Res 16(19):4769–4778
2. Junutula JR, Raab H, Clark S, Bhakta S, Leipold DD, Weir S, Chen Y, Simpson M, Tsai SP, Dennis MS, Lu Y, Meng YG, Ng C, Yang J, Lee CC, Duenas E, Gorrell J, Katta V, Kim A, McDorman K, Flagella K, Venook R, Ross S, Spencer SD, Lee WW, Lowman HB, Vandlen R, Sliwkowski MX, Scheller RH, Polakis P, Mallet W (2008) Site-specific conjugation of a cytotoxic drug to an antibody improves the therapeutic index. Nat Biotechnol 26(8):925–932
3. Sunbul M, Yin J (2009) Site specific protein labeling by enzymatic posttranslational modification. Org Biomol Chem 7(17):3361–3371
4. Rabuka D (2010) Chemoenzymatic methods for site-specific protein modification. Curr Opin Chem Biol 14(6):790–796
5. Boeggeman E, Ramakrishnan B, Pasek M, Manzoni M, Puri A, Loomis KH, Waybright TJ, Qasba PK (2009) Site specific conjugation of fluoroprobes to the remodeled Fc N-glycans of monoclonal antibodies using mutant glycosyltransferases: application for cell surface antigen detection. Bioconjug Chem 20(6): 1228–1236
6. Solomon B, Koppel R, Schwartz F, Fleminger G (1990) Enzymic oxidation of monoclonal antibodies by soluble and immobilized bifunctional enzyme complexes. J Chromatogr 510: 321–329

7. Jeger S, Zimmermann K, Blanc A, Grunberg J, Honer M, Hunziker P, Struthers H, Schibli R (2010) Site-specific and stoichiometric modification of antibodies by bacterial transglutaminase. Angew Chem Int Ed Engl 49(51): 9995–9997
8. Mindt TL, Jungi V, Wyss S, Friedli A, Pla G, Novak-Hofer I, Grunberg J, Schibli R (2008) Modification of different IgG1 antibodies via glutamine and lysine using bacterial and human tissue transglutaminase. Bioconjug Chem 19 (1):271–278
9. Mehta K, Eckert R (2005) Transglutaminases: family of enzymes with diverse functions, vol 38. Progress in experimental tumor research. Karger, Basel
10. Fontana A, Spolaore B, Mero A, Veronese FM (2008) Site-specific modification and PEGylation of pharmaceutical proteins mediated by transglutaminase. Adv Drug Deliv Rev 60 (1):13–28
11. Knogler K, Grünberg J, Novak-Hofer I, Zimmermann K, Schubiger PA (2006) Evaluation of 177Lu-DOTA-labeled aglycosylated monoclonal anti-L1-CAM antibody chCE7: influence of the number of chelators on the in vitro and in vivo properties. Nucl Med Biol 33(7):883–889

Chapter 13

Formulation Development of Antibody–Drug Conjugates

William J. Galush and Aditya A. Wakankar

Abstract

Formulation development of an ADC resembles that of a conventional antibody, but the conjugated form introduces new molecular attributes such as drug-to-antibody ratio and stability of the drug itself that need to be considered. An extended set of analytical tools, coupled with understanding of how ADCs and conventional antibodies differ in terms of their stability, guides formulation selection.

Key words Quality attributes, Physical stability, Chemical stability, Stability-indicated methods, Biophysical characterization

1 Introduction

Formulation development of antibody–drug conjugates (ADCs) aims to ensure that stable, high-quality products are dosed to patients. Though this goal is common to all pharmaceutical formulations, ADCs present a unique set of physicochemical properties that can impact safety, quality, and efficacy as compared to traditional therapeutic proteins. While there is a body of literature that outlines which product attributes affect the safety, quality, and efficacy for conventional, unconjugated monoclonal antibodies (mAbs) [1], an understanding of attributes important to ADCs is only now emerging.

Quality attributes of ADCs can be broken down into three categories. These include those associated with (1) the antibody–small molecule conjugate form, (2) the small molecule drug moiety, and (3) the antibody itself. Table 1 lists attributes and their potential clinical impact on the ADC, as well as a categorization within this scheme. For instance, the drug-to-antibody ratio (DAR) is considered to be a quality attribute unique to an ADC. A high DAR could potentially affect the safety profile of the ADC, whereas a low DAR could lead to decrease in efficacy. Similarly, the release of free drug species is another attribute that affects safety and bioactivity. In addition to these ADC- and drug-specific attributes,

Laurent Ducry (ed.), *Antibody-Drug Conjugates*, Methods in Molecular Biology, vol. 1045,
DOI 10.1007/978-1-62703-541-5_13, © Springer Science+Business Media, LLC 2013

Table 1
Quality attributes specific for ADCs

Attribute	Impact	Category	Applicable analytical techniques
Aggregates	Immunogenicity Pharmacokinetics Potency	mAb, conjugate	• Size-exclusion chromatography • CE-SDS • Analytical ultracentrifugation
Charge variants	Pharmacokinetics Potency Safety	mAb, conjugate	• Ion exchange chromatography • Isoelectric focusing
Chemical stability of conjugated drug	Potency Pharmacokinetics Safety	Drug	• Depends on the mechanism of degradation[a]
Cross-linked species	Immunogenicity Pharmacokinetics	mAb, conjugate	• CE-SDS
Drug-to-antibody ratio (low, high)	Potency Pharmacokinetics Safety	Conjugate	• Absorption spectrophotometry • Hydrophobic interaction chromatography • Reversed-phase chromatography • Mass spectrometry
Drug distribution	Potency Pharmacokinetics Safety	Conjugate	• Mass spectrometry • Hydrophobic interaction chromatography with capillary electrophoresis or reversed-phase HPLC • Imaged capillary isoelectric focusing
Free drug	Safety	Drug	• Reversed-phase chromatography

[a]In certain cases a functionality assay may be used as a surrogate measure

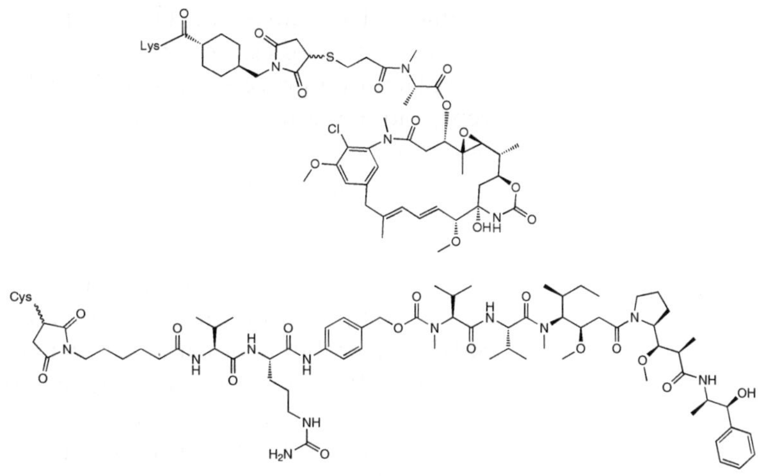

Fig. 1 (*Top*) Maytansinoid DM1 conjugated to a lysine residue. (*Bottom*) The auristatin analog vcMMAE conjugated to a cysteine residue

there are also those that are intrinsic to the mAb portion of the molecule. These attributes—such as aggregates, fragments, charge heterogeneities, and chemical instabilities such as deamidation and oxidation—can affect clinical aspects such as bioactivity, immunogenicity, pharmacokinetics, and safety.

Each of these quality attributes may be affected by process parameters of ADC manufacturing. Each may also change over the shelf life of the product. An understanding of attributes that are inherited from ADC manufacturing and those that are important to assess during formulation development is important. Formulation strategies for ADCs should include a fundamental understanding of both the ADC-specific and mAb-related attributes. The following sections discuss various ADC-related attributes and formulation parameters that must be considered to attain a desirable drug product profile, highlighted with examples from ADCs utilizing maytansinoid- and auristatin-based toxins, two prominent examples of the toxins and linkage chemistries currently in development across the biopharmaceutical industry [2]. Chemical structures of these two molecules are shown in Fig. 1. Pathways of ADC degradation are discussed in the sections below, along with an overview of analytical technique interpretation in the context of formulation studies.

2 Process Considerations for ADC Quality Attributes

Classes of antibody–drug conjugates vary based on the sites of conjugation and drug–linker combination used. In typical examples, conjugation of a cytotoxin occurs at either disulfide-derived or engineered cysteines [3, 4] or naturally occurring lysine [5, 6] residues. Regardless of the site of conjugation, the ADC manufacturing process exposes the mAb to pH, temperature, solvent, and physical stresses that may alter the physicochemical attributes of the mAb.

The conjugation process in the case of the ADC T-DM1 (trastuzumab emtansine) results in generation of intermediates such as T-MCC [7]. This intermediate is an activated form of the mAb intended for conjugation to the cytotoxic drug DM1 and is composed of the trastuzumab antibody modified with a SMCC heterobifunctional linker. A free maleimide group remains on the SMCC once it is conjugated to a lysine residue. Studies have demonstrated that this activated form of the mAb can react with other T-MCC molecules depending on the process hold times, which can result in formation of intermolecular cross-linked species. Such changes to product quality mean that these cross-linked species are an attribute that needs to be monitored and controlled during the conjugation process. Process control of the cross-linked forms was achieved in case of T-DM1. However, if these species are not controlled during conjugation, then the activated forms may be present in the final drug product and may represent a formulation stability challenge that needs to be minimized during process development efforts. As shown in Table 1, cross-linked species may impact immunogenicity and pharmacokinetics of the conjugate.

The conjugation process may also drive certain types of protein degradation. For instance, aggregation may be driven by the conjugation process conditions, and, depending on size, these may not be removed by downstream steps such as filtration. Depending on their physicochemical nature, aggregates may catalyze the growth of yet more aggregated species in stored drug substance or drug product.

Another class of process-related impurities includes those related to the small molecule drug itself. The drug may be added to the antibody conjugation mixture by first solubilizing it in organic solvents. Sufficient clearance of these solvents during processing needs to be demonstrated from both a product stability and safety standpoint. Remaining unconjugated drugs are also a potential concern, given the high potency and toxicity of ADC cytotoxins of the maytansine, auristatin, and calicheamicin families as compared to standard chemotherapeutics [3, 5, 8]. The final formulated drug product may inherit some of the process-related quality attributes discussed above. Knowledge of process-related quality attributes, their impacts, and levels helps define product quality expectations for formulation development.

3 Considerations for ADC Formulation Development

The choice of formulation has the potential to affect all categories of ADC quality attributes. Because conjugation of an ADC requires an unconjugated antibody as an intermediate, the formulation development process for a conjugate necessarily involves formulating a mAb at some stage, likely as an intermediate for manufacturing of the final ADC form. The formulation optimization for the antibody portion of the ADC follows a similar course to that of an unconjugated antibody and therefore can leverage the biotechnology industry's considerable experience developing this class of molecule. Many examples of successful commercial antibody formulations, both liquid and lyophilized, have been reported [9–11]. However, the complexity of the formulation development process potentially increases when quality attributes of the small molecule drug and those of the conjugated form are taken into account.

The formulation development process for an ADC requires an understanding of what modes of instability are intrinsic to the molecule and which are influenced by the choice of formulation components. The design of a formulation screen is determined by the known physical and chemical attributes of the ADC coupled to how formulation parameters such as pH, buffering species, and excipients may affect molecule attributes. Many of these attributes are discussed below, but the list may not be exhaustive and depends on the ADC technology platform used.

3.1 Physical Stability

Monoclonal antibodies are typically susceptible to noncovalent aggregation upon storage. Aggregation is driven by the minimization of free energy achieved when antibodies come into close contact—for instance, at relatively hydrophobic sites on the molecules. Dimerization may be thought of as the first step in aggregation, and sometimes the process proceeds no further. Dimers may be reversible [12] or not, but growth can lead to larger and larger oligomers and even potentially insoluble particulates, as time progresses [11]. Because ADCs are decorated with one or more small molecule drug moieties, they have a different set of biophysical properties compared with the unconjugated antibody, leading to new or altered intermolecular interactions. An antibody that exhibits acceptable aggregation behavior in its unconjugated form may have different physical behavior in its conjugated form, either because of changes in surface properties such as hydrophobicity due to drug attachment or because the drugs have altered the higher-order structure of the antibody such that new modes of antibody–antibody interactions are possible. These factors could contribute to a substantially different propensity for aggregation. This effect is most readily observed in a formulation screen designed to test both conjugated and unconjugated forms in parallel and subjected to the same assays. Such a study does not automatically reveal the exact cause of the effect; only that it is related to the conjugated form or conjugation process. The degree to which the molecule has been physically altered by conjugation may be assessed by techniques such as differential scanning calorimetry (DSC) [7], with physical perturbations manifested as changes (likely decreases) in the onset of melting or melting temperature, T_m, of the conjugated mAb as compared to the unconjugated antibody. This decrease in thermodynamic stability may translate to a decreased colloidal stability of the conjugate compared to an unconjugated antibody. Consequences of aggregates, covalent or not, can include a variety of safety and efficacy effects, as mentioned in Table 1.

3.2 Chemical Stability

Part of ADC chemical stability is inherited from the unconjugated antibody. For instance, if the unconjugated antibody is susceptible to deamidation or isomerization with known pH dependence, this degradation mode is also likely to be present in the ADC. These types of degradations may impact product potency, especially if the affected residues are found in the complementarity-determining region. Much has been learned through years of experience with unconjugated antibodies about the susceptibility of various amino acid residues to chemical degradations, allowing substantial insights to be gained from examination of the protein primary sequence alone, coupled to available information about local solvent exposure and flexibility [13, 14]. It may be expected that most chemical modifications to the primary sequence of the unconjugated antibody will also occur in the ADC form.

Fragmentation is another possible chemical degradation pathway for ADCs, driven by the breakage of covalent bonds between chains or within the peptide backbone. The altered physical state of the molecule following addition of the small molecule drug may result in some differences in the susceptibility of the ADC to fragmentation, but the fundamental susceptibility of the ADC to fragmentation is likely derived mostly from the mAb. A common unconjugated antibody degradation mode involves breaking of the heavy chain peptide NOT heavy chain-peptide backbone near the hinge region, leading to free F_{ab} and F_{ab} + F_c products [15]. This is still a feasible degradation pathway for ADCs as well. Comparison of fragmentation rates between conjugated and unconjugated antibodies can reveal whether the ADC form has different stability towards fragmentation.

Some antibody conjugation methods rely on linking drugs to interchain disulfides [4], which disrupts particular covalent bonds holding the antibody quaternary structure together. This can, in principle, affect the propensity to fragment into heavy chain + light chain fragments, or individual free chains, but significant noncovalent interactions still hold together antibodies in standard aqueous buffers. With covalent interchain bonds broken, however, fragmentation is readily driven under denaturing conditions such as in the presence of SDS [16]. Thus, some fragmentation assays that apply to an unconjugated antibody, such as SDS-PAGE or CE-SDS, are not useful for assessing fragmentation of molecules with purposefully disrupted interchain disulfides. A non-denaturing technique, such as size-exclusion HPLC (SE-HPLC), remains the primary tool to detect ADC fragmentation in stability studies and though the presence of aggregating fragments can confound accurate quantification.

Conjugation adds a new set of chemical properties on the resulting ADC molecule that leads to new possible routes of chemical degradation specific to the drug and conjugate. The exact chemical degradation products depend on the drug being used, but some insights can be gathered by the examination of non-therapeutic examples of bioconjugation using similar chemistries. For instance, succinimido rings similar to that left from the reaction of a maleimide linker with the free thiol of a cysteine have long been known to be capable of opening via aminolysis [17] and hydrolysis in a pH-dependent manner [18–20]. Interestingly, antibodies modified with similarly altered forms of linked drugs have been shown to possess different in vivo stability and activity compared to intact succinimido forms [20]. Degradation pathways such as these should be examined and controlled in a manner appropriate to the developmental phase of the ADC.

The covalent bonds linking drugs to antibodies may be broken by a variety of mechanisms over the shelf life of the product and under stressed storage conditions. One example of bond breakage that can happen is where the drug moiety is bound to the protein. Disulfides, hydrazones, and thioethers have all been used to link drugs and antibodies for preclinical or clinical ADCs [2], and each has different intrinsic stabilities in formulation conditions as well as in vivo (hydrazone linkers were also used for the first FDA-approved ADC, gemtuzumab ozogamicin, which has subsequently been withdrawn from the market, though not on account of hydrazone stability). Reactive linkers may also undergo side reactions during the conjugation process, leading to unstable covalent bonds to the antibody. For instance, one study has shown that lysine-reactive succinimidyl esters may also form bonds to several other residue side chains, including cysteine and tyrosine [19]. Being chemically labile, drugs conjugated to these residues quickly hydrolyze and fall off the antibody. Regardless of the source, a comprehensive set of possible liberated drug forms must be considered for monitoring on a stability program. Given the generally hydrophobic nature of most chemotherapeutics like those in Fig. 1, these species may often be detected using reversed-phase HPLC methods [21].

A related attribute concerning the small molecule portion of the ADC is the chemical stability of the bound small molecule drug [22]. For instance, stereoisomeric forms of the drug–linker may racemize at chiral centers. Alternatively, chemical moieties such as the succinimide ring found on conjugated vcMMAE are somewhat labile and can open with time. These factors are an analytical challenge, and some features may most readily be assessed in solution conditions, without the protein portion of the ADC.

Any drug that becomes unconjugated from the antibody also changes the drug-to-antibody ratio of the parent molecule. The drug-to-antibody ratio may be monitored as a bulk property, expressed as the overall drug-to-antibody ratio of the entire population within the sample, or in some cases may be broken down into abundances of individual drug-to-antibody ratios. The drug-to-antibody ratio of T-DM1 is an example of an easily measured bulk property, in this case by UV/Vis spectrometry. Conjugates based on MMAE, on the other hand, may be chromatographically separated to reveal the number of antibodies with 0, 2, 4, 6, or 8 drugs per mAb, and the bulk average drug-to-antibody ratio reconstructed from this. Release of free drug is not the only factor that affects the drug-to-antibody ratio, however, since chemical changes of the drug or linker can change the potency of the small molecule. Thus, the drug-to-antibody ratio can be thought of as the number of fully active drugs per mAb, which may or may not be the same as the total number of detectable small molecule moieties conjugated to the mAb, since drug degradation products may or may not be measurable by a given detection method, such as absorbance.

4 Stability-Indicating Methods

Robust analytical techniques that can measure antibody, drug, and conjugate-related attributes are required for formulation development. Because ADCs retain the quality concerns of a conventional monoclonal antibody, the analytical tools required for characterization of conventional mAb [23] typically also apply to the ADC form. These include methods to detect charge variants, covalent and non-covalent aggregates, fragments, and potency in addition to standard solution measurements of pH, concentration/strength, and particulates. It may not always be possible to directly transfer methods from an unconjugated mAb to an ADC, however. There may be changes to the physical and chemical characteristics of a mAb upon conjugation with a small molecule drug that require different characterization techniques compared to the unconjugated mAb.

From a formulation development perspective, availability of appropriate analytical methods is important for ensuring selection of a robust formulation. The following section discusses ADC-specific assay issues that are relevant to formulation development. A detailed discussion on many analytical methodologies is available elsewhere in this volume.

4.1 Assays for DAR

The drug-to-antibody ratio, as previously discussed, is a critical attribute for an ADC. The simplest technique for stability monitoring involves use of the UV/Vis spectra of the ADC [21]. This method requires that the spectra of the antibody and the drug each have different maximum absorbance wavelengths so that the concentrations of both can be separately calculated. This, in turn, allows the determination of average DAR.

Hydrophobic interaction chromatography (HIC) is another technique that also provides information about the average DAR of an ADC [24]. In contrast to UV/Vis spectrometry, HIC may also directly measure individual drug-to-antibody ratio species by chromatographically separating them from each other. This is useful in the context of a stability program, because individual drug-to-antibody ratio species are monitored. The breakdown of covalent bonds between linker and mAb or linker and drug may lead to generation of unbound drug species. The release of unbound drug could lead to a decrease in DAR of an ADC. Chemical changes to the drug may also affect the assay, potentially complicating analysis. In case of UV/Vis, the generation of unbound drug species may not necessarily lead to a decrease in measured DAR as the unbound drug may demonstrate similar absorbance as the bound fraction. In such cases, orthogonal methods such as HIC or RP-HPLC are used to confirm release of unbound drug species. Mass spectrometry, though more laborious to execute than UV/Vis or HIC, can also provide or confirm DAR measurements [25].

4.2 RP-HPLC for Unconjugated Drug Species

Unconjugated drugs are typically hydrophobic and have low molecular weights, thus reversed-phase HPLC (RP-HPLC) has become the method of choice during formulation screens to monitor generation of unconjugated drug species. One of the issues with monitoring for unconjugated drug is the presence of mAb in the sample analyte. The procedure, as a result, requires removal of the protein from the formulation sample to prevent irreversible binding of the protein to the stationary phase. The sample is typically treated with organic solvents like methanol and centrifuged. The protein is precipitated out and the supernatant containing the hydrophobic drug is injected into the RP-HPLC column. The extraction procedure may be influenced by the choice of buffer and excipient in the formulation sample, and additional development work may be necessary where incomplete protein precipitation is observed.

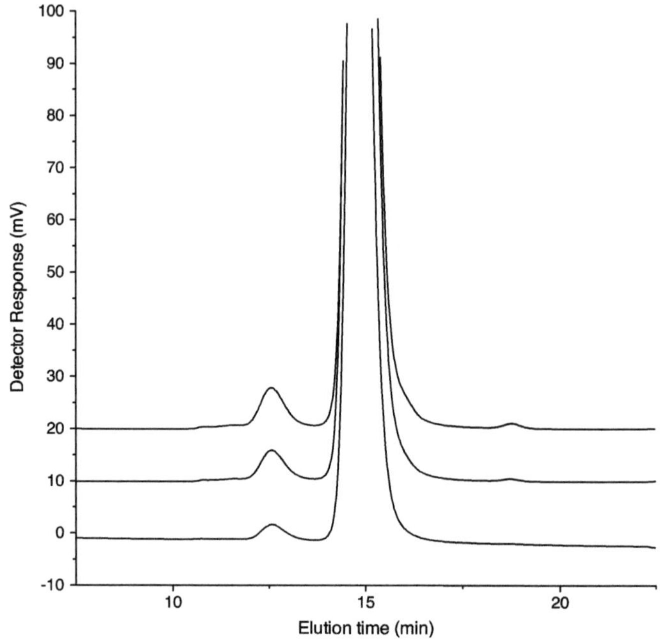

Fig. 2 SEC chromatograms of an ADC linked via Lys residues. The chromatograms of reference samples of a liquid formulation stored over 3 months at 25 °C depicting high-molecular-weight species and fragments at 12 and 18 min retention times, respectively, are shown

4.3 SE-HPLC for Size Variant Analysis

Similar to other biologics, it is important to monitor high-molecular-weight species in an ADC, as such species have potential to elicit an anti-therapeutic antibody response (ATA) and may have altered potency. SE-HPLC is a long-established method to measure size variants of proteins, especially high-molecular-weight species. A representative SE-HPLC profile of an ADC is shown in Fig. 2. It is possible to employ the same technique with ADCs. Due to the greater hydrophobic character of the ADC as compared to the parent mAb, however, SE-HPLC must sometimes include addition of an organic solvent to the chromatography mobile phase to potentiate nonideal interactions with the stationary phase caused by hydrophobic drugs [21]. The addition of a modifier such as these to the mobile phase may potentially disrupt high-molecular-weight species formed during storage and interfere with quantitation. Orthogonal techniques such as analytical ultracentrifugation (AUC) can be used to verify the ability of the SE-HPLC to accurately quantify monomeric and high-molecular-weight species with organic mobile phase additives. Careful titration of organics into the mobile phase coupled to consistent HPLC integration areas with stressed and unstressed materials can also be an indicator that an assay is not altering stability data from a formulation screen. Similar to experience with mAbs, SE-HPLC can also generally detect the presence of fragments in addition to HMWS for ADCs.

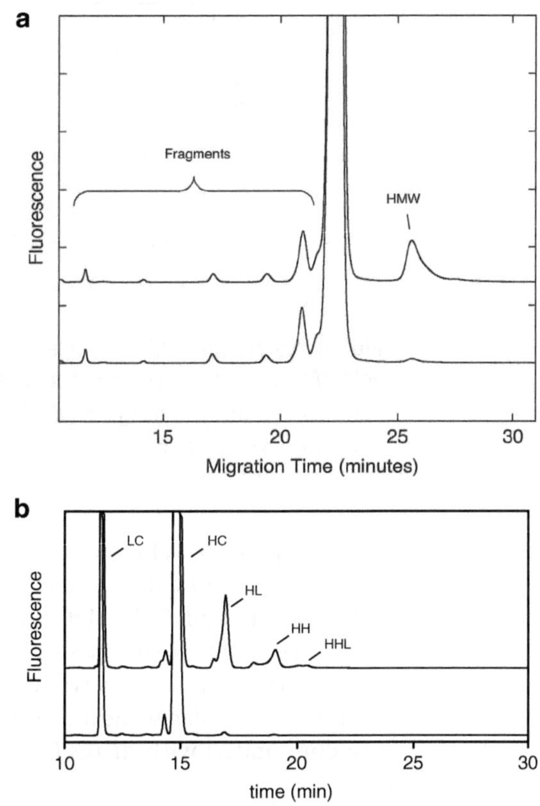

Fig. 3 (**a**) Nonreduced CE-SDS electropherogram of an ADC conjugated with DM1 via Lys residues showing the fragments and the high-molecular-weight species. The offscale peak is monomer. A comparison between the conjugated antibody (the top trace) and the unconjugated antibody (the bottom trace) is depicted (courtesy of Fred Jacobson). (**b**) Reduced CE-SDS electropherogram of an ADC conjugated with DM1 via Lys residues. The peak elution time correlates with increasing molecular weight from *LC* (light chain), *HC* (heavy chain), *HL*, *HH*, and *HHL*. It was demonstrated that the *HL*, *HH*, and *HHL* forms result from intermolecular interchain cross-links that are mediated via Lys residues. Profile shows comparison between the conjugated antibody (the top trace) and the unconjugated antibody (bottom trace) (courtesy of Fred Jacobson)

4.4 CE-SDS Nonreduced for Size Variants

This technique due to its speed, reproducibility, resolution, robustness, and ease of automation has become a preferred technique for monitoring size variants in mAbs [26]. As in the case of mAbs, CE-SDS can monitor fragments and aggregates that are linked via covalent bonds. Aggregates mediated via covalent mechanisms such as intermolecular cross-links involving the unconjugated linker have been studied using nonreduced CE-SDS [7]. These cross-links have been shown to increase on stability for the intermediate, T-MCC, in synthesis of T-DM1. However, increase in covalent aggregates was minimal in case of T-DM1. Nonreduced CE-SDS (Fig. 3a) in conjunction with reduced CE-SDS (Fig. 3b)

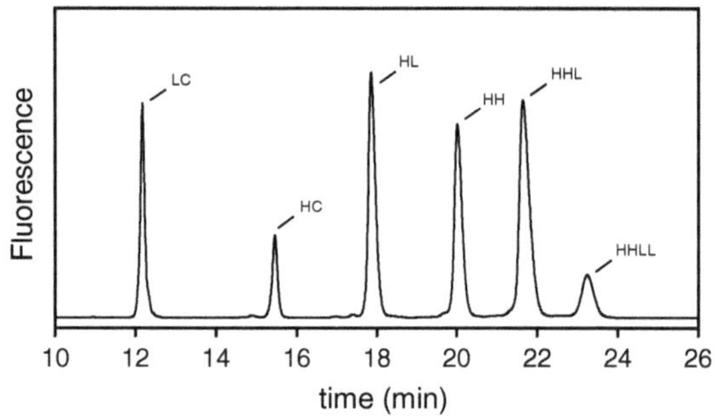

Fig. 4 Nonreduced CE-SDS electropherogram of an ADC conjugated with vcMMAE via interchain disulfide cysteine residues. The peak elution time correlates with increasing molecular weight from *LC* (light chain), *HC* (heavy chain), *HL*, *HH*, *HHL*, to *HHLL*

can also provide valuable information for interchain (combinations of heavy and light chains) cross-links. A different situation arises for CE-SDS analysis of ADCs conjugated via interchain disulfide cysteines. Due to the loss of disulfide linkages between light and heavy chains, the ADCs will dissociate in the presence of SDS into various molecular weight fragments as a function of what residues are conjugated with drugs (Fig. 4).

4.5 Potency

Assays that appropriately measure the biological activity, or potency, of the ADC are important to show that the function of the product remains uncompromised over its shelf life. They also play an important role in screening of formulations, since changes in biological activity can occur preferentially at one set of solution conditions over another due to factors such as pH or oxidative potential of various formulation ingredients. Constant potency over a stability study implies, however, that the overall biofunctionality of the ADC is retained despite whatever measurable physicochemical changes occurred. In the context of ADCs, two obvious categories of functional assays include those based on epitope-binding and cell-killing ability. Specifics of choosing and developing such assays are beyond the scope of this chapter, but such assays are critical components for formulation development.

5 Biophysical Considerations of ADCs Affecting Formulation Development

Antibody–drug conjugates may be expected to have altered biophysical properties, such as conformation and structural stability, as compared to the corresponding unconjugated antibody. This accounts for the specific process and formulation considerations already discussed. Linked drugs represent new chemical moieties that must be properly solvated or buried in the protein surface, and they may also alter the distribution of charge across the protein, such as with the lysine-linked chemotoxins used with T-DM1. This latter case is brought about by virtue of the fact that the terminal ε-amine on the side chain does not remain in an ionizable form upon drug conjugation. Cysteine-linked drugs introduce another range of biophysical perturbations in a slightly different manner. Formation of these ADCs, such as brentuximab vedotin, requires the breaking of interchain disulfides and removes covalent bonds that hold together the antibody quaternary structure.

The effects of biophysical perturbations associated with the conjugated form are most readily captured by comparison of the behavior of the unconjugated antibody to the ADC. This can take the form of comparative physical stability by SEC (as discussed above), capillary electrophoresis, and analytical ultracentrifugation (AUC), for instance. The standard catalog of higher-order structure-sensitive tools such as differential scanning calorimetry (DSC), ultraviolet circular dichroism (UV-CD), and Fourier transform infrared spectroscopy (FTIR) is as applicable to ADCs as they are to unconjugated antibodies. This class of tools also has the same limitations as are seen when analyzing unconjugated antibodies, namely, that they simultaneously probe an entire ensemble of biophysical states of large, complicated molecules. In the case of ADCs, sample heterogeneity is multiplied by the fact that many samples include a population of molecules with different drug-to-antibody ratios.

These factors notwithstanding, the conjugation process imparts several resolvable changes to the biophysical characteristics of the molecules, which may inform formulation development of an ADC. For instance, Wakankar et al. showed that the melting temperature of the trastuzumab antibody CH_2 domain in T-DM1 decreased first upon addition of the heterobifunctional linker SMCC and then further upon conjugation of the DM1 chemotoxin [7], implying reduced structural stability of the ADC CH_2 domain as compared to the unconjugated form. The apparent alteration in the onset of melting of the domains may vary with the antibody and type of drug used for conjugation. This may be seen in example thermograms of an IgG1 antibody conjugated with vcMMAE at the interchain disulfides, as compared to the unconjugated antibody (Fig. 5). In this case, the onset of melting temperature is lower for the conjugated versus unconjugated antibody. Formulation conditions, such as pH, also affect the thermal stability of the ADC, also shown in Fig. 5.

The implications of data such as these must be carefully considered. On the one hand, a decreased melting temperature means lower structural stability, especially in stressed conditions. On the other hand, this does not automatically translate to unacceptable shelf life for a drug product stored at refrigerated temperatures.

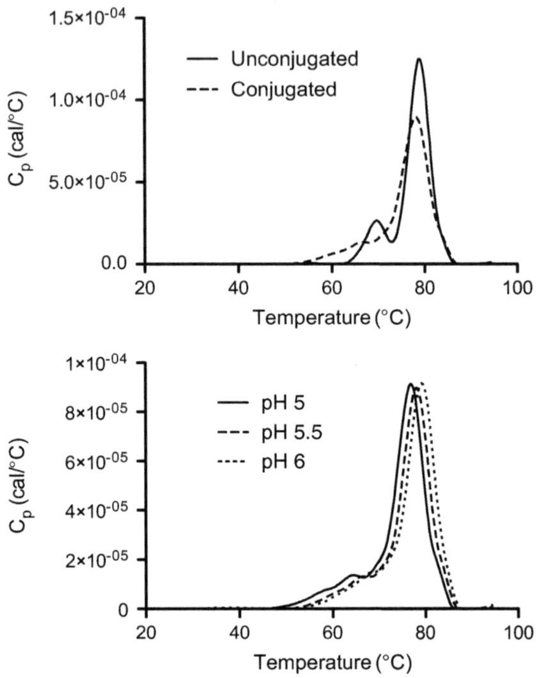

Fig. 5 (*Top*) DSC thermograms of a vcMMAE-conjugated ADC as well as its unconjugated precursor. (*Bottom*) DSC thermograms of the same ADC in different pH conditions in the same buffer system

However, DSC thermogram data may have utility in understanding results from experiments run under stress conditions, such as during formulation screening. As an example, a screening stress condition temperature close to a melting transition may mean that degradation seen under such stress is not representative of that expected in real storage conditions. Thus, caution must be applied during the choice of stressed screen temperatures or during the analysis of data from relatively high-temperature stresses.

In a similar fashion, spectroscopic tools like CD-UV and FTIR may be used with ADCs, but information content and value should be critically analyzed. Some groups have applied methods like these towards the analysis of unconjugated antibodies, though the implementation of qualified methods and interpretation of the data can be challenging [27]. Analysis of a conjugated antibody would not be simpler, and the existing difficulties may be compounded by the spectral contributions of the drug component. The field awaits more fruitful methods to analyze the higher-order structure of compounds such as these, and tools such as hydrogen/deuterium exchange mass spectrometry (HDX-MS) [28, 29] may eventually prove useful for ADCs in the same way they are emerging in the conventional therapeutic antibody field.

6 In-Use Studies and Administration

The final development stage relevant to ADC formulation is administration to the patient. This may be supported by experiments simulating in-use conditions that take into account ADC diluent and dilution factor, product-contacting materials like IV bags, and hold times and temperatures necessary for pharmacists to prepare solutions and nurses to administer them. Again, the additional hydrophobic nature of the ADC as compared to the unconjugated antibody due to the linker–drug moiety may affect in-use stability of the molecule. Also, the higher the drug load in an ADC, the greater the hydrophobicity of the ADC molecule. ADCs with higher drug load may be particularly susceptible to formation of soluble aggregates and/or insoluble precipitates in the presence of saline due to salting-out effects. It is important to evaluate the compatibility of the ADC in solutions representative of dosing solution conditions. Formulation approaches that not only maintain stability during drug product storage but also during administration, and possibly shipping post-dilution, need to be implemented. In situations where formulation fixes are not attainable, use of alternate solutions for administration (e.g., dextrose, half saline) or excipient-containing diluents can be considered.

7 Making ADC Formulation Decisions

Formulation decisions are based on choosing a product profile that best ensures the quality of the drug, guided using the behavior of attributes like those in Table 1 in screening experiments. The same set of formulation decisions required for conventional antibody–drug substance and product is relevant for ADCs, such as pH, buffering species, concentration, stabilizing excipients, container closure, and liquid versus lyophilized format. Examples from unconjugated antibodies are readily found [11]. Choice of these parameters is based on the considerations discussed above. However, given the current limited state of clinical knowledge and experience with ADCs, the understanding of the safety and efficacy effects of the various quality attributes is still evolving, along with regulatory expectations. Formulation development strikes a balance between the antibody-, drug-, and conjugate-specific attributes, which encompasses more factors than are encountered with standard, unconjugated antibody therapeutics.

Successful formulation development ensures that the product quality is maintained during storage, shipping, handling, and administration. Formulation development for an ADC requires understanding of the chemical degradative mechanisms of the drug–linker species in addition to the physicochemical instabilities of the mAb. The former aspect is especially challenging in terms of preparing aqueous formulations of ADCs. Also, conditions that may render optimal stability to the drug–linker species may not necessarily be stable for the mAb portion of the ADC. This suggests that lyophilized formulations would be preferred, as evidenced by the commercial and clinical formulations of brentuximab vedotin and T-DM1, respectively. However, there are still potential practical limitations of this development path, such as availability of lyophilization manufacturing suites that can handle cytotoxic biologics. Assessments based on clinical experience that involve identifying quality attributes that are truly critical will facilitate formulation choices in the future.

References

1. Goetze AM, Schenauer MR, Flynn GC (2010) Assessing monoclonal antibody product quality attribute criticality through clinical studies. MAbs 2(5):500–507. doi:10.4161/mabs.2.5.12897
2. Ducry L, Stump B (2010) Antibody–drug conjugates: linking cytotoxic payloads to monoclonal antibodies. Bioconjug Chem 21(1):5–13. doi:10.1021/bc9002019
3. Doronina SO, Toki BE, Torgov MY, Mendelsohn BA, Cerveny CG, Chace DF, DeBlanc RL, Gearing RP, Bovee TD, Siegall CB, Francisco JA, Wahl AF, Meyer DL, Senter PD (2003) Development of potent monoclonal antibody auristatin conjugates for cancer therapy. Nat Biotechnol 21(7):778–784. doi:10.1038/nbt832
4. Junutula JR, Raab H, Clark S, Bhakta S, Leipold DD, Weir S, Chen Y, Simpson M, Tsai SP, Dennis MS, Lu Y, Meng YG, Ng C, Yang J, Lee CC, Duenas E, Gorrell J, Katta V, Kim A, McDorman K, Flagella K, Venook R, Ross S, Spencer SD, Lee Wong W, Lowman HB, Vandlen R, Sliwkowski MX, Scheller RH, Polakis P, Mallet W (2008) Site-specific conjugation of a cytotoxic drug to an antibody improves the therapeutic index. Nat Biotechnol 26 (8):925–932. doi:10.1038/nbt.1480
5. Chari RV, Martell BA, Gross JL, Cook SB, Shah SA, Blättler WA, McKenzie SJ, Goldmacher VS (1992) Immunoconjugates containing novel maytansinoids: promising anticancer drugs. Cancer Res 52(1):127–131
6. Kovtun YV, Audette CA, Ye Y, Xie H, Ruberti MF, Phinney SJ, Leece BA, Chittenden T, Blattler WA, Goldmacher VS (2006) Antibody–drug conjugates designed to eradicate tumors with homogeneous and heterogeneous expression of the target antigen. Cancer Res 66(6):3214–3221. doi:10.1158/0008-5472.CAN-05-3973
7. Wakankar AA, Feeney MB, Rivera J, Chen Y, Kim M, Sharma VK, Wang YJ (2010) Physicochemical stability of the antibody–drug conjugate Trastuzumab-DM1: changes due to modification and conjugation processes. Bioconjug Chem 21(9):1588–1595. doi:10.1021/bc900434c
8. Hinman L, Hamann P, Wallace R, Menendez A, Durr F, Upeslacis J (1993) Preparation and characterization of monoclonal-antibody conjugates of the calicheamicins – a novel and potent family of antitumor antibiotics. Cancer Res 53(14):3336–3342
9. Daugherty AL, Mrsny RJ (2006) Formulation and delivery issues for monoclonal antibody therapeutics. Adv Drug Deliv Rev 58(5–6):686–706. doi:10.1016/J.Addr.2006. 03.011
10. Wang W, Singh S, Zeng DL, King K, Nema S (2007) Antibody structure, instability, and formulation. J Pharm Sci 96(1):1–26. doi:10.1002/Jps.20727
11. Wang W, Singh S, Zeng DL, King K, Nema S (2006) Antibody structure, instability, and formulation. J Pharm Sci 96(1):1–26. doi:10.1002/jps.20727
12. Moore J, Patapoff T, Cromwell M (1999) Kinetics and thermodynamics of dimer formation and dissociation for a recombinant humanized monoclonal antibody to vascular endothelial growth factor. Biochemistry 38 (42):13960–13967
13. Kosky AA, Dharmavaram V, Ratnaswamy G, Manning MC (2009) Multivariate analysis of the sequence dependence of asparagine deamidation rates in peptides. Pharm Res 26 (11):2417–2428. doi:10.1007/s11095-009-9953-8

14. Robinson NE (2001) Molecular clocks. Proc Natl Acad Sci 98(3):944–949. doi:10.1073/pnas.98.3.944
15. Cordoba A, Shyong B, Breen D, Harris R (2005) Non-enzymatic hinge region fragmentation of antibodies in solution. J Chromatogr B Anal Technol (Biomed Life Sci) 818(2):115–121. doi:10.1016/j.jchromb.2004. 12.033
16. Sun MMC, Beam KS, Cerveny CG, Hamblett KJ, Blackmore RS, Torgov MY, Handley FGM, Ihle NC, Senter PD, Alley SC (2005) Reduction–alkylation strategies for the modification of specific monoclonal antibody disulfides. Bioconjug Chem 16(5):1282–1290. doi:10.1021/bc050201y
17. Wu CW, Yarbrough LR (1976) N-(1-pyrene) maleimide: a fluorescent cross-linking reagent. Biochemistry 15(13):2863–2868
18. Baldwin AD, Kiick KL (2011) Tunable degradation of maleimide–thiol adducts in reducing environments. Bioconjug Chem 22 (10):1946–1953. doi:10.1021/bc200148v
19. Chih H-W, Gikanga B, Yang Y, Zhang B (2011) Identification of amino acid residues responsible for the release of free drug from an antibody–drug conjugate utilizing lysine-succinimidyl ester chemistry. J Pharm Sci. doi:10.1002/jps.22485
20. Shen B-Q, Xu K, Liu L, Raab H, Bhakta S, Kenrick M, Parsons-Reponte KL, Tien J, Yu S-F, Mai E, Li D, Tibbitts J, Baudys J, Saad OM, Scales SJ, McDonald PJ, Hass PE, Eigenbrot C, Nguyen T, Solis WA, Fuji RN, Flagella KM, Patel D, Spencer SD, Khawli LA, Ebens A, Wong WL, Vandlen R, Kaur S, Sliwkowski MX, Scheller RH, Polakis P, Junutula JR (2012) Conjugation site modulates the in vivo stability and therapeutic activity of antibody-drug conjugates. Nat Biotechnol 1–8. doi:10.1038/nbt.2108
21. Wakankar A, Chen Y, Gokarn Y, Jacobson FS (2011) Analytical methods for physicochemical characterization of antibody drug conjugates. MAbs 3(2):161–172. doi:10.4161/mabs.3.2.14960
22. Suchocki JA, Sneden AT (1987) Characterization of decomposition products of maytansine. J Pharm Sci 76(9):738–743. doi:10.1002/jps.2600760913
23. Harris RJ, Shire SJ, Winter C (2004) Commercial manufacturing scale formulation and analytical characterization of therapeutic recombinant antibodies. Drug Dev Res 61 (3):137–154. doi:10.1002/ddr.10344
24. Hamblett KJ, Senter PD, Chace DF, Sun MMC, Lenox J, Cerveny CG, Kissler KM, Bernhardt SX, Kopcha AK, Zabinski RF, Meyer DL, Francisco JA (2004) Effects of drug loading on the antitumor activity of a monoclonal antibody drug conjugate. Clin Cancer Res J Am Assoc Cancer Res 10 (20):7063–7070. doi:10.1158/1078-0432.CCR-04-0789
25. Siegel MM, Hollander IJ, Hamann PR, James JP, Hinman L, Smith BJ, Farnsworth APH, Phipps A, King DJ et al (1991) Matrix-assisted UV-laser desorption/ionization mass spectrometric analysis of monoclonal antibodies for the determination of carbohydrate, conjugated chelator, and conjugated drug content. Anal Chem 63(21):2470–2481. doi:10.1021/ac00021a016
26. Hunt GG, Nashabeh WW (1999) Capillary electrophoresis sodium dodecyl sulfate nongel sieving analysis of a therapeutic recombinant monoclonal antibody: a biotechnology perspective. Anal Chem 71(13):2390–2397
27. Jiang Y, Li C, Nguyen X, Muzammil S, Towers E, Gabrielson J, Narhi L (2011) Qualification of FTIR spectroscopic method for protein secondary structural analysis. J Pharm Sci 100 (11):4631–4641. doi:10.1002/jps.22686
28. Houde D, Peng Y, Berkowitz S, Engen J (2010) Post-translational modifications differentially affect IgG1 conformation and receptor binding. Mol Cell Proteomics 9:1716–1728
29. Konermann L, Pan J, Liu Y-H (2011) Hydrogen exchange mass spectrometry for studying protein structure and dynamics. Chem Soc Rev 40(3):1224. doi:10.1039/c0cs00113a

Chapter 14

Conjugation Process Development and Scale-Up

Bernhard Stump and Jessica Steinmann

Abstract

Manufacturing highly potent antibody–drug conjugates (ADCs) is a demanding task—combining conventional organic synthesis with biotechnological manufacturing. Hence a series of new and unique engineering and chemistry challenges have to be addressed to support clinical trials and commercial manufacturing. These include the development of reliable processes leading to uniform product properties, as well as establishment of ADC-specific analytical methods and safe strategies for handling cytotoxic compounds. This review focuses on process development and scale-up for the production of ADCs and highlights the most important features in such a process.

Key words Antibody–drug conjugates, Process development, Design of experiments (DoE), Scale-up, Cytotoxic compounds

1 ADC Process Development: Why and How?

Antibody–drug conjugates (ADCs) represent a new and promising class of drugs for cancer treatment [1–3]. An ADC consists of three components, a monoclonal antibody (mAb) specific for a tumor antigen, a linker species, and a cytotoxic payload. The antibody portion allows the targeted delivery of cytotoxic drugs that otherwise often would not be suitable for patient treatment due to their narrow therapeutic windows. The highly potent drug needs to be attached to the antibody without disturbing the biological attributes of the latter [4]. The highly different biophysical properties of the antibody compared to the cytotoxic payload such as their size and level of hydrophobicity can pose a great challenge for the manufacturing of an ADC. The antibody has to be handled with special care since it is susceptible to high temperatures and temperature fluctuations as well as high stirring rates [5, 6]. The cytotoxic drug is usually very hydrophobic, which requires the use of organic co-solvents that have to be tolerable for the antibody portion too. This exemplifies just a few of the challenges which are encountered during the synthesis of an ADC.

Laurent Ducry (ed.), *Antibody-Drug Conjugates*, Methods in Molecular Biology, vol. 1045,
DOI 10.1007/978-1-62703-541-5_14, © Springer Science+Business Media, LLC 2013

Familiari-zation	Process Development			Clilincal supply	Process characterization	Commercial supply
Reagent Titration	DoE	Verification runs	Purification development	batches for toxicology / clinical studies	process design	commercial batches
	mg scale		g scale	> 100 g scale	g / mg scale	> 1 kg scale

Fig. 1 Typical process development activities for an ADC process

Typically, a procedure for the synthesis of a new and promising ADC is devised during the drug discovery phase. So why is it necessary to spend time and money for an extensive process development? The value of the process development work becomes visible in later phases of projects. A project where the main process parameters are already set, before producing material for toxicology and clinical studies, reduces the risk associated with the implementation of process changes in the further life cycle. This allows that material of well-comparable quality can be used throughout all stages.

How can a process development program be designed? First of all, the objectives of the development have to be defined. Ensuring a reliable and safe process that fits into the available production facilities is an obvious goal. But how is the success of the process development assessed even before preparing the biopharmaceutical at manufacturing scale? A thorough control of the ADC characteristics at the molecular level during the whole development phase can give confidence that a reliable, robust process has been set up. Properties such as the drug-to-antibody ratio [7] (DAR), the monomer content, and as far as possible the linkage sites need to be controlled by the process. In addition, these analytically traceable features can be key indicators of the product quality. Furthermore, the ADCs have to be active as shown by cell killing assays and have to be recognized by the target antigen, as proven by antigen binding assays such as ELISA.

Typically, a development program starts with a familiarization phase in order to test and assess the initial set of process parameters, which are then refined in the actual process development phase (*see* Fig. 1). In this phase, a variety of process parameters are investigated in detail, e.g., in the so-called design of experiments (DoE) setup. In a next step, the optimized process parameters are checked in a number of verification runs. All these operations can be performed at mg-scale if a representative scale down model is available. Thereafter, a first up-scaling to gram quantities of antibody starting material can be ventured, and purification steps can be explored. The process is then typically ready to be scaled up to >100 g scale to supply toxicology and early clinical studies. On the way to a commercial process, a process qualification phase where ADC manufacturing is thoroughly investigated will be necessary to meet all regulatory needs [8] leading to a well-characterized process that can be executed at a 1 kg scale or more.

2 Familiarize with the Process

In a typical ADC process, only a handful of reaction parameters influence the DAR. For cysteine conjugations like in *Seattle Genetic*'s maleimide-based conjugation technology, the DAR defining step is classically the partial reduction of the antibody. More specifically, the stoichiometry of the reducing agent such as tris(2-carboxyethyl) phosphine (TCEP) controls the number of free thiols generated [9]. In a next step, the free thiol groups are then conjugated to the drug–linker molecule of choice (*see* Fig. 2). In case of the lysine conjugation-based ADCs, as used in *Immunogen*'s targeted antibody payload (TAP) technology [10], the modification of the antibody with the respective linker typically defines the loading ratio. Thus, these antibody modification steps prior to the actual drug conjugation need to be addressed with special care for both types of conjugation technologies. It is therefore necessary to become familiar with the effect of the above-mentioned key parameters on the drug loading in order to gain a good starting point for further ADC process development. An initial titration of the mAb with the antibody-modifying agent by simply altering the reagent stochiometries, followed by conjugation to the drug and analysis of the resulting ADCs for their DAR value, gives valuable information on how to direct a process towards the desired drug loading characteristics. Normally, such an experiment reveals the relationship between the mAb-modifying agent and the DAR. A first set of standard reaction conditions results from such a process familiarization phase that

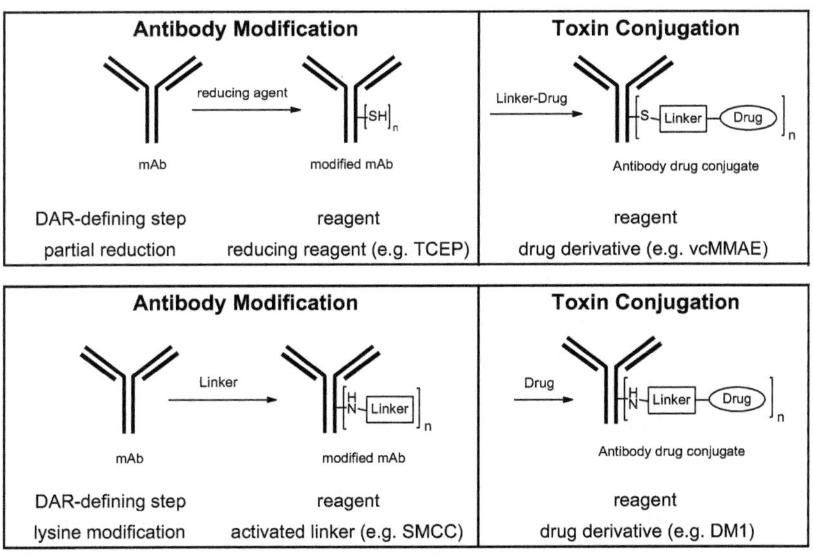

Fig. 2 Typical ADC process steps involving antibody modification prior to the conjugation reactions. The two examples involve cysteine-based (*above*) and lysine-based (*below*) conjugations

allows production of the ADC with a reproducible, predefined drug loading ratio.

The material prepared during the familiarization phase can be further utilized to establish preliminary data on the stability of the conjugate, which is certainly helpful to judge the validity of analytical results in the upcoming process phases if, e.g., no immediate analytical investigation can be performed when experiments are run in parallel.

3 Finding the Ideal Process Parameters: DoE as a Tool

Having gained initial knowledge with the conjugation process through the familiarization phase, a more detailed investigation is desirable. Investigating the effect of the reaction parameters on the ADC quality attributes allows designing a tailor-made process.

The potentially vast number of parameters that can be varied renders an approach where each possible combination of reaction conditions is studied in single experiments ineffective. Such a "one-factor-at-a-time" (OFAT) approach would result in a hardly manageable number of experiments to be conducted. The extensive number of experiments would consume precious raw materials, prolong the process development phase by running and analyzing all these conjugation experiments, and hence cause considerable costs and delays for a preclinical program. Furthermore, no information on interaction between the parameters is gained by single experiments. Approaches that reach the same readout with fewer individual experiments are therefore preferred.

A well-established and reliable tool for a systematic investigation of process parameters is the so-called "DoE" [11]. The underlying principle of a DoE is to systematically plan the experiments with a statistical background, allowing extrapolation of the obtained results to the non-investigated parameter combinations. The effect on the properties of a conjugate can then be calculated within the investigated parameter ranges. As only certain statistically selected combinations are experimentally analyzed, the number of experiments to be carried out is considerably reduced compared to an OFAT approach.

A DoE can only be carried out for a process that reproducibly delivers the conjugate in a defined and measurable quality. Only then, the effect of the parameters changed vs. the parameters held constant can be interpreted. The conjugations carried out during the familiarization phase should give confidence that the process itself is already stable enough to be further investigated in a DoE. Then, the next task is to select the parameters that shall be investigated. Some choices are obvious and valid for most biotechnological manufacturing processes such as reaction temperature and time, protein concentration, and reagent stoichiometries.

Furthermore, the pH of the reaction solution as well as buffer salt concentrations, addition times of reagent solutions, stirring rates, and many more parameters can be considered. As mentioned earlier, the analytically traceable ADC properties that define the product quality are typically DAR, drug distribution, monomer content, cell killing activity, or antigen-recognition. All these features can be chosen as output measures in a DoE. In addition, properties of process intermediates such as linker-to-antibody ratio (LAR), free thiol-to-antibody ratio (FTAR), or monomer content can be assessed within a DoE of a single process step. It is crucial that these methods are accurate enough to generate precise data that can be further interpreted in the statistical model. This means that they have to be accurate and precise with minimal scattering, thereby allowing the detection of even minor differences of product quality as a result of process parameter changes.

3.1 Setting Up the Experimental Plan

Computer programs such as *Design Expert* [12], *MODDE* [13], or *Statistica* [14] provide tremendous help for setting up an appropriate experimental plan for a DoE investigation, as well as for the data analysis after the execution of the designed experiments in the laboratory. For a project entering the early clinical phases, a parameter screening DoE typically provides the necessary information about a process, in particular, a good understanding of which parameters have a significant effect on the process outcome and which values for these parameters are adequate to reach the desired product characteristics. For each parameter chosen, the upper and lower limits that shall be investigated have to be selected. Manufacturability considerations and process experience from the familiarization phase, from related conjugation processes, or from literature examples shape the “corners” of the chosen parameter space.

3.2 Parameter Screening by DoE: An Example

For example, in a lysine conjugation process (Fig. 3), the effects of concentration, pH, modification agent stoichiometry, reaction temperature, reaction time, and organic co-solvent content on the LAR and monomer content were investigated. A parameter screening was chosen, in the form of a fractional factorial design for a parameter screening DoE. For all parameters, a setpoint as well as a lower (−) and higher (+) boundary were defined. In order to investigate if the nature of the co-solvent has an effect on the process outcome, two sub-blocks were defined based on two different organic solvents (*see* Table 1).

In the experimental plan, the order of the experiments was randomized to avoid any grouping of parameters during the execution in the laboratory. In addition, three “center point” experiments for each co-solvent block (runs 1, 4, 8, 12, 16, and 22 in Table 1) with all variables on setpoint were defined to check the reproducibility of the process using standard conditions and to find out whether a linear model could be applied to describe the conjugation process or due to

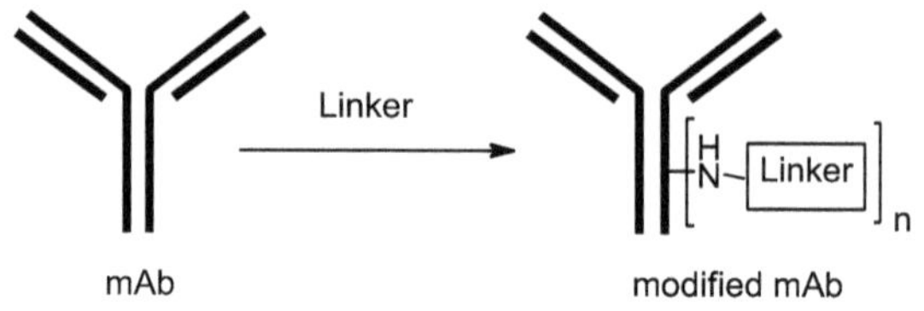

Fig. 3 Investigated lysine conjugation process

observation of a curvature, a more complex response surface model should be considered. These six runs with identical parameters were randomly distributed over the experimental plan.

The execution of the conjugation experiments is performed at mg scale. In order to have an optimal level of control over the investigated parameters, adequate equipment is needed. *Lonza* is using scale down models of glass reactors as they are utilized in the manufacturing of clinical material in the manufacturing suites. Jacketed 10 mL glass reactors provide a tight temperature control and permit stirring using magnetic stir bars (*see* Fig. 4). In order to carry out a DoE investigation for a conjugation reaction, well-trained technicians or scientists are required who can safely handle highly potent compounds. In addition, the analytical investigations need to be performed within a short period of time and therefore the corresponding equipment, procedures, and personnel have to be readily available. For this study, two output readings were chosen: monomer content, as determined by size exclusion chromatography, as well as the loading of the antibody. Additionally, the concentration of the conjugate as well as the amount of free linker in the solution were analytically assessed.

After having collected all data of the completed DoE, the effects of single-parameter changes as well as interactions between multiple parameters are analyzed with the support of the DoE software. The center point experiments give a measure of the reproducibility of the process using these standard conditions. The parameters that significantly influence the nature of the output are identified, in this case the LAR as well as the monomer content of the modified antibody. In addition, the DoE approach also allows to rate the effect of single parameters as well as parameter combinations such as temperature and pH (*see* Fig. 5). Typically, the number of statistically significant parameters in a conjugation process is considerably smaller than the number of investigated parameters. This means that only a handful of parameters determine the success of the conjugation within the selected ranges. These inputs have to be well controlled in the ADC manufacturing process.

Apart from the ability to identify process parameters or combinations thereof that control the process outcome, the power of the DoE approach lies in the option to extrapolate the process outcome on values that were not experimentally investigated. The obtained DoE dataset can be presented as two- or three-dimensional plots

Table 1
Experimental plan for a fractional factorial design with two blocks and three center points per block, as proposed by *Design Expert*. Italic: "center point" experiments

Run # (randomized)	Block (co-solvent)	Temperature [°C]	pH	Time [h]	mAb conc [g/L]	Org solv content [% v/v]	Linker [eq]
1	A	*setpoint*	*setpoint*	*setpoint*	*setpoint*	*setpoint*	*setpoint*
2	A	**setpoint +**	setpoint –	**setpoint +**	setpoint –	setpoint –	**setpoint +**
3	B	**setpoint +**	**setpoint +**	**setpoint +**	**setpoint +**	**setpoint +**	**setpoint +**
4	B	*setpoint*	*setpoint*	*setpoint*	*setpoint*	*setpoint*	*setpoint*
5	A	setpoint –	setpoint –	setpoint –	setpoint –	setpoint –	setpoint –
6	B	setpoint –	**setpoint +**	setpoint –	**setpoint +**	**setpoint +**	setpoint –
7	A	setpoint –	**setpoint +**	**setpoint +**	**setpoint +**	setpoint –	setpoint –
8	A	*setpoint*	*setpoint*	*setpoint*	*setpoint*	*setpoint*	*setpoint*
9	A	setpoint –	setpoint –	**setpoint +**	**setpoint +**	**setpoint +**	**setpoint +**
10	B	setpoint –	setpoint –	**setpoint +**	setpoint –	**setpoint +**	setpoint –
11	B	**setpoint +**	setpoint –	**setpoint +**	**setpoint +**	setpoint –	setpoint –
12	B	*setpoint*	*setpoint*	*setpoint*	*setpoint*	*setpoint*	*setpoint*
13	A	**setpoint +**	**setpoint +**	setpoint –	**setpoint +**	setpoint –	**setpoint +**
14	B	**setpoint +**	**setpoint +**	setpoint –	setpoint –	setpoint –	setpoint –
15	A	**setpoint +**	**setpoint +**	**setpoint +**	setpoint –	**setpoint +**	setpoint –
16	A	*setpoint*	*setpoint*	*setpoint*	*setpoint*	*setpoint*	*setpoint*
17	B	setpoint –	**setpoint +**	**setpoint +**	setpoint –	setpoint –	**setpoint +**
18	A	setpoint +	**setpoint +**	setpoint +	setpoint –	**setpoint –**	**setpoint +**

(continued)

Table 1
(continued)

Run # (randomized)	Block (co-solvent)	Temperature [°C]	pH	Time [h]	mAb conc [g/L]	Org solv content [% v/v]	Linker [eq]
19	A	**setpoint +**	setpoint –	setpoint –	**setpoint +**	**setpoint +**	setpoint –
20	B	setpoint –	setpoint –	setpoint –	**setpoint +**	setpoint –	**setpoint +**
21	B	**setpoint +**	setpoint –	setpoint –	setpoint –	**setpoint +**	**setpoint +**
22	B	*setpoint –*	*setpoint –*	*setpoint +*	*setpoint –*	*setpoint +*	*setpoint –*

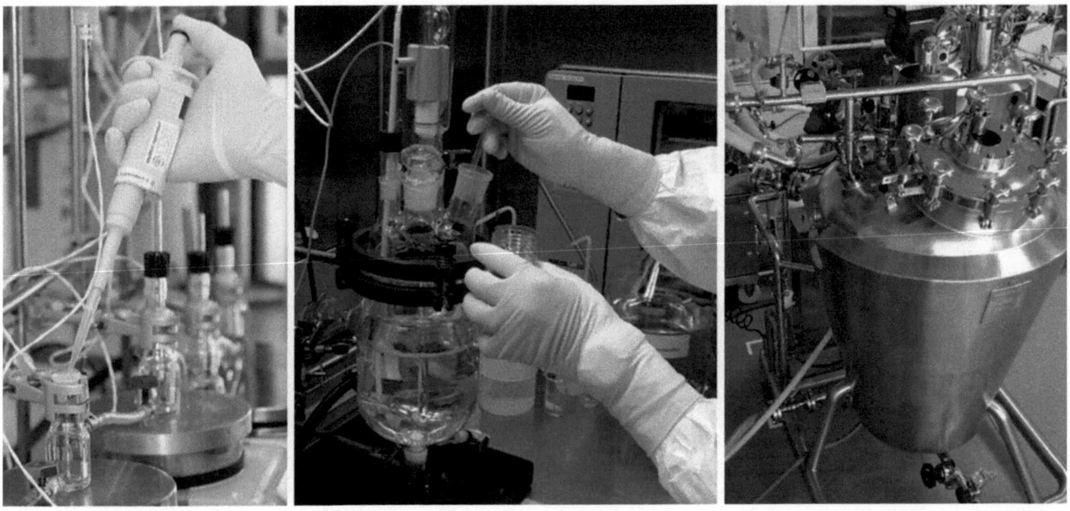

Fig. 4 ADC process equipment at Lonza Visp: mg-scale jacketed glass reactors, g-scale glass reactor, kg-scale stainless steel reactor

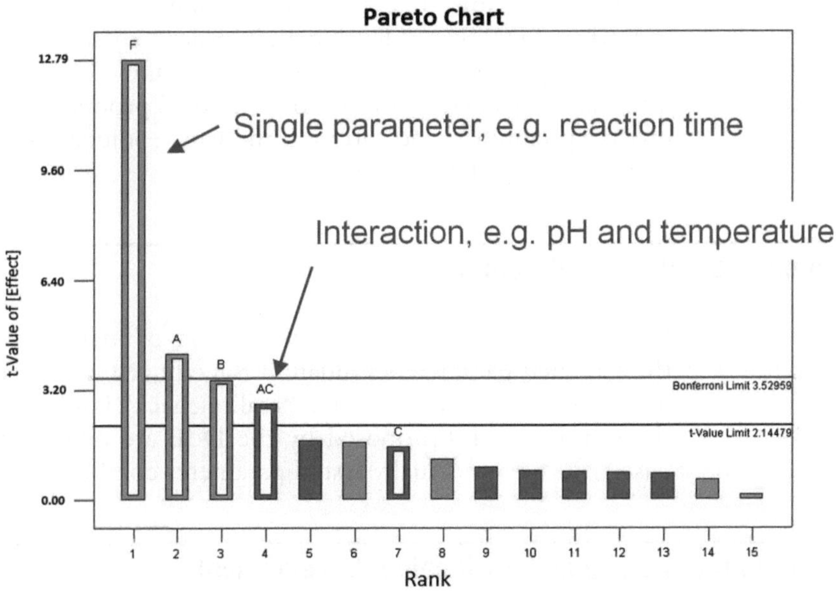

Fig. 5 Pareto chart deciphering the significance of the effect of single parameters (A, B, C, . . .) and parameter combinations (AB, AC, . . .) on the LAR

if multiple parameters are investigated. The statistical model for the whole process now provides the identification of the most suitable set of parameters to reach the desired output values if the data supports a linear model. If the data analysis gives hints for a nonlinear behavior of the process output based on the parameter variations, additional experiments will be needed to obtain a response-surface model describing the process (*see* Fig. 6 for an example of a dataset with a curvature).

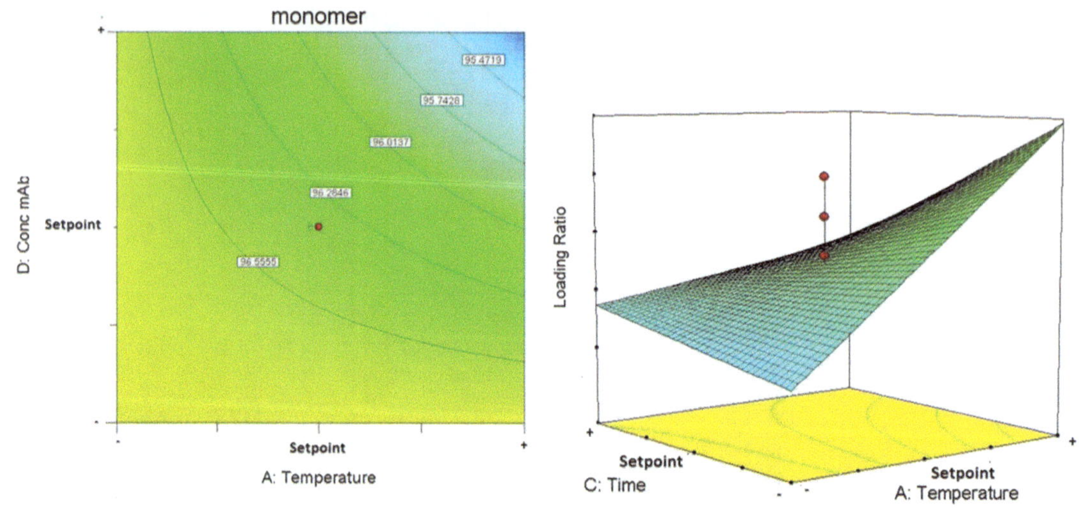

Fig. 6 2D plot of the influence of mAb concentration and temperature on the monomer content (*left*). 3D plot of time and temperature on the loading ratio (LAR, *right*)

It is advisable to carry out a parameter screening for each individual ADC that is developed, in order to gain full understanding of the process. If time or resources are limited, transposing the information gained in a DoE for one ADC process to another can provide preliminary indications if the same conjugation technology is applied for different antibodies.

4 Verification of the Process Parameters

Verification runs using the combination of identified values for the screened parameters validate if they indeed reliably deliver the desired product quality. Such a "reality check" is advisable because the optimal values proposed by the DoE are only extrapolations based on the few actually tested parameter combinations.

5 Up-Scaling to Gram Scale and Purification Development

After having identified the significant parameters and having defined and verified their setpoints in order to reach the desired product quality, the process is ready to be scaled up from milligram to gram scale. Thereby, additional data about the process robustness and scalability are gained. At this point, the purification techniques [15] are explored that will be used when clinical material is prepared.

Techniques that can be scaled up such as tangential flow filtration (TFF) shall be favored. TFF is a method to concentrate and purify proteins [16–18]. It allows efficient buffer exchanges and

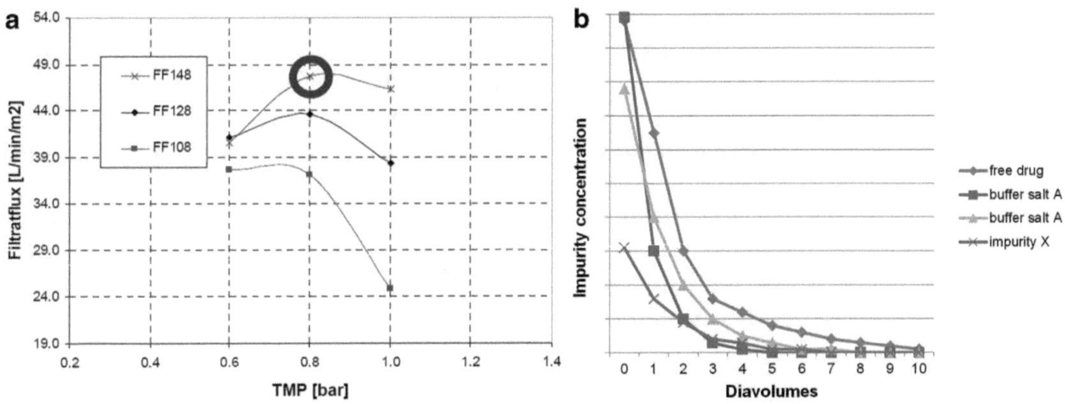

Fig. 7 Example of the influence of TMP and FF on TFF flux rate (*left*) and low-molecular-weight impurity clearance (*right*)

small-molecule impurity clearance steps that are typically needed for an antibody modification process. In particular the clearance of free drug derivatives is crucial for an ADC process to avoid any unconjugated residue of the highly toxic drug in the bulk ADC end product. While the process solution volumes at mg scale are typically too small to establish a technique like TFF, the volumes of gram-scale conjugation are large enough for proper screening of TFF parameters.

In TFF systems, operating parameter selection has a considerable impact on the process performance. A goal for the TFF step within a conjugation process consists of an optimized flux leading to an efficient buffer exchange, but also to gain an improved impurity clearance simultaneously. To achieve a reproducible and optimized process flux and time, several membrane types and suppliers can be screened and key TFF parameters should be optimized at the earliest convenience in the process development phase. For a rapid optimization of the key parameters, a first screen of different feed flow (FF) rates while simultaneously varying the transmembrane pressure (TMP) delivers data for the maximization of the flux rates (*see* Fig. 7) (e.g., *see* ref. 19).

High flux rates are preferred as they allow a short TFF process time. After having determined the optimal TMP and FF, the influence of the protein concentration on the TFF performance is investigated in a second step (*see* Fig. 7, left).

In order to determine the necessary number of diavolumes in a TFF step, analytical methods for quantifying the amount of the impurities of interest are needed. By analyzing samples pulled from the recycle tank, the decrease of the impurity level can be traced and the amounts of diavolumes for the process are defined. The selected buffer volume needs to secure that the concentration for these substances go below the threshold values (*see* Fig. 7, right).

At the end of the TFF purification development, the membrane type, FF, TMP, and number of diavolumes have been established. If the development shows that TFF is not a suitable technique to remove the impurities of the ADC process or that it has an inacceptable negative impact on product attributes (e.g., monomer content), alternative strategies such as chromatography need to be considered. Unless protein aggregation cannot be controlled during the conjugation process, chromatography purification is generally not needed which is advantageous both in terms of yield and cost of goods.

6 Clinical Supply

When producing material for toxicological or clinical studies, a robust bioburden control concept must be available for the whole process. Bioburden control starts with the selection of the appropriate high-quality raw material supplier and the rigorous release testing at the manufacturing site of the ADC. The installation of an appropriate production equipment to ensure running the process as closed and aseptic as possible, together with a rigorous bioburden awareness training of the plant operators, further minimizes the contamination risk for ADC batches. Tracking endotoxin levels and bioburden throughout the process via in-process controls gives additional data and know-how of potential sources of contaminations. In addition, the definition of bioburden reduction steps such as 0.2 μm filtrations during a process is crucial to avoid unnecessary risks. Typically, an ADC process starts with the transfer of the naked mAb via a filter into a closed reaction vessel. After prolonged reaction times, additional in-process filtrations might be necessary. Certainly, a final fill filtration will be performed before the formulated ADC solution is stored. In addition, buffers might be filtered post manufacturing and/or point of use, and the acceptable storage times and temperatures of these solutions need to be critically assessed.

After definition of the process parameters using a DoE parameter screening approach and a purification development, followed by the definition of a production concept, the process is ready to be scaled up typically to a >50 g scale that allows the production material to support toxicity studies as well as early clinical phases. A reproducible product quality should be achieved over different batches equal to the material obtained earlier in the laboratory.

7 Challenges on the Way to Commercial Processes

When a process moves forward through the clinical phases, it has to be further characterized in order to finally pass validation, a necessity to produce ADCs for the commercial supply [8]. During the so-called process design phase, the parameters of the future commercial process are defined based on additional laboratory experiments and the knowledge gained through the scale-up activities of the ADC manufacturing for the early clinical phases. In this phase of the process life cycle, the DoE methodology again allows gaining deep process knowledge with comparable limited number of experiments.

After having identified the significant process parameters to ensure the desired product quality by an initial factorial screening DoE in the earlier phase of the process, these factors can be further optimized during the "process design" phase in an even more comprehensive DoE. If required, an observed curvature of the output in the initial screening DoE can be further investigated using a response-surface model for nonlinear systems. Thereby, a model can be established that accurately describes the behavior of the conjugation process and visualizes the interactions of all relevant variables. This allows the definition of a design space for the process parameters. Within the borderlines of the design space, a process performs as expected. This can be verified by additional experiments that prove the robustness of the conjugation process. These investigations lead to the identification of critical process parameters (CPPs) and definition of proven acceptable ranges (PARs) for all relevant process parameters, which have to be followed in order to achieve the production of the ADC in equivalent quality from batch to batch.

Due to the fact that the change to commercial production often involves a further up-scaling compared to the earlier clinical phases, any potential impact on the product quality should be considered. For example, power input through stirring, tip speeds of agitators, and times to homogeneity upon reagent addition can hardly be kept constant (e.g., *see* ref. 20). Therefore, it has to be assured that the values chosen for these variables do not affect any ADC properties. If contact materials change in this further up-scaling, additional laboratory investigations might be needed to prove their compatibility with the process stream. Furthermore, filter sizing experiments help choosing the appropriate 0.2 μm filter sizes for the commercial process. With all the information collected and a deep knowledge acquired through the manufacturing process, the ADC is now ready to be produced at large scale for commercial applications.

Acknowledgements

We thank Dr. Nikolaus Bieler for helpful discussions regarding the application of the DoE approach to bioconjugation reactions.

References

1. Polson AG, Ho WY, Ramakrishnan Y (2011) Investigational antibody-drug conjugates for hematological malignancies. Expert Opin Investig Drugs 20:75–85
2. Pasquetto MV, Vecchia L, Covini D, Digillio R, Scotti C (2011) Targeted drug delivery using immunoconjugates: principles and applications. J Immunother 34:611–628
3. Fitzgerald DJ, Wayne AJ, Kreitman RJ, Pastan I (2011) Treatment of hematologic malignancies with immunotoxins and antibody-drug conjugates. Cancer Res 71:6300–6309
4. Hughes B (2010) Antibody–drug conjugates for cancer: poised to deliver? Nat Rev Drug Discov 9:665–667
5. Vermeer AWP, Norde W (2000) The thermal stability of immunoglobulin: unfolding and aggregation of a multi-domain protein. Biophys J 78:394–404
6. Shire SJ, Gombotz W, Bechtold-Peters K, Andya J (2010) Current trends in monoclonal antibody development and manufacturing. Springer, New York
7. Hamblett KJ, Senter PD, Chace DF, Sun MMC, Lenox J, Cerveny CG, Kissler KM, Bernhardt SX, Kopcha AK, Zabinski RF, Meyer DL, Francisco JA (2004) Effects of drug loading on the antitumor activity of a monoclonal antibody drug conjugate. Clin Cancer Res 10:7063–7070
8. Guidance for industry—process validation: general principles and practices, U.S. Department of Health and Human Services Food and Drug Administration, Jan 2011
9. McDonagh CF, Kim KM, Turcott E, Brown LL, Westendorf L, Feist T, Sussman D, Stone I, Anderson M, Miyamoto J, Lyon R, Alley SC, Gerber H-P, Carter PJ (2008) Engineered anti-CD70 antibody-drug conjugate with increased therapeutic index. Mol Cancer Ther 7:2913–2923
10. Chari RVJ (2008) Targeted cancer therapy: conferring specificity to cytotoxic drugs. Acc Chem Res 41:98–107
11. Eriksson L, Johansson E, Kettaneh-Wold N, Wikström C, Wohl S (2008) Design of experiments—principles and applications. Umetrics Academy, Umea
12. Design Expert, Stat-Ease, Inc. 2021 E. Hennepin Avenue, Suite 480 Minneapolis, MN 55413-2726
13. MODDE, Umetrics Inc./MKS Inst., 70 W. Rio Robles Drive, San Jose, CA 95134, USA
14. Statistica, StatSoft Inc., 2300 East 14th Street, Tulsa, OK 74104, USA
15. Gagnon P (2012) Technology trends in antibody purification. J Chromatogr 1221:57–70
16. Van Reis R, Gadam S, Frautschy LN, Orlando S, Goodrich EM, Saksena S, Kuriyel R, Simpson CM, Pearl S, Zydney AL (1997) High performance tangential flow filtration. Biotechnol Bioeng 56:71–82
17. Van Reis R, Zydney A (2001) Membrane separations in biotechnology. Curr Opin Biotechnol 12:208–212
18. Van Reis R, Zydney A (1997) Bioprocess membrane technology. J Membr Sci 297:16–50
19. (2008) A hands-on guide to ultrafiltration/diafiltration optimizing using Pellicon® Cassettes. Application note, Millipore http://www.millipore.com/publications.nsf/a73664f9f981af8c852569b9005b4eee/08773250551d1562852574e0007d4570/$FILE/an2700en00.pdf
20. (1990) Mixing band agitation. In: Walas SM (ed) Chemical process equipment—selection and design. Elsevier See http://www.sciencedirect.com/science/book/9780123725066. Chemical Process Equipment (Third Edition), Author(s):James R. Couper, W. Roy Penney, James R. Fair and Stanley M. Walas, therein "Chapter 10 - MIXING AND AGITATION, 273–324"

Chapter 15

Methods for Conjugating Antibodies to Nanocarriers

Anil Wagh and Benedict Law

Abstract

Antibodies are one of the most commonly used targeting ligands for nanocarriers, mainly because they are specific, have a strong binding affinity, and are available for a number of disease biomarkers. The bioconjugation chemistry can be a crucial factor in determining the targeting efficiency of drug delivery and should be chosen on a case-by-case basis. An antibody consists of a number of functional groups which offer many flexible options for bioconjugation. This chapter focuses on discussing some of the approaches including periodate oxidation, carbodiimide, maleimide, and heterofunctional linkers, for conjugating antibodies to different nanocarriers. The advantages and limitations are described herein. Specific examples are selected to demonstrate the experimental procedures and to illustrate the potential for applying to other nanocarrier system.

Key words Nanocarriers, Nanoparticles, Bioconjugation, Antibodies, Targeting ligands

1 Introduction

Nanocarriers are nanometer-sized materials that have the capacity to deliver therapeutic agents at the disease site [1, 2]. They are designed to possess unique physicochemical properties, aiming to improve the pharmacokinetic and biodistribution of a drug molecule [3, 4] and to deliver a significant amount of drug molecules. Examples of some therapeutic nanocarriers are lipid-based particles [5], micelles [6], nanoparticles [7], dendrimers [8], and polymersomes [9]. Some of these have been proposed for the treatment of various diseases including cancer [10, 11], coronary artery diseases [12, 13], and rheumatoid arthritis [14, 15]. In particular cancer, the unique anatomy, i.e., the leakiness of the tumoral vasculatures, concedes a passive transport of the nanocarriers by enhanced permeability and retention (EPR) effect [16]. However, the porosity of the tumor blood vessels may vary with the tumor type [17, 18]. Even with a successful delivery by the EPR effect, the nanocarriers must be able to internalize into the cancer cells [19, 20].

Laurent Ducry (ed.), *Antibody-Drug Conjugates*, Methods in Molecular Biology, vol. 1045,
DOI 10.1007/978-1-62703-541-5_15, © Springer Science+Business Media, LLC 2013

A new paradigm in drug delivery embroils a combination of active and passive targeting. Targeting ligands such as antibodies [21], peptides [22], small molecules [23], or aptamers [10] can be attached onto the surface of a nanocarrier. The carriers recognize and bind to the cell-surface receptors and are subsequently taken by the cells via receptor-mediated endocytosis for releasing the therapeutic payloads [24]. The binding affinity of targeted nanocarriers can also be increased several orders of magnitude by the multivalent effect [25].

Among all the targeting ligands, antibodies are well known for their high binding affinity, specificity, and availability for a number of disease biomarkers [26]. An antibody can be simply absorbed on the surface of a nanocarrier via hydrophobic and/or electrostatic interaction [27]. However, using this approach, the absorbed antibody may orient randomly on the surface and result in losing the binding affinity. Furthermore, the antibody may exchange with other endogenous protein in vivo [28]. Therefore, antibodies are generally preferred to attach to the nanocarriers covalently [29].

An antibody consists of a number of functional groups that provides many options for bioconjugation [26]. In this chapter, we describe the general approaches for conjugating multiple antibodies to therapeutic nanocarriers. Based on the modifications of the functional groups, the conjugation methods are categorized into carbohydrate modification, amine or carboxylic acid modification, and conjugation via the sulfhydryl group [26, 28]. It is important to note that there is not a universal method that is superior to the others. The differences in the amino acid composition and sequence in the polypeptide chains should be taken into an account, as they may affect the reactivity of the antibody [30]. The method should be chosen with an aim to preserve the binding affinity of the antibody, and the chemistry should be selected in accordance to the type as well as the availability of the functional group on the carrier surface.

2 Materials

2.1 Carbohydrate Modification Components

1. All the chemicals and reagents were analytical grade ($\geq$95 % purity).
2. Sodium cyanoborohydride ($NaBH_3(CN)$) and sodium periodate ($NaIO_4$) were purchased from Sigma-Aldrich (St. Louis, MO).
3. Sephadex G-25 was purchased from GE Healthcare Biosciences (Piscataway, NJ).
4. Mouse anti-HRP antibody was obtained from Santa Cruz Biotechnology, Inc. (Santa Cruz, CA).

5. Rat anti-CC52 antibody was purchased from Thermo Fisher Scientific, Inc. (Rockford, USA).
6. Phosphate buffer (10 mM, pH 7.0): sodium phosphate monobasic monohydrate (0.059 g, 0.43 mmoL) and sodium phosphate dibasic heptahydrate (0.16 g, 0.60 mmoL) in deionized water (100 mL).
7. Phosphate buffer (10 mM, pH 8.0): sodium phosphate monobasic monohydrate (0.01 g, 0.08 mmoL) and sodium phosphate dibasic heptahydrate (0.25 g, 0.94 mmoL) in deionized water (100 mL).
8. 2-Morpholinoethanesulfonic acid (MES) saline buffer (10 mM, pH 6.1): MES monohydrate (0.196 g, 1 mmoL) and NaCl (0.87 g, 15 mmoL) in deionized water (100 mL).

2.2 Amine or Carboxylic Acid Modification Components

1. All the chemicals and reagents were analytical grade (≥95 % purity).
2. 1-Ethyl-3-(3-dimethylaminopropyl)carbodiimide hydrochloride (EDC) and *N*-hydroxysuccinimide (NHS) were obtained from Sigma-Aldrich (St. Louis, MO).
3. Anti-EGFR antibody and Herceptin were supplied by Imgenex Corporation (San Diego, CA) and Genentech, Inc. (San Francisco, CA), respectively.
4. Phosphate buffer saline (100 mM, pH 5.8): sodium phosphate monobasic monohydrate (1.28 g, 9.3 mmoL), sodium phosphate dibasic heptahydrate (0.22 g, 0.82 mmoL), and NaCl (0.87 g, 15 mmoL) in deionized water (100 mL).
5. Phosphate buffer saline (100 mM, pH 7.4): sodium phosphate monobasic monohydrate (0.32 g, 2.3 mmoL), sodium phosphate dibasic heptahydrate (2.1 g, 7.9 mmoL), and NaCl (0.87 g, 15 mmoL) in deionized water (100 mL).

2.3 Sulfhydryl Conjugation Components

1. All the chemicals and reagents were analytical grade (≥95 % purity).
2. Dithiothreitol (DTT) was obtained from Sigma-Aldrich (St. Louis, MO).
3. P-10 desalting columns and Sephadex CL-4B were purchased from GE Healthcare Biosciences (Piscataway, NJ).
4. Herceptin and antihuman DEC-205 antibody were purchased from Genentech, Inc. (San Francisco, CA) and BioLegend, Inc. (San Diego, CA), respectively.
5. Dextran desalting column, *N*-succinimidyl 3-(2-pyridyldithio) propionate (SPDP), and Traut's reagent (2-iminothiolane) were purchased from Thermo Fisher Scientific, Inc. (Rockford, USA).

6. *N*-(2-hydroxyethyl)piperazine-*N'*-(2-ethanesulfonic acid) (HEPES)-buffered saline (25 mM, pH 6.6): HEPES (0.6 g, 2.5 mmoL) and NaCl (0.87 g, 15 mmoL) in deionized water (100 mL).
7. Sodium acetate-buffered saline (100 mM, pH 4.5): sodium acetate (0.82 g, 10 mmoL) and NaCl (0.87 g, 15 mmoL) in deionized water (100 mL).
8. Phosphate buffer (100 mM, pH 8.0): sodium phosphate monobasic monohydrate (0.095 g, 0.69 mmoL) and sodium phosphate dibasic heptahydrate (2.5 g, 9.3 mmoL) in deionized water (100 mL).

3 Methods

3.1 Carbohydrate Modification by Periodate Oxidation

Periodate oxidation is a friendly approach for bioconjugation of an antibody [31–34]. A typical IgG antibody consists of oligosaccharides covalently attached to the asparagine residue (Asp297) at the constant region (F_c) of the heavy chains [35]. The oligosaccharides are usually presented in a diantennary complex form which consists of a core heptasaccharide attached with a variable outer arm of sugar residues, including fucose, galactose, bisecting *N*-acetylglucosamine, sialic acid, and *N*-acetylneuraminic acid [36]. The pyranose rings of the sugars containing the vicinal diols can be oxidized by sodium periodate ($NaIO_4$) to generate reactive dialdehydes (Fig. 1a and Subheading 2.2, **item 1**) [37], and the oxidized antibody (IgG-*CHO*) can react with the nanocarriers that consist of primary amine or hydrazide functional groups via reductive amination (Fig. 1b and Subheading 2.2, **item 2**) [38, 39]. The advantage of this approach is that it is specific, since a modification of oligosaccharides would not affect the antibody–antigen binding [40]. For example, multiple of IgG antibodies were conjugated to the surface of hydrazide-terminated liposomes (LP-$NHNH_2$) [41] and the amino-terminated magnetic nanoparticles (MNP-NH_2) [42]. However, a comparative study has shown that fewer antibodies were conjugated to the same nanocarrier as compared to using the sulfhydryl-maleimide chemistry (17 % vs. 63 %) [39]. Two examples were chosen to demonstrate periodate oxidation chemistry for conjugating antibodies to nanocarriers [41, 42].

3.1.1 Oxidation of the Antibody

1. An antibody (1 mg, 6.67 nmoL) was dissolved in phosphate buffer pH 7.0 (1 mL) and was stored at 4 °C (*see* **Notes 1–3**).
2. Periodate solution was prepared by dissolving $NaIO_4$ (21.4 mg, 0.1 mmoL) in deionized water (1 mL) (*see* **Note 4**).
3. An aliquot of the periodate solution (100 μL) was added to the antibody solution (1 mL) and further incubated for 2 h at 4 °C.

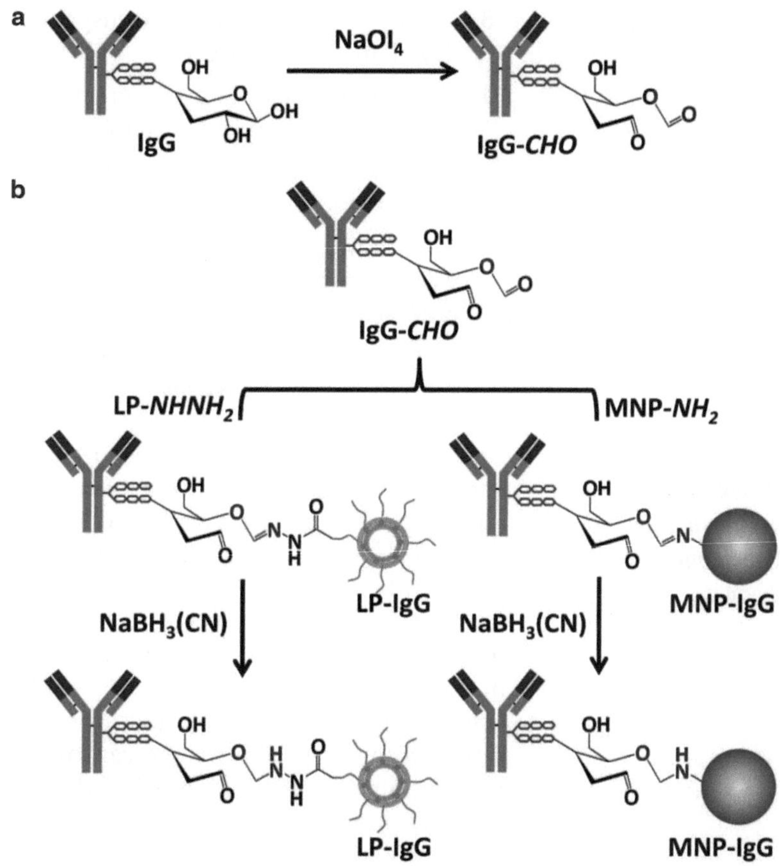

Fig. 1 Synthetic schemes for conjugating antibodies to the nanocarriers using periodate oxidation. (**a**) The oligosaccharides of an IgG antibody could be oxidized to dialdehydes by $NaIO_4$. (**b**) The resulting antibody (IgG-*CHO*) reacted with the hydrazide-terminated liposomes (LP-*$NHNH_2$*) or amino-terminated magnetic nanoparticles (MNP-*NH_2*) to form the Schiff base intermediates, which are further reduced to the corresponding secondary amines in the presence of $NaBH_3(CN)$

4. The reaction mixture was purified by size exclusion chromatography (Sephadex G-25) using phosphate buffer pH 8.0 as the eluent (*see* **Notes 5** and **6**).
5. The stock IgG-*CHO* solution (0.1 mg/mL) was used immediately for the conjugation (*see* **Note 7** and Subheading 3.1.2).

3.1.2 Conjugation of IgG-CHO to the Hydrazide- or Amino-Terminated Nanocarrier

1. LP-*$NHNH_2$* were synthesized by a lipid hydration method [41]. The particles were encapsulated with 5-fluorodeoxyuridine.
2. MNP-*NH_2* were synthesized as previously described [42]. The particles were encapsulated with doxorubicin.

3. The particles (10 mg) were suspended in phosphate buffer pH 8.0 (1 mL) (*see* **Note 1**).
4. The nanoparticles (1 mL) were mixed with the stock IgG-*CHO* solution (1 mL) and further incubated for 2 h at 37 °C.
5. $NaBH_3(CN)$ (31.5 mg, 0.5 mmoL) was added to the reaction mixture and further incubated for 30 min at 37 °C (*see* **Note 8**).
6. The resulting particles were purified by centrifugation and washed with the phosphate buffer pH 8.0 (3 × 2 mL) to remove the unbound antibody (*see* **Note 9**).
7. The antibody-conjugated nanoparticles were stored in MES buffer at 4 °C (*see* **Notes** 7 and **10**).

3.2 Amine or Carboxylic Acid Modification by Carbodiimide Chemistry

Antibodies can be conjugated to the nanoparticles via the free amino or carboxylic acid groups from the side chains of lysine and aspartic acid or glutamic acid residues, respectively [26, 28]. These functional groups are usually exposed towards the outside of the antibody because of the ionic charges and, thus, are easily accessible for bioconjugation. However, the carboxylic acid groups are known to be nonreactive. Carbodiimides such as 1-ethyl-(3-dimethylaminopropyl)carbodiimide (EDC), *N,N'*-dicyclohexylcarbodiimide (DCC), and *N,N'*-diisopropylcarbodiimide (DIC) (Fig. 2) are often required to activate the carboxylic acids to form the active *O*-acylisourea intermediates [43], which can be further reacted with the amino groups at the nanoparticle surface to form stable amide bonds (Fig. 3 and Subheading 3.2.1) [44, 45].

Since the *O*-acylisourea intermediates can rapidly undergo hydrolysis to regenerate the original carboxylic acids, the chemistry is usually performed with the addition of *N*-hydroxysuccinimide (NHS) to generate a more stable but activated complex (i.e., the succinimidyl ester) with a slower hydrolytic rate (Fig. 3) [46]. For example, EDC, in the presence of NHS, has been employed for conjugating Herceptin, a monoclonal antibody against HER2

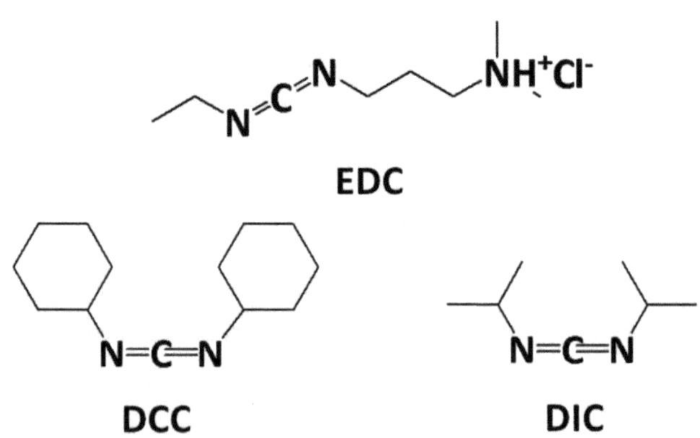

Fig. 2 Examples of some carbodiimides

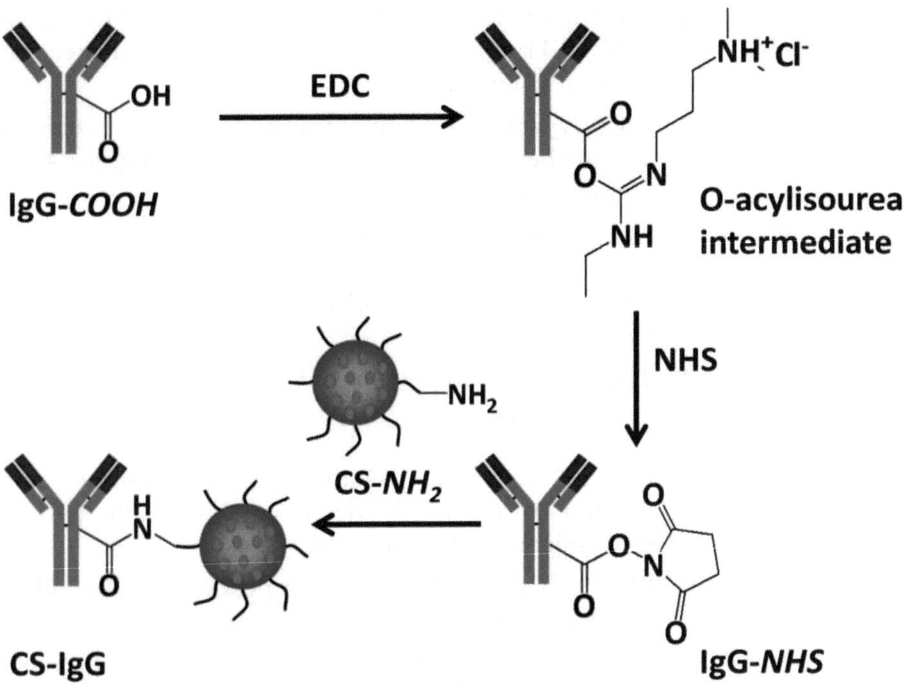

Fig. 3 Synthetic scheme for conjugating antibodies to the nanocarriers using carbodiimide chemistry. The carboxylic acid groups of the antibodies were first activated by EDC to form the *O*-acylisourea intermediates, which were then reacted with NHS to form the activated NHS ester. The activated antibodies (IgG-*NHS*) were then conjugated to the amino-terminated nanoparticles (CS-NH_2) via the formation of stable amide bonds

receptor, to the amino-terminated chitosan nanoparticles (CS-NH_2) (Fig. 3) [47]. Similarly, the carboxylic acid-terminated poly (D,L-lactide-*co*-glycolide) nanoparticles (PLGA-*COOH*) can be activated by EDC prior conjugating to antibody via the amino groups (Subheading 3.2.2) [48]. The later approach offers the advantages of minimizing the denaturation and the loss of binding affinity of the antibody, since the activation chemistry is performed on the nanocarriers rather than the antibodies [26].

The following two examples illustrate the methods to conjugate antibodies to the nanocarriers using carbodiimide chemistry [47, 48].

3.2.1 Conjugation of Antibodies to the Amino-Terminated Nanocarrier

1. CS-NH_2 were synthesized by an ionic gelation method as previously described [49]. The particles were encapsulated with gemcitabine (*see* **Note 1**).
2. CS-NH_2 (10 mg) was suspended in PBS buffer pH 5.8 (1 mL).
3. EDC (40 mg, 208 μmoL) and NHS (9.7 mg, 84.5 μmoL) were dissolved in PBS buffer pH 5.8 (4 mL) (*see* **Note 11**).
4. Herceptin (1 mg, 6.67 nmoL) was dissolved in PBS buffer pH 7.4 (1 mL) (*see* **Note 1**).

5. An aliquot of the antibody solution (250 μL) was added to EDC/NHS solution (4 mL) and further incubated for 30 min at room temperature.
6. CS-NH_2 solution (1 mL) was added to the reaction mixture and further incubated with magnetic stirring for 4 h at room temperature (*see* **Notes 12** and **13**).
7. The resulting particles (CS-IgG) were purified by ultracentrifugation (40,000 × *g*, 20 min) at 4 °C and washed with PBS buffer pH 5.8 (3 × 5 mL) to remove the unbound antibody (*see* **Note 9**).
8. The CS-IgG were lyophilized and kept at 4 °C before further use (*see* **Note 7**).

3.2.2 Conjugation of Antibodies to the Carboxylic Acid-Terminated Nanocarrier

1. PLGA-*COOH* were synthesized by a solvent evaporation method as previously described [48]. The particles were encapsulated with rapamycin.
2. PLGA-*COOH* (10 mg) was suspended in PBS buffer pH 7.4 (5 mL) (*see* **Note 1**).
3. EDC (1 mg, 5.2 μmoL) was dissolved in PBS buffer pH 7.4 (1 mL) (*see* **Note 11**).
4. NHS (1 mg, 8.7 μmoL) was dissolved in PBS buffer pH 7.4 (1 mL) (*see* **Note 11**).
5. Anti-EGFR antibody (100 μg, 0.67 nmoL) was dissolved in PBS buffer pH 7.4 (1 mL) (*see* **Note 1**).
6. PLGA-*COOH* (5 mL) was activated by incubating with excess EDC (250 μL) and NHS (250 μL) with moderate agitation for 4 h at room temperature (*see* **Note 12**).
7. The resulting particles (PLGA-*NHS*) were purified by ultracentrifugation (40,000 × *g*, 20 min) at 4 °C and further washed with PBS buffer pH 7.4 (3 × 1 mL) to remove the unreacted EDC and NHS (*see* **Notes 9** and **14**).
8. PLGA-*NHS* (10 mg) was then diluted with PBS buffer pH 7.4 (2 mL).
9. An aliquot of the anti-EGFR antibody solution (500 μL) was added to the PLGA-*NHS* solution (2 mL). The reaction mixture was kept at moderate agitation for 2 h at room temperature and further incubated for 12 h at 4 °C.
10. The resulting particles (PLGA-IgG) were purified by ultracentrifugation (40,000 × *g*, 20 min) and washed with PBS buffer pH 7.4 to remove the unbound antibody (*see* **Note 9**).
11. The PLGA-IgG were kept at 4 °C before further use (*see* **Note 7**).

3.3 Conjugation via the Sulfhydryl Moiety

Antibodies can be conjugated to nanoparticles via the sulfhydryl group of cysteine residues [50]. Theoretically, an antibody does not have any free sulfhydryl group, as all the cysteines are engaged in forming disulfide bonds [51]. However, a number of free sulfhydryls can be found in a mature antibody as a result of incomplete formation of disulfide bond during posttranslational modification [52] or breakage of the disulfide bond during storage by β-elimination [53], but the number of sulfhydryls is much lower when compared to the free amines or carboxylic acids.

Free sulfhydryls can be generated through partial or complete reduction of the antibody interchain disulfide bonds using dithiothreitol (DTT) [54], 2-mercaptoethylamine [55], or tris (2-carboxyethyl)phosphine (TCEP) [56]. Nanocarriers containing maleimide [57, 58] or iodoacetyl [59] functional groups can be conjugated to the antibody fragments via the formation of thioether linkages. For example, TCEP was employed to reduce a monoclonal antibody against carcinoembryonic antigen (CEA) into half antibodies, which were subsequently used for attaching to the maleimide-terminated lipid particles [60].

Additional sulfhydryl groups can also be introduced to an antibody by employing various heterobifunctional linkers such as *N*-succinimidyl-3-(2-pyridyldithio) propionate (SPDP), 4-succinimidyloxycarbonyl-alpha-methyl-alpha(2-pyridyldithio) toluene (SMPT), *N*-succinimidyl-*S*-acetylthiopropionate (SATP), and *N*-succinimidyl-*S*-acetylthioacetate (SATA) (Fig. 4). Each linker consists of a *N*-hydroxysuccinimide ester on one side, so that it can be conjugated to the antibody at the lysine residues using carbodiimide chemistry [61]. The other side of the linker is

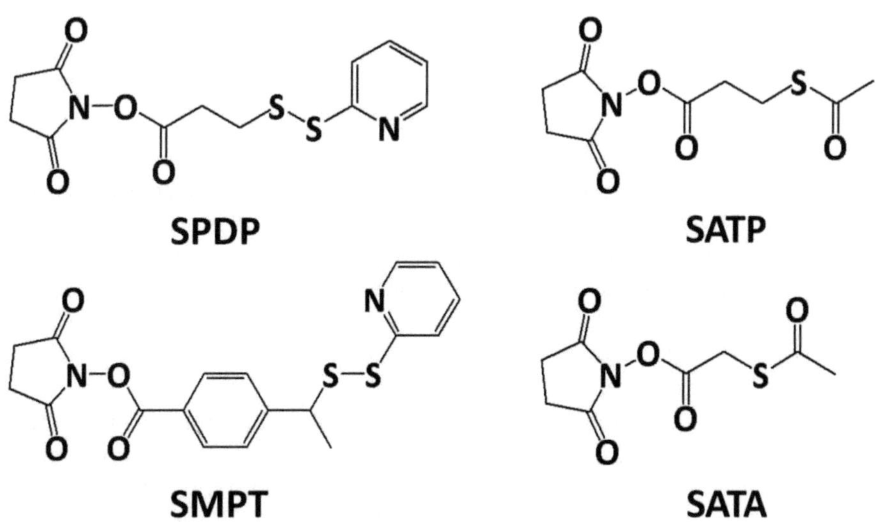

Fig. 4 Examples of the heterobifunctional linkers

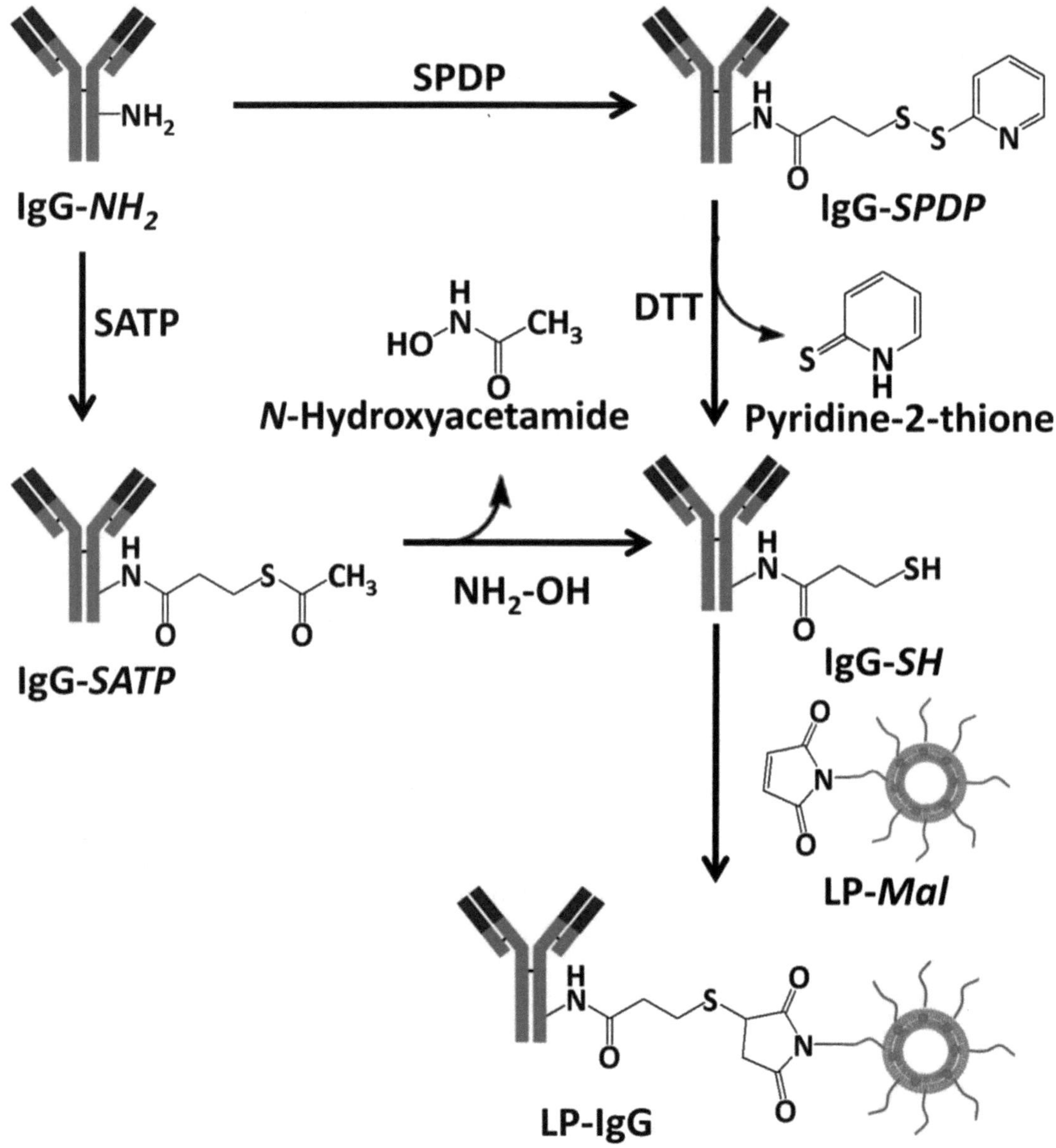

Fig. 5 Synthetic scheme for conjugating antibodies to the nanocarriers using heterobifunctional linkers. The amino groups of the antibody were modified by SPDP or SATP, and the terminal protected groups were subsequently deprotected by DTT or hydroxylamine (NH_2OH), respectively, to generate free sulfhydryl groups. The modified antibody (IgG-*SH*) was conjugated to maleimide-terminated liposomes (LP-*Mal*)

attached with a sulfhydryl that is protected by a pyridylthiol or an acetyl group.

The function of pyridylthiol and acetyl is to protect the terminal sulfhydryl, which can be readily deprotected by DTT and hydroxylamine, respectively, to obtain the free sulfhydryl group and further react with the maleimide-terminated nanoparticles (Fig. 5 and Subheading 3.3.2) [26, 28, 62]. However, this

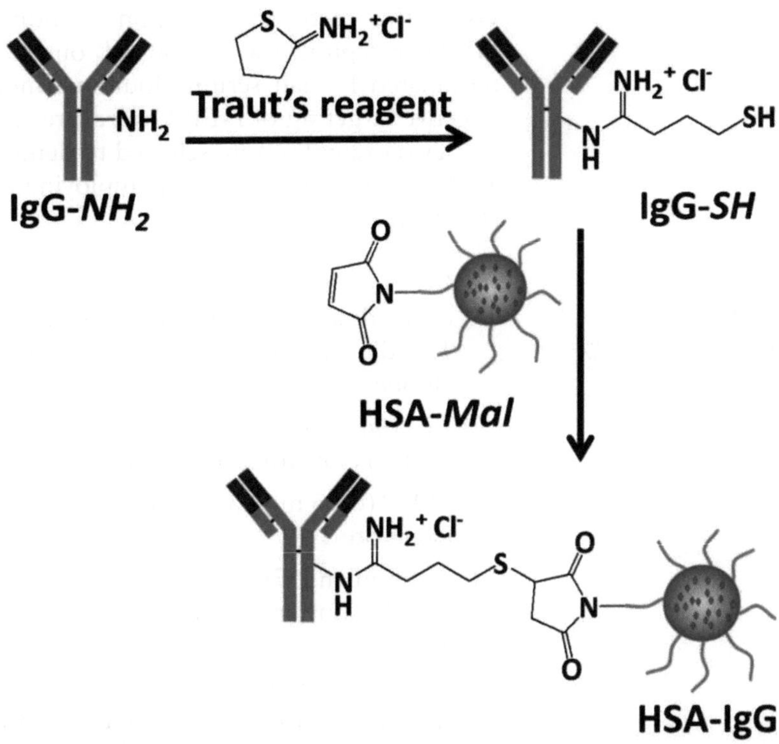

Fig. 6 Synthetic scheme for conjugation of nanoparticles to the antibody using Traut's reagent as a linker. The Traut's reagent was reacted with the amino groups of the antibodies to generate free sulfhydryls. The modified antibodies (IgG-*SH*) could be anchored to the surface of maleimide-terminated human serum albumin nanoparticles (HSA-*Mal*) via thioether bonds

approach requires multiple purification steps in order to remove the excess linkers and deprotecting reagents. In the case of using pyridylthiol as the protecting group, the antibody can directly attach to the sulfhydryl-terminated nanoparticle, since the pyridylthiol is reactive towards the free sulfhydryl group and forms a disulfide bond [63]. To develop an antibody-nanoparticle conjugate for in vivo application, a thioether linkage is generally preferred because the disulfide bond is not stable in systematic circulation [64].

Another approach to introduce free sulfhydryl groups to an antibody is by using 2-iminothiolane (Traut's reagent). 2-Iminothiolane is a cyclic imidothioester that can react with the primary amine of an antibody and results in the opening of thiophene ring to generate a terminal free sulfhydryl group (Fig. 6 and Subheading 3.3.2) [65]. When compared to using heterobifunctional linkers, this approach does not require the deprotection step and, thus, minimizes a number of purification steps. More importantly, the original positive charge of the antibody is retained after conjugation because of the presence of the amidine group [65].

Using this method, Herceptin, a monoclonal antibody against HER2 receptor, was decorated on the surface of maleimide-terminated human serum albumin nanoparticles (HSA-*Mal*) for selective targeting of HER2 overexpressing cancer cells [66].

Two examples were selected to demonstrate how to conjugate antibodies to nanocarriers by employing SPDP and Traut's reagent [66, 67].

3.3.1 Conjugation of Antibodies to the Nanocarrier Using SPDP

1. LP-*Mal* were synthesized by lipid hydration method as previously described [67]. The particles were encapsulated with 1,1'-dioctadecyl-3,3,3',3'-tetramethylindocarbocyanineperchlorate.
2. LP-*Mal* (1.6 mg, 2 μmoL) was suspended in HBS buffer (1 mL) (*see* **Notes 1** and **15**).
3. SPDP (6.25 mg, 20 μmoL) was dissolved in HBS buffer (1 mL) (*see* **Note 16**).
4. Antihuman DEC-205 antibody (5 mg, 33 nmoL) was dissolved in HBS buffer (1 mL) and was stored at 4 °C (*see* **Notes 1** and **2**).
5. An aliquot of SPDP solution (17 μL) was added to the antibody solution (1 mL) and then incubated for 30 min at room temperature.
6. The reaction mixture was purified by size exclusion chromatography (P-10 desalting column, GE Healthcare Biosciences) using SAS buffer as the eluent.
7. The purified IgG-*SPDP* (5 mg) was diluted in SAS buffer (1 mL) (*see* **Note 7**).
8. DTT (7.7 mg, 50 μmoL) was added to the IgG-*SPDP* solution (1 mL) and incubated for 20 min at room temperature (*see* **Notes 17** and **18**).
9. The reaction mixture was purified by size exclusion chromatography (P-10 desalting column) using HBS buffer as the eluent.
10. The stock IgG-*SH* (1 mg/mL) was used immediately (*see* **Notes 6**, **7**, and **19**).
11. An aliquot of antibody solution (300 μL) was added to the LP-*Mal* solution (1 mL), and the reaction mixture was further incubated in dark for 12 h at room temperature (*see* **Note 18**).
12. The product (LP-IgG) was then purified by size exclusion chromatography (Sephadex CL-4B) using HBS buffer as the eluent.
13. The LP-IgG were stored in HBS buffer at 4 °C (*see* **Notes 7** and **10**).

3.3.2 Conjugation of Antibody to the Nanocarrier Using Traut's Reagent

1. HSA-*Mal* were synthesized by desolvation method as previously described [66]. The particles were encapsulated with doxorubicin.
2. HSA-*Mal* (40 mg) was diluted in phosphate buffer (1 mL) (*see* **Notes 1** and **15**).
3. Traut's reagent (1.14 mg, 8.3 μmoL) was dissolved in phosphate buffer (1 mL).
4. Herceptin (1 mg, 6.67 nmoL) was diluted in phosphate buffer (1 mL) (*see* **Notes 1** and **2**).
5. An aliquot of Traut's reagent (40 μL) was added to the antibody solution (1 mL) and incubated for 2 h at room temperature (*see* **Note 18**).
6. The reaction mixture was purified by a dextran desalting column using phosphate buffer as the eluent.
7. The stock IgG-*SH* (0.5 mg/mL) was used immediately (*see* **Notes** 7 and **19**).
8. HSA-*Mal* solution (1 mL) was mixed with the IgG-*SH* solution (1 mL) and further incubated with constant shaking for 12 h at 20°C (*see* **Note 18**).
9. The resulting particles (HSA-IgG) were purified by centrifugation (16,100 × *g*, 10 min) at 4 °C and washed with phosphate buffer (3 × 2 mL) (*see* **Note 9**).
10. The HSA-IgG were stored in deionized water at 4°C (*see* **Notes** 7 and **10**).

4 Notes

1. Depending on the stability of the antibody and the physiochemical properties of the nanocarriers, the reaction conditions, including the pH and the choice of buffer, may vary.
2. IgG antibody may precipitate in the buffer during storage. It should be centrifuged (10,000 × *g*, 10 min) to remove any visible aggregates.
3. The level of glycosylation can be different, depending on the source and type of the antibody. The presence of oligosaccharides should be confirmed prior to performing the reaction [36].
4. The periodate solution should be freshly prepared and protected from light. Periodate can be reduced to iodine by light.
5. Excess $NaIO_4$ may be quenched by the addition of ethylene glycol (0.25 mL). The ethylene glycol gets oxidized by the excess $NaOI_4$ to form formaldehyde and iodate (IO_3^-) [68].

6. SDS-PAGE gel can be performed to verify the integrity of the antibody. SDS-PAGE should be performed under nonreducing conditions in order to prevent reduction of the endogenous disulfide bonds of the antibody.
7. The amount of antibody can be determined by standard protein assays such as the microBCA™ and Bradford protein assay [69, 70]. Alternatively, the antibody can be quantified by absorbance at 280 nm ($\varepsilon_{280\ \mathrm{nm}} = 210{,}000\ \mathrm{M}^{-1}\ \mathrm{cm}^{-1}$) [71].
8. $NaBH_3(CN)$ is a mild reducing agent that reduces the intermediate imines to give the secondary amines. Sodium borohydride or pyridine borane can be used as alternatives [72, 73].
9. In the case of nanocarriers that cannot be purified by centrifugation, the impurities can be removed by dialysis or size exclusion chromatography (Sephadex CL-4B) [31, 74].
10. The conjugated nanoparticles may not be suitable for long-term storage. Depending on the drug delivery system, the drug may release from the particles with time.
11. Both the EDC and NHS can undergo hydrolysis in an aqueous environment. They should be freshly prepared for immediate use.
12. In absence of NHS, the *O*-acylisourea intermediate can undergo spontaneous rearrangement via an intramolecular acyl transfer to form a nonreactive *N*-acylurea derivative and thus significantly reduces the conjugation efficiency [75].
13. The NHS ester of one antibody can react with the free amino groups from the other antibody. If necessary, the endogenous amino groups can be reversibly blocked by citraconic or maleic anhydride to prevent antibody cross-linking or precipitation [76].
14. The particles should be used immediately, since NHS esters are susceptible to hydrolysis in an aqueous environment.
15. Maleimide can undergo hydrolysis in an aqueous environment. The maleimide-terminated particles should be freshly prepared.
16. SPDP is not completely soluble in the buffer. It should be dissolved in a small amount of water-miscible polar organic solvent such as dimethylsulfoxide (DMSO) or dimethylformamide (DMF) prior dilution with buffer. A water-soluble derivative such as sulfo-LC-SPDP can be used as a substitute [77].
17. The reaction can be monitored by the release of pyridine-2-thione, which can be indicated by an increase in the absorbance at 343 nm ($\varepsilon = 8{,}080\ \mathrm{M}^{-1}\ \mathrm{cm}^{-1}$). The number of SPDP molecules conjugated to the antibody can be determined by this method [65].
18. The reaction should be performed in an inert atmosphere or a chelating agent such as ethylenediaminetetraacetic acid

(EDTA) (2–5 mM) can be added to the buffer to prevent the metal-catalyzed oxidation. Alternatively, the oxygen in the buffer can be removed by bubbling with nitrogen gas for 20 min [78].

19. The number of free sulfhydryl groups in the antibody can be quantified by various assays using Ellman's reagent or *N*-(1-pyrenyl)maleimide [79, 80].

Acknowledgments

The authors would like to thank Elango Kumarasamy for editorial assistance. This research was supported in part by North Dakota EPSCoR Program, Department of Pharmaceutical Sciences (NDSU), Darryle and Clare Schoepp Research Fund, and American Association of Colleges of Pharmacy (AACP) NIA award to B.L.

References

1. Schroeder A, Heller DA, Winslow MM, Dahlman JE, Pratt GW, Langer R, Jacks T, Anderson DG (2012) Treating metastatic cancer with nanotechnology. Nat Rev Cancer 12:39–50
2. Arias JL (2011) Advanced methodologies to formulate nanotheragnostic agents for combined drug delivery and imaging. Expert Opin Drug Deliv 8:1589–1608
3. Alexis F, Pridgen E, Molnar LK, Farokhzad OC (2008) Factors affecting the clearance and biodistribution of polymeric nanoparticles. Mol Pharm 5:505–515
4. Li SD, Huang L (2008) Pharmacokinetics and biodistribution of nanoparticles. Mol Pharm 5:496–504
5. Al-Jamal WT, Kostarelos K (2011) Liposomes: from a clinically established drug delivery system to a nanoparticle platform for theranostic nanomedicine. Acc Chem Res 44:1094–1104
6. Kedar U, Phutane P, Shidhaye S, Kadam V (2010) Advances in polymeric micelles for drug delivery and tumor targeting. Nanomedicine 6:714–729
7. Shi J, Votruba AR, Farokhzad OC, Langer R (2010) Nanotechnology in drug delivery and tissue engineering: from discovery to applications. Nano Lett 10:3223–3230
8. Svenson S (2009) Dendrimers as versatile platform in drug delivery applications. Eur J Pharm Biopharm 71:445–462
9. Levine DH, Ghoroghchian PP, Freudenberg J, Zhang G, Therien MJ, Greene MI, Hammer DA, Murali R (2008) Polymersomes: a new multi-functional tool for cancer diagnosis and therapy. Methods 46:25–32
10. Farokhzad OC, Cheng J, Teply BA, Sherifi I, Jon S, Kantoff PW, Richie JP, Langer R (2006) Targeted nanoparticle-aptamer bioconjugates for cancer chemotherapy in vivo. Proc Natl Acad Sci USA 103:6315–6320
11. Dhar S, Kolishetti N, Lippard SJ, Farokhzad OC (2011) Targeted delivery of a cisplatin prodrug for safer and more effective prostate cancer therapy in vivo. Proc Natl Acad Sci USA 108:1850–1855
12. Chan JM, Zhang L, Tong R, Ghosh D, Gao W, Liao G, Yuet KP, Gray D, Rhee JW, Cheng J, Golomb G, Libby P, Langer R, Farokhzad OC (2010) Spatiotemporal controlled delivery of nanoparticles to injured vasculature. Proc Natl Acad Sci USA 107:2213–2218
13. Chan JM, Rhee JW, Drum CL, Bronson RT, Golomb G, Langer R, Farokhzad OC (2011) In vivo prevention of arterial restenosis with paclitaxel-encapsulated targeted lipid-polymeric nanoparticles. Proc Natl Acad Sci USA 108:19347–19352
14. Thomas TP, Goonewardena SN, Majoros IJ, Kotlyar A, Cao Z, Leroueil PR, Baker JR Jr (2011) Folate-targeted nanoparticles show efficacy in the treatment of inflammatory arthritis. Arthritis Rheum 63:2671–2680

15. Bosch X (2011) Dendrimers to treat rheumatoid arthritis. ACS Nano 5:6779–6785
16. Maeda H, Fang J, Inutsuka T, Kitamoto Y (2003) Vascular permeability enhancement in solid tumor: various factors, mechanisms involved and its implications. Int Immunopharmacol 3:319–328
17. Hobbs SK, Monsky WL, Yuan F, Roberts WG, Griffith L, Torchilin VP, Jain RK (1998) Regulation of transport pathways in tumor vessels: role of tumor type and microenvironment. Proc Natl Acad Sci USA 95:4607–4612
18. Bae YH (2009) Drug targeting and tumor heterogeneity. J Control Release 133:2–3
19. Northfelt DW, Dezube BJ, Thommes JA, Miller BJ, Fischl MA, Friedman-Kien A, Kaplan LD, Du Mond C, Mamelok RD, Henry DH (1998) Pegylated-liposomal doxorubicin versus doxorubicin, bleomycin, and vincristine in the treatment of AIDS-related Kaposi's sarcoma: results of a randomized phase III clinical trial. J Clin Oncol 16:2445–2451
20. Gradishar WJ, Tjulandin S, Davidson N, Shaw H, Desai N, Bhar P, Hawkins M, O'Shaughnessy J (2005) Phase III trial of nanoparticle albumin-bound paclitaxel compared with polyethylated castor oil-based paclitaxel in women with breast cancer. J Clin Oncol 23:7794–7803
21. Mamot C, Drummond DC, Noble CO, Kallab V, Guo Z, Hong K, Kirpotin DB, Park JW (2005) Epidermal growth factor receptor-targeted immunoliposomes significantly enhance the efficacy of multiple anticancer drugs in vivo. Cancer Res 65:11631–11638
22. Srinivasan R, Marchant RE, Gupta AS (2009) In vitro and in vivo platelet targeting by cyclic RGD-modified liposomes. J Biomed Mater Res A 93:1004–1015
23. Kukowska-Latallo JF, Candido KA, Cao Z, Nigavekar SS, Majoros IJ, Thomas TP, Balogh LP, Khan MK, Baker JR Jr (2005) Nanoparticle targeting of anticancer drug improves therapeutic response in animal model of human epithelial cancer. Cancer Res 65:5317–5324
24. Shi J, Xiao Z, Kamaly N, Farokhzad OC (2011) Self-assembled targeted nanoparticles: evolution of technologies and bench to bedside translation. Acc Chem Res 44:1123–1134
25. Wang J, Tian S, Petros RA, Napier ME, Desimone JM (2010) The complex role of multivalency in nanoparticles targeting the transferrin receptor for cancer therapies. J Am Chem Soc 132:11306–11313
26. Manjappa AS, Chaudhari KR, Venkataraju MP, Dantuluri P, Nanda B, Sidda C, Sawant KK, Murthy RS (2011) Antibody derivatization and conjugation strategies: application in preparation of stealth immunoliposome to target chemotherapeutics to tumor. J Control Release 150:2–22
27. Sokolov K, Follen M, Aaron J, Pavlova I, Malpica A, Lotan R, Richards-Kortum R (2003) Real-time vital optical imaging of precancer using anti-epidermal growth factor receptor antibodies conjugated to gold nanoparticles. Cancer Res 63:1999–2004
28. Nobs L, Buchegger F, Gurny R, Allemann E (2004) Current methods for attaching targeting ligands to liposomes and nanoparticles. J Pharm Sci 93:1980–1992
29. Arruebo M, Valladares M, González-Fernández A (2009) Antibody-conjugated nanoparticles for biomedical applications. J Nanomaterials. Article ID 439389
30. Soga S, Kuroda D, Shirai H, Kobori M, Hirayama N (2010) Use of amino acid composition to predict epitope residues of individual antibodies. Protein Eng Des Sel 23:441–448
31. Simard P, Leroux JC (2009) pH-sensitive immunoliposomes specific to the CD33 cell surface antigen of leukemic cells. Int J Pharm 381:86–96
32. Pereira M, Lai EP (2008) Capillary electrophoresis for the characterization of quantum dots after non-selective or selective bioconjugation with antibodies for immunoassay. J Nanobiotechnol 6:10
33. Simard P, Leroux JC (2010) In vivo evaluation of pH-sensitive polymer-based immunoliposomes targeting the CD33 antigen. Mol Pharm 7:1098–1107
34. Yokoyama T, Tam J, Kuroda S, Scott AW, Aaron J, Larson T, Shanker M, Correa AM, Kondo S, Roth JA, Sokolov K, Ramesh R (2011) EGFR-targeted hybrid plasmonic magnetic nanoparticles synergistically induce autophagy and apoptosis in non-small cell lung cancer cells. PLoS One 6:e25507
35. Jefferis R (2009) Glycosylation as a strategy to improve antibody-based therapeutics. Nat Rev Drug Discov 8:226–234
36. Jefferis R (2005) Glycosylation of recombinant antibody therapeutics. Biotechnol Prog 21:11–16
37. Kristiansen KA, Potthast A, Christensen BE (2010) Periodate oxidation of polysaccharides for modification of chemical and physical properties. Carbohydr Res 345:1264–1271
38. Goren D, Horowitz AT, Zalipsky S, Woodle MC, Yarden Y, Gabizon A (1996) Targeting of stealth liposomes to erbB-2 (Her/2) receptor: in vitro and in vivo studies. Br J Cancer 74:1749–1756

39. Hansen CB, Kao GY, Moase EH, Zalipsky S, Allen TM (1995) Attachment of antibodies to sterically stabilized liposomes: evaluation, comparison and optimization of coupling procedures. Biochim Biophys Acta 1239:133–144
40. Domen PL, Nevens JR, Mallia AK, Hermanson GT, Klenk DC (1990) Site-directed immobilization of proteins. J Chromatogr 510:293–302
41. Koning GA, Kamps JA, Scherphof GL (2002) Efficient intracellular delivery of 5-fluorodeoxyuridine into colon cancer cells by targeted immunoliposomes. Cancer Detect Prev 26:299–307
42. Puertas S, Batalla P, Moros M, Polo E, Del Pino P, Guisan JM, Grazu V, de la Fuente JM (2011) Taking advantage of unspecific interactions to produce highly active magnetic nanoparticle-antibody conjugates. ACS Nano 5:4521–4528
43. Valeur E, Bradley M (2009) Amide bond formation: beyond the myth of coupling reagents. Chem Soc Rev 38:606–631
44. McCarron PA, Marouf WM, Quinn DJ, Fay F, Burden RE, Olwill SA, Scott CJ (2008) Antibody targeting of camptothecin-loaded PLGA nanoparticles to tumor cells. Bioconjug Chem 19:1561–1569
45. Bullous AJ, Alonso CM, Boyle RW (2011) Photosensitiser-antibody conjugates for photodynamic therapy. Photochem Photobiol Sci 10:721–750
46. Grabarek Z, Gergely J (1990) Zero-length crosslinking procedure with the use of active esters. Anal Biochem 185:131–135
47. Liu Y, Li K, Liu B, Feng SS (2010) A strategy for precision engineering of nanoparticles of biodegradable copolymers for quantitative control of targeted drug delivery. Biomaterials 31:9145–9155
48. Acharya S, Dilnawaz F, Sahoo SK (2009) Targeted epidermal growth factor receptor nanoparticle bioconjugates for breast cancer therapy. Biomaterials 30:5737–5750
49. Arya G, Vandana M, Acharya S, Sahoo SK (2011) Enhanced antiproliferative activity of Herceptin (HER2)-conjugated gemcitabine-loaded chitosan nanoparticle in pancreatic cancer therapy. Nanomedicine 7:859–870
50. Mamot C, Drummond DC, Greiser U, Hong K, Kirpotin DB, Marks JD, Park JW (2003) Epidermal growth factor receptor (EGFR)-targeted immunoliposomes mediate specific and efficient drug delivery to EGFR- and EGFRvIII-overexpressing tumor cells. Cancer Res 63:3154–3161
51. Chumsae C, Gaza-Bulseco G, Liu H (2009) Identification and localization of unpaired cysteine residues in monoclonal antibodies by fluorescence labeling and mass spectrometry. Anal Chem 81:6449–6457
52. Zhang W, Czupryn MJ (2002) Free sulfhydryl in recombinant monoclonal antibodies. Biotechnol Prog 18:509–513
53. Cohen SL, Price C, Vlasak J (2007) Beta-elimination and peptide bond hydrolysis: two distinct mechanisms of human IgG1 hinge fragmentation upon storage. J Am Chem Soc 129:6976–6977
54. Ji T, Muenker MC, Papineni RV, Harder JW, Vizard DL, McLaughlin WE (2010) Increased sensitivity in antigen detection with fluorescent latex nanosphere-IgG antibody conjugates. Bioconjug Chem 21:427–435
55. Kausaite-Minkstimiene A, Ramanaviciene A, Kirlyte J, Ramanavicius A (2010) Comparative study of random and oriented antibody immobilization techniques on the binding capacity of immunosensor. Anal Chem 82:6401–6408
56. Humphreys DP, Heywood SP, Henry A, Ait-Lhadj L, Antoniw P, Palframan R, Greenslade KJ, Carrington B, Reeks DG, Bowering LC, West S, Brand HA (2007) Alternative antibody Fab' fragment PEGylation strategies: combination of strong reducing agents, disruption of the interchain disulphide bond and disulphide engineering. Protein Eng Des Sel 20:227–234
57. Mamot C, Ritschard R, Kung W, Park JW, Herrmann R, Rochlitz CF (2006) EGFR-targeted immunoliposomes derived from the monoclonal antibody EMD72000 mediate specific and efficient drug delivery to a variety of colorectal cancer cells. J Drug Target 14:215–223
58. Brignole C, Marimpietri D, Gambini C, Allen TM, Ponzoni M, Pastorino F (2003) Development of Fab' fragments of anti-GD(2) immunoliposomes entrapping doxorubicin for experimental therapy of human neuroblastoma. Cancer Lett 197:199–204
59. Hashimoto K, Loader JE, Kinsky SC (1986) Iodoacetylated and biotinylated liposomes: effect of spacer length on sulfhydryl ligand binding and avidin precipitability. Biochim Biophys Acta 856:556–565
60. Hu CM, Kaushal S, Tran Cao HS, Aryal S, Sartor M, Esener S, Bouvet M, Zhang L (2010) Half-antibody functionalized lipid-polymer hybrid nanoparticles for targeted drug delivery to carcinoembryonic antigen presenting pancreatic cancer cells. Mol Pharm 7:914–920

61. East DA, Mulvihill DP, Todd M, Bruce IJ (2011) QD-antibody conjugates via carbodiimide-mediated coupling: a detailed study of the variables involved and a possible new mechanism for the coupling reaction under basic aqueous conditions. Langmuir 27:13888–13896
62. Kozlova D, Chernousova S, Knuschke T, Buer J, Westendorf AM, Epple M (2012) Cell targeting by antibody-functionalized calcium phosphate nanoparticles. J Mater Chem 22:396–404
63. Mercadal M, Domingo JC, Petriz J, Garcia J, de Madariaga MA (2000) Preparation of immunoliposomes bearing poly(ethylene glycol)-coupled monoclonal antibody linked via a cleavable disulfide bond for ex vivo applications. Biochim Biophys Acta 1509:299–310
64. Saito G, Swanson JA, Lee KD (2003) Drug delivery strategy utilizing conjugation via reversible disulfide linkages: role and site of cellular reducing activities. Adv Drug Deliv Rev 55:199–215
65. Jue R, Lambert JM, Pierce LR, Traut RR (1978) Addition of sulfhydryl groups to *Escherichia coli* ribosomes by protein modification with 2-iminothiolane (methyl 4-mercaptobutyrimidate). Biochemistry 17:5399–5406
66. Anhorn MG, Wagner S, Kreuter J, Langer K, von Briesen H (2008) Specific targeting of HER2 overexpressing breast cancer cells with doxorubicin-loaded trastuzumab-modified human serum albumin nanoparticles. Bioconjug Chem 19:2321–2331
67. Badiee A, Davies N, McDonald K, Radford K, Michiue H, Hart D, Kato M (2007) Enhanced delivery of immunoliposomes to human dendritic cells by targeting the multilectin receptor DEC-205. Vaccine 25:4757–4766
68. Wu Y-P, Miller LG, Danielson ND (1985) Determination of ethylene glycol using periodate oxidation and liquid chromatography. Analyst 110:1073–1076
69. Puertas S, Moros M, Fernández-Pacheco R, Ibarra MR, Grazú V, de la Fuente JM (2010) Designing novel nano-immunoassays: antibody orientation versus sensitivity. J Phys D: Appl Phys 43:474012
70. Lin PC, Chen SH, Wang KY, Chen ML, Adak AK, Hwu JR, Chen YJ, Lin CC (2009) Fabrication of oriented antibody-conjugated magnetic nanoprobes and their immunoaffinity application. Anal Chem 81:8774–8782
71. Grimsley GR, Pace CN (2004) Spectrophotometric determination of protein concentration. Curr Protoc Protein Sci Chapter 3:Unit 3.1
72. Peng L, Calton GJ, Burnett JW (1987) Effect of borohydride reduction on antibodies. Appl Biochem Biotechnol 14:91–99
73. Wong WS, Osuga DT, Feeney RE (1984) Pyridine borane as a reducing agent for proteins. Anal Biochem 139:58–67
74. Tiwari DK, Tanaka S, Inouye Y, Yoshizawa K, Watanabe TM, Jin T (2009) Synthesis and characterization of Anti-HER2 antibody conjugated CdSe/CdZnS quantum dots for fluorescence imaging of breast cancer cells. Sensors (Basel) 9:9332–9364
75. Hermanson G (2008) Bioconjugate techniques, 2nd edn. Academic, London
76. Freedman MH, Grossberg AL, Pressman D (1968) The effects of complete modification of amino groups on the antibody activity of antihapten antibodies. Reversible inactivation with maleic anhydride. Biochemistry 7:1941–1950
77. Lee J, Choi Y, Kim K, Hong S, Park HY, Lee T, Cheon GJ, Song R (2010) Characterization and cancer cell specific binding properties of anti-EGFR antibody conjugated quantum dots. Bioconjug Chem 21:940–946
78. Vinci F, Catharino S, Frey S, Buchner J, Marino G, Pucci P, Ruoppolo M (2004) Hierarchical formation of disulfide bonds in the immunoglobulin Fc fragment is assisted by protein-disulfide isomerase. J Biol Chem 279:15059–15066
79. Riener CK, Kada G, Gruber HJ (2002) Quick measurement of protein sulfhydryls with Ellman's reagent and with 4,4'-dithiodipyridine. Anal Bioanal Chem 373:266–276
80. Woodward J, Tate J, Herrmann PC, Evans BR (1993) Comparison of Ellman's reagent with N-(1-pyrenyl)maleimide for the determination of free sulfhydryl groups in reduced cellobiohydrolase I from *Trichoderma reesei*. J Biochem Biophys Methods 26:121–129

Chapter 16

Drug-to-Antibody Ratio (DAR) by UV/Vis Spectroscopy

Yan Chen

Abstract

UV/Vis spectroscopy is a simple and convenient method to determine protein concentrations as well as the average number of drugs that are conjugated to the antibody in an antibody–drug conjugate (ADC). Using the measured absorbances of the ADC and the extinction coefficients of the antibody and the drug, the average drug-to-antibody ratio (DAR) can be determined.

Key words Antibody–drug conjugate, Drug-to-antibody ratio, UV/Vis, Extinction coefficient

1 Introduction

Drug-to-antibody ratio (DAR) is an important quality attribute of an ADC as it determines the amount of "payload" that can be delivered to the tumor cell and can directly affect both safety and efficacy [1]. Various methods that are available to determine DAR include spectrophotometric assays [2], radiometric methods [3], hydrophobic interaction chromatography [2], and mass spectrometric methods [4, 5]. Here, we describe the simplest technique, which relies on the UV/Vis spectroscopic analysis of the ADC.

UV/Vis spectroscopy is routinely used for the quantitative determination of different analytes, such as transition metal ions [6], highly conjugated organic compounds [7], and biological macromolecules [8]. The basis for quantitative analysis in the UV/Vis spectrophotometric assay is the Beer–Lambert law, a direct proportional relationship between the absorbance and concentration of a substance:

$$A = \varepsilon c \ell,$$

where A is the absorbance, ε is the extinction coefficient (a physical constant of the substance), ℓ is the path length through the cell containing the analyte (usually 1 cm), and c is the concentration.

Laurent Ducry (ed.), *Antibody-Drug Conjugates*, Methods in Molecular Biology, vol. 1045,
DOI 10.1007/978-1-62703-541-5_16,

The Beer–Lambert law can also apply to a multicomponent system if these components have different absorption spectra and there are no interactions among these components. In this case, the absorption of light by these components of the sample solution is additive. The total absorbance of the solution at a given wavelength, λ, is the sum of the individual absorbance for each species:

$$A_\lambda = (\varepsilon_1^\lambda c_1 + \varepsilon_2^\lambda c_2 + \ldots + \{\varepsilon_n^\lambda c_n +)\ell,$$

where n is the number of different absorbing species in the sample solution, ε_n^λ is the extinction coefficient of the nth species, and c_n is the concentration of the nth species.

By measuring the absorbances of a multicomponent system at a number of wavelengths equal to or greater than n, it is possible to write a series of simultaneous equations using the absorbances, path lengths, extinction coefficients, and concentrations of these different components. If the path length and extinction coefficients are known, it is possible to solve the simultaneous equations for the concentration of each of the components in the sample.

This principle can be applied to determine the average DAR in an ADC sample. It requires that (a) the drug has a UV/Vis chromophore, (b) the drug and the antibody exhibit distinct absorption maxima in their UV/Vis spectra, and (c) the presence of the drug does not affect the light-absorbing properties of the antibody moiety in the ADC sample and vice versa. If these requirements are met, one can consider the ADC sample as a two-component mixture and apply the Beer–Lambert law to determine individual concentrations of the antibody and the drug [2]. Thus, the average DAR (moles of drug per mole of antibody) can be subsequently calculated.

This technique has been used widely for various ADCs with different drugs including the maytansinoid DM1 ((N2′-deacetyl-N2′-(3-mercapto-1-oxopropyl)-maytansine)) [9], methotrexate [10], CC-1065 analogues [11], adriamycin [12, 13], calicheamicin analogues [3, 14], and dipeptide-linked auristatins such as vc-MMAE [2]. Most of these cytotoxic drugs show absorption maxima significantly different from 280 nm, the commonly observed absorption maximum of a protein containing tryptophan or tyrosine residues. Figure 1 shows an example of the UV absorption spectra of (a) DM1, a cytotoxic drug; (b) trastuzumab, a humanized anti-HER2 IgG1 antibody; and (c) trastuzumab emtansine, an ADC that contains trastuzumab linked to the microtubule inhibitory DM1 via the thioether bond of MCC (maleido-cyclohexane-1-carboxylate). Because DM1 has an absorption maximum at 252 nm and the MCC linker does not have significant absorbance at either 252 or 280 nm, the amount of drug bound to the antibody can be determined by differential absorption measurements at 252 and 280 nm. It was reported [15] that similar spectroscopic analysis

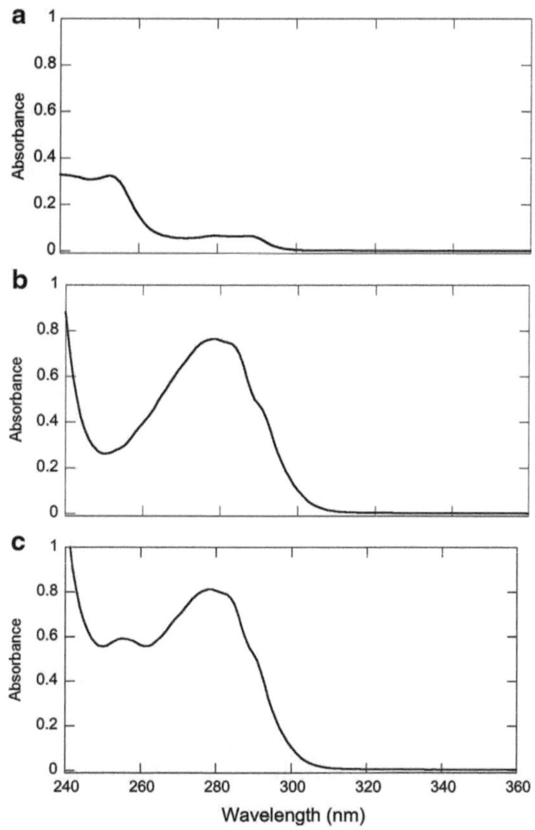

Fig. 1 UV absorbance spectra of DM1 (**a**), trastuzumab (**b**), and trastuzumab emtansine (**c**)

was applied even for ADCs with a relatively small difference in the absorption maxima between protein and drug, such as with the conjugated vinca alkaloid 4-desacetylvinblastine where the absorption maximum of the drug is 270 nm. In all cases, contributions from both the antibody and the drug were considered for the determination of the average DAR using the UV/Vis spectrophotometric method.

2 Materials

1. Any dual-beam or single-beam spectrophotometer capable of baseline subtraction and measurement in the UV/Vis range would be suitable.
2. Quartz crystal cuvettes are routinely used for measurement (*see* **Note 1**). Blank samples should be measured using the sample buffer solution but with no protein or drug present (*see* **Note 2**).

3 Methods

1. Determine the absorption maximum, $\lambda(D)$, of the drug.
   Follow the operating instructions for the UV/Vis spectrophotometer. Turn on the spectrophotometer and allow enough time for warm up of the instrument before use. Select the appropriate wavelength range, i.e., 200–500 nm. Insert a clean cuvette containing the appropriate blank solution into the holder. Since cytotoxic drugs are typically low molecular weight, hydrophobic molecules, organic solvents such as dimethylacetamide or methanol are commonly used to dissolve them. Be sure that the cuvette is clean and free of fingerprints. Use the blank solution to zero the spectrophotometer. To read a sample, simply insert the same or matched cuvettes holding the test solution. Obtain the spectra for the drug. At high concentrations, the absorption bands might saturate and show absorption flattening. Dilute the sample to avoid saturation if required. Identify the $\lambda(D)$ of the cytotoxic drug by inspecting the spectra.
2. Determine the extinction coefficients (ε) of the antibody and the drug at 280 nm and $\lambda(D)$.
   Accurate determination of the extinction coefficients of the antibody and the drug at both 280 nm and $\lambda(D)$ is required for this method (*see* **Note 2**).

   The extinction coefficient of the antibody at any given wavelength can be determined based on the Beer–Lambert law using a solution of the antibody product having a known protein concentration as determined by techniques such as amino acid compositional analysis [16] or nitrogen determination [17].

   If the amino acid composition of the antibody is known, extinction coefficients can also be predicted. At 280 nm, the absorbance of protein is mainly due to the amino acids tryptophan, tyrosine, and cystine (disulfide-bonded cysteine residues) with their molar extinction coefficients decreasing in that order. The molar extinction coefficient of a particular protein can be approximated by the weighted sum of the molar extinction coefficients of these three constituent amino acids at 280 nm. Differences in buffer type, ionic strength, and pH will impact the absorptivity of these amino acids. The most widely used molar extinction coefficients of tryptophan, tyrosine, and cystine used in estimating the extinction coefficients of proteins were determined by Pace et al. [18]. The average error in determining the protein concentration using the predicted extinction coefficients was found to be less than 4 % [18].

The extinction coefficients of the drug at 280 nm and $\lambda(D)$ can be determined using a solution of the drug with a known concentration. Dissolve a small amount (accurately weighed) of a high-purity material with appropriate solvent or buffer. Calculate the concentration of the solution based on the weight and the purity of the material. Measure the absorbances of the solution at 280 nm and $\lambda(D)$. Calculate the extinction coefficients based on the Beer–Lambert law.

3. Obtain the absorption spectrum of the ADC sample; record the absorbances at both 280 nm and $\lambda(D)$ (*see* **Notes 3** and **4**).

   If required, the ADC sample may be diluted to obtain solutions with absorbance values in the linear range of detection.

4. Calculate the average DAR of the ADC sample.
   Using the measured absorbances (from **step 3**) of the ADC and the extinction coefficients determined from **step 2**, the individual concentrations of antibody and drug, c_{mAb} and c_{drug}, can be determined by the solution of two simultaneous equations described below.

   In Equation 1, the absorbance at 280 nm of the drug and the antibody contributes to the total absorbance (A_{280}):

$$A_{280} = \left(\varepsilon_{\text{drug}}^{280} c_{\text{drug}} + \varepsilon_{\text{mAb}}^{280} c_{\text{mAb}}\right)\ell, \tag{1}$$

   where $\varepsilon_{\text{drug}}^{280}$ is the extinction coefficient of the drug at 280 nm, c_{drug} is the concentration of the drug, $\varepsilon_{\text{mAb}}^{280}$ is the extinction coefficient of the antibody at 280 nm, and c_{mAb} is the concentration of the antibody.

   Equation 2 is a parallel equation for the total absorbance at the absorption maximum, $\lambda(D)$, of the drug:

$$A_{\lambda(D)} = \left(\varepsilon_{\text{drug}}^{\lambda(D)} c_{\text{drug}} + \varepsilon_{\text{mAb}}^{\lambda(D)} c_{\text{mAb}}\right)\ell, \tag{2}$$

   where $\varepsilon_{\text{drug}}^{\lambda(D)}$ is the extinction coefficient of the drug at $\lambda(D)$, c_{drug} is the concentration of the drug, $\varepsilon_{\text{mAb}}^{\lambda(D)}$ is the extinction coefficient of the antibody at $\lambda(D)$, and c_{mAb} is the concentration of the antibody.

   Solving the above two equations simultaneously will give the individual concentrations of antibody and drug:

$$c_{\text{mAb}} = \left(A_{280}\,\varepsilon_{\text{drug}}^{\lambda(D)} - A_{\lambda(D)}\,\varepsilon_{\text{drug}}^{280}\right)\Big/\left[\left(\varepsilon_{\text{mAb}}^{280}\,\varepsilon_{\text{drug}}^{\lambda(D)} - \varepsilon_{\text{mAb}}^{\lambda(D)}\,\varepsilon_{\text{drug}}^{280}\right)\ell\right]$$

$$c_{\text{drug}} = \left(A_{280}\,\varepsilon_{\text{mAb}}^{\lambda(D)} - A_{\lambda(D)}\,\varepsilon_{\text{mAb}}^{280}\right)\Big/\left[\left(\varepsilon_{\text{drug}}^{280}\,\varepsilon_{\text{mAb}}^{\lambda(D)} - \varepsilon_{\text{drug}}^{\lambda(D)}\,\varepsilon_{\text{mAb}}^{280}\right)\ell\right].$$

   Dividing c_{drug} by c_{mAb} gives the average drug-to-antibody ratio (DAR) expressed as moles of drugs to moles of antibody:

$$\text{DAR} = c_{\text{drug}}/c_{\text{mAb}}.$$

4 Notes

1. Quartz crystal cuvettes are routinely used for UV/Vis methods. Cuvettes made with optical glass are not suitable for analysis of drug with $\lambda(D)$ at or below 320 nm. Currently several manufacturers offer disposable cuvettes made from various plastics including polystyrene and acrylic. No cleaning between samples is required when using the disposable cuvettes, which is convenient when handling cytotoxic ADCs. However, they often have a restricted wavelength range that may not be suitable for analysis of certain ADCs.
2. The absorbance spectra from various amino acids (tryptophan and tyrosine) are environmentally sensitive; therefore, ε, derived for a protein in one buffer, may not be the same for another buffer if there is a significant change in pH or solvent polarity. Excipient components with strong UV absorbance (e.g., the detergent Triton X-100) will interfere with this method and should be avoided. Blank samples should be measured using the sample buffer solution but with no protein present. Similarly, different solvents may impact the extinction coefficient of the cytotoxic drug if it contains acidic or basic groups.
3. The Beer–Lambert law may not be applicable to solutions with high turbidity which causes light to be scattered due to the presence of microscopic particles. As a result, less light will fall on the detector and a falsely high absorbance reading will be observed. Corrections can be performed by subtracting the absorbance at 320 nm (or 340 nm), assuming the protein or the drug does not display significant absorbance at these wavelengths.
4. Another key element in an ADC besides the antibody and the cytotoxic drug is the chemical linker which allows the covalent attachment of the drug to the antibody. The method described above applies to ADCs in which the chemical linker does not contribute significantly to the absorbances at either 280 nm or $\lambda(D)$. If the linker absorbs at one or both of these two wavelengths but has a different absorption maximum compared with the antibody and the drug, it is possible to treat the ADC sample as a three-component system and obtain quantitative determination of DAR.

Acknowledgements

We thank Pat Rancatore, Richard Seipert, Boyan Zhang, and Andrea Ji for comments and help in preparing this review.

References

1. Wakankar A, Chen Y, Gokarn Y (2011) Analytical methods for physicochemical characterization of antibody drug conjugates. MAbs 3:161–172
2. Hamblett KJ, Senter PD, Chace DF et al (2004) Effects of drug loading on the antitumor activity of a monoclonal antibody drug conjugate. Clin Cancer Res 10:7063–7070
3. Hinman LM, Hamann PR, Wallace R et al (1993) Preparation and characterization of monoclonal antibody conjugates of the calicheamicins: a novel and potent family of antitumor antibiotics. Cancer Res 53:3336–3342
4. Siegel MM, Hollander IJ, Hamann PR et al (1991) Matrix-assisted UV-laser desorption/ionization mass spectrometric analysis of monoclonal antibodies for the determination of carbohydrate, conjugated chelator and conjugated drug content. Anal Chem 63:2470–2481
5. Lazar AC, Wang L, Blattler WA et al (2005) Analysis of the composition of immunoconjugates using size-exclusion chromatography coupled to mass spectrometry. Rapid Commun Mass Spectrom 19:1806–1814
6. Schoonheydt RA (2010) UV-VIS-NIR spectroscopy and microscopy of heterogeneous catalysts. Chem Soc Rev 39:5051–5066
7. Pretsch E, Bühlmann P, Badertscher M (2009) Structure determination of organic compounds, tables of spectral data, 4th edn. Springer, New York, pp 401–420
8. Schmid F (2001) Biological macromolecules: UV-visible spectrophotometry. Encyclopedia Life sci. doi:10.1038/npg.els.0003142
9. Wang L, Amphlett G, Blattler WA et al (2005) Structural characterization of the maytansinoid-monoclonal antibody immunoconjugate, huN901-DM1, by mass spectrometry. Protein Sci 14:2436–2446
10. Hudecz F, Garnett MC, Khan T et al (1992) The influence of synthetic conditions on the stability of methotrexate-monoclonal antibody conjugates determined by reversed phase high performance liquid chromatography. Biomed Chromatogr 6:128–132
11. Chari RV, Jackel KA, Bourret LA et al (1995) Enhancement of the selectivity and antitumor efficacy of a CC-1065 analogue through immunoconjugate formation. Cancer Res 55:4079–4084
12. Greenfield RS, Kaneko T, Daues A et al (1990) Evaluation in vitro of adriamycin immunoconjugates synthesized using an acid-sensitive hydrazone linker. Cancer Res 50:6600–6607
13. Willner D, Trail PA, Hofstead SJ et al (1993) (6-Maleimidocaproyl)hydrazone of doxorubicin—a new derivative for the preparation of immunoconjugates of doxorubicin. Bioconjug Chem 4:521–527
14. Moran J (2002) Presentation at 224th American Chemical Society National Meeting, 18–22 Aug, Boston, MA
15. Laguzza BC, Nichols CL, Briggs SL et al (1989) New antitumor monoclonal antibody-vinca conjugates LY203725 and related compounds: design, preparation and representative in vivo activity. J Med Chem 32:548–555
16. Benson AM, Suruda AJ, Talalay P (1975) Concentration-dependent association of A-3-ketosteroid isomerase of *Pseudomonas testosteroni*. J Biol Chem 250:276–280
17. Jaenicke L (1974) A rapid micromethod for the determination of nitrogen and phosphate in biological material. Anal Biochem 61:623–627
18. Pace CN, Vajdos F, Fee L et al (1995) How to measure and predict the molar absorption coefficient of a protein. Protein Sci 4:2411–2423

Chapter 17

Drug-to-Antibody Ratio (DAR) and Drug Load Distribution by Hydrophobic Interaction Chromatography and Reversed Phase High-Performance Liquid Chromatography

Jun Ouyang

Abstract

Hydrophobic interaction chromatography (HIC) is the method of choice for determination of the drug-to-antibody ratio (DAR) and drug load distribution for cysteine (Cys)-linked antibody–drug conjugates (ADCs). The drug-loaded species are resolved based on the increasing hydrophobicity with the least hydrophobic, unconjugated form eluting first and the most hydrophobic, 8-drug form eluting last. The area percentage of a peak represents the relative distribution of the particular drug-loaded ADC species. The weighted average DAR is then calculated using the percentage peak area information and the drug load numbers. Reversed phase high-performance liquid chromatography (RP-HPLC) offers an orthogonal method to obtain DAR for Cys-linked ADCs. The method involves, first, a reduction reaction to completely dissociate the heavy and light chains of the ADC, then separation of the light and heavy chains and their corresponding drug-loaded forms on an RP column. The percentage peak area from integration of the light chain and heavy chain peaks, combined with the assigned drug load for each peak, is used to calculate the weighted average DAR.

Key words Drug-to-antibody ratio, Drug load distribution, Hydrophobic interaction chromatography, Reversed phase high-performance liquid chromatography, Cysteine-linked antibody–drug conjugate

1 Introduction

The Cys-linked ADC described here utilizes the linker maleimidocaproyl-valine-citrulline-*para*-aminobenzyloxycarbonyl (MC-VC-PABC) to attach the hydrophobic cytotoxic drug monomethyl auristatin E (MMAE) to a monoclonal antibody (Fig. 1) [1]. To make the ADC, the antibody is partially reduced to convert the interchain disulfides to free cysteine residues. The sulfhydryl (SH) group of the free cysteine residue is then reacted with the maleimidyl group of the linker-drug to form the ADC which is a heterogeneous mixture of drug-loaded antibody species with 0 to 8 drugs [2, 3].

Laurent Ducry (ed.), *Antibody-Drug Conjugates*, Methods in Molecular Biology, vol. 1045,
DOI 10.1007/978-1-62703-541-5_17, © Springer Science+Business Media, LLC 2013

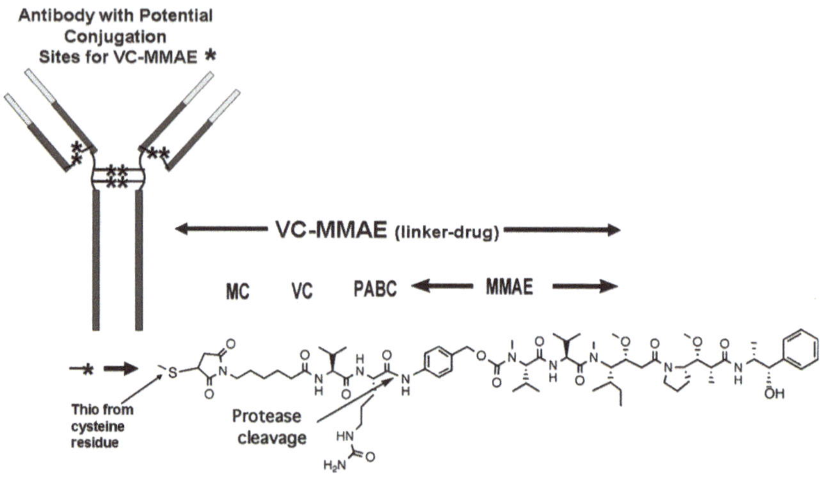

Fig. 1 Schematic illustration of MC-VC-PABC-MMAE ADC

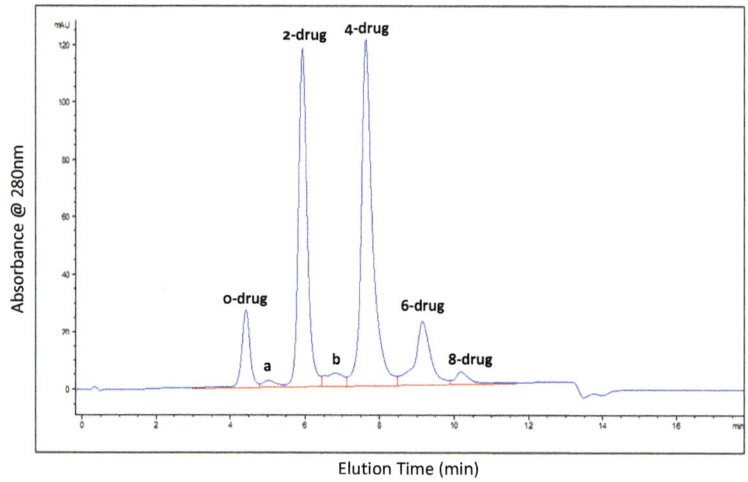

Fig. 2 A representative HIC chromatogram

The HIC method has been developed to resolve the drug-loaded species of Cys-linked ADCs [2, 4]. The addition of the hydrophobic linker-drug to the antibody increases its retention on a hydrophobic stationary phase such as TOSOH Bioscience Butyl-NPR. Elution with a gradient of decreasing salt concentration and an increasing organic modifier impacts the column retention of the drug-loaded species with the least hydrophobic, unconjugated form eluting first and the most hydrophobic, 8-drug form eluting last (Fig. 2). Although the more highly loaded species contain linker-drugs at cysteine residues of the interchain disulfides (such as between heavy and light chains and between the two heavy chains), the non-denaturing and relatively mild conditions used for HIC do not result in dissociation of these forms into the antibody components such as light and heavy chains. The percentage peak area from the HIC represents the relative proportion of a particular drug-loaded form. The weighted average DAR can be calculated from both peak percentage and drug load.

RP-HPLC is another separation technique based on hydrophobicity that has been developed for Cys-linked ADC analysis [3, 4]. However, as RP-HPLC uses organic solvent and a small amount of organic acid, the method proves to be too disruptive for the intact Cys-linked ADC. When analyzed directly, the ADC cannot withstand the highly denaturing conditions and will dissociate into antibody fragments. This is because some of the interchain disulfides are no longer present but replaced with the linker-drugs during conjugation, and the ADC is held together through noncovalent hydrophobic interactions. Treatment of the Cys-linked ADC with reductants such as dithiothreitol (DTT) fully reduces the remaining interchain disulfides and yields six species: light chain, light chain with one drug attached, heavy chain, and heavy chains with one, two, or three drugs attached. These species are stable in the denaturing organic environment and can be well resolved on an RP column such as Varian PLRP-S. The weighted average DAR is obtained by integration of the light and heavy chain peaks and calculation of the percentage peak area taking into account the assigned drug load for each peak.

2 Materials

All solutions and reagents should be prepared using high purity salts, buffers, HPLC grade solvents, and ultrapure water (HPLC grade or double deionized), as appropriate. In general, the mobile phase solutions are stored at room temperature and can be used for a month.

2.1 Equipment

1. High-performance liquid chromatography (HPLC) system: Agilent 1100 or 1200 HPLC system equipped with a binary pump, a thermostat autosampler, a column compartment with temperature control and a diode array detector (Agilent Technologies, Santa Clara, CA), or other HPLC systems with equivalent modules.
2. Water bath capable of controlling temperature at 37 ± 2 °C.

2.2 HIC

1. HIC column: nonporous TSKgel Butyl-NPR column (Tosoh Bioscience, part # 14947) with 2.5 μm particle size in a dimension of 4.6 mm (inner diameter) by 35 mm (length).
2. Mobile phases: mobile phase A is an aqueous solution of 1.5 M ammonium sulfate, 25 mM sodium phosphate at pH 6.95; mobile phase B is 75 % (v/v) aqueous solution of 25 mM sodium phosphate at pH 6.95 and 25 % (v/v) isopropyl alcohol (IPA).

2.3 RP-HPLC

1. RP column: polymer-based PLRP-S column (Varian, part # PL1912-1502) column with 5 μm particle size and 1,000 Å pore size in a dimension of 2.1 mm (inner diameter) by 50 mm (length).
2. Mobile phases: mobile phase A is an aqueous solution with 0.1 % (v/v) formic acid and 0.025 % (v/v) trifluoroacetic acid (TFA); mobile phase B is an acetonitrile (ACN) solution with 0.1 % (v/v) formic acid and 0.025 % (v/v) TFA.
3. Tris(hydroxymethyl)aminomethane (Tris) buffer: 50 mM, pH 8.0.
4. Dithiothreitol (DTT) stock solution: 1 M DTT solution in water is made fresh prior to use.

3 Methods

3.1 HIC

Experimental Conditions

1. Follow the instrument manufacturer's instructions for system start-up and basic operations.
2. Connect the column and set the column compartment temperature at 24 °C. Turn on the diode array detector.
3. Equilibrate the column with 100 % mobile phase A at 0.8 mL/min flow rate for about 20 min or until the baseline (monitored at 280 nm) is stable (*see* **Note 1**).
4. Inject 50–100 μg of the ADC sample in a volume of 5–10 μL. A larger volume (>10 μL) is not recommended because it may cause early breakthrough peak(s).
5. The loaded sample is eluted with a linear gradient as described in Table 1.
6. Diode array detector is set to acquire UV spectrum from 220 to 350 nm as well as absorbance at 280 nm (and 248 nm, optional).

Table 1
Gradient conditions of HIC

Time (min)	%B
0.0	0
12.0	100
12.1	0
18.0	0

Table 2
Example of drug load distribution and DAR calculation from HIC analysis

Peak name	Drug load	Percentage peak area (%)[a]	Weighted peak area (drug load × peak area%)
0-drug	0	4.7	0.0
(a)[b]	1	0.4	0.4
2-drug	2	28.7	57.4
(b)[b]	3	1.5	4.5
4-drug	4	48.8	195.2
6-drug	6	13.2	79.2
8-drug	8	2.8	22.4
Weighted average DAR			3.6

[a]Percentage peak area (%) represents the distribution of drug-loaded species (drug load distribution), for example, 2-drug species in this ADC accounts for 28.7 %
[b]*See* **Note 2**

7. A typical chromatogram with UV detection at 280 nm is shown in Fig. 2.
8. The ADC species are eluted according to the increasing hydrophobicity conferred from the hydrophobic linker-drug, with 0-drug (unconjugated species) eluting first and 8-drug species eluting last (*see* **Note 2**).

Data Analysis

1. Integrate peaks using either manual or automatic integration tools (Fig. 2) (*see* **Note 3**).
2. Calculate the peak area in percentage and transcribe the information in a table. As an example, Table 2 is shown: this information is transcribed in the 3rd column of Table 2.
3. Calculate weighted peak area by multiplying the percentage peak area by the corresponding drug load and transcribe the information in the table (as an example, this information is shown in the 4th column of Table 2).
4. Calculate the weighted average DAR by summing the weighted peak area column and dividing the sum by 100. That is,

$$\mathrm{DAR} = \sum(\text{Weighted Peak Area})/100.$$

5. The assignments of the HIC peak identity can be confirmed by examining the UV spectra from 220 to 350 nm. Figure 3 shows the stacked UV spectra of the corresponding HIC peaks with

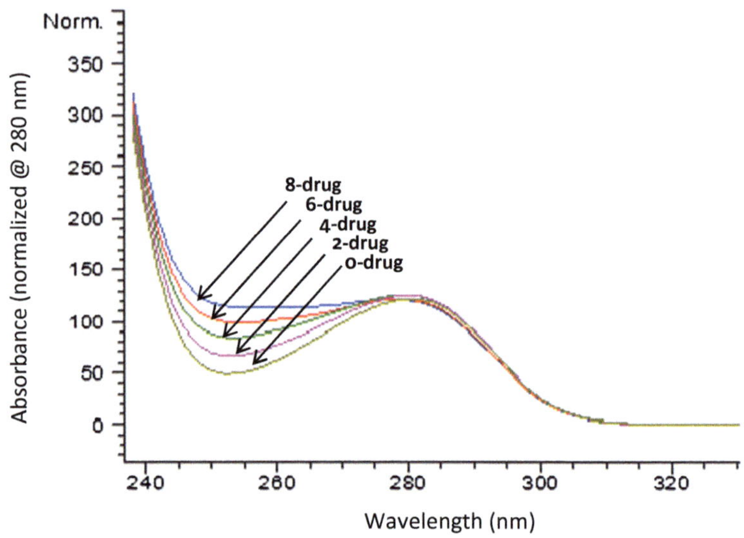

Fig. 3 UV spectra of drug-loaded species

the absorbance signal normalized at 280 nm, the maximum absorbance of the antibody portion of the ADC. As reported in the literature [2], the linker-drug portion of the ADC has maximum UV absorbance at 248 nm. As seen in Fig. 3, the relative absorbance around 250 nm of the major peaks in HIC increases with the drug load.

3.2 RP-HPLC

Experimental Conditions

1. Preparation of reduced ADC sample: Dilute ADC sample to 1 mg/mL using 50 mM Tris buffer at pH 8, and add freshly made DTT stock solution to a final concentration of 50 mM. Incubate the sample at 37 °C for 20–30 min for the reduction reaction (*see* **Note 4**).
2. Connect the column and set the column compartment temperature at 70 °C. Turn on the diode array detector and set it to acquire UV absorbance at 280 nm (and 248 nm, optional).
3. Equilibrate the column with 73 % mobile phase A (27 % mobile phase B) at 0.25 mL/min flow rate for about 30 min or until the baseline (monitored at 280 nm) is stable (*see* **Note 5**).
4. Inject 10–20 μg of the reduced ADC sample (from **step 1**).
5. Elute the sample with a linear gradient as described in Table 3 (*see* **Note 6**).
6. A typical chromatogram with UV detection at 280 nm is shown in Fig. 4 (*see* **Note 7**).
7. The light chain peaks usually elute first followed by the heavy chain peaks (*see* **Note 8**).

Table 3
Gradient conditions of RP-HPLC (*see* Note 6)

Time (min)	%B
0.0	27
3.0	27
25.0	49
26.0	95
31.0	95
31.5	27
45.0	27

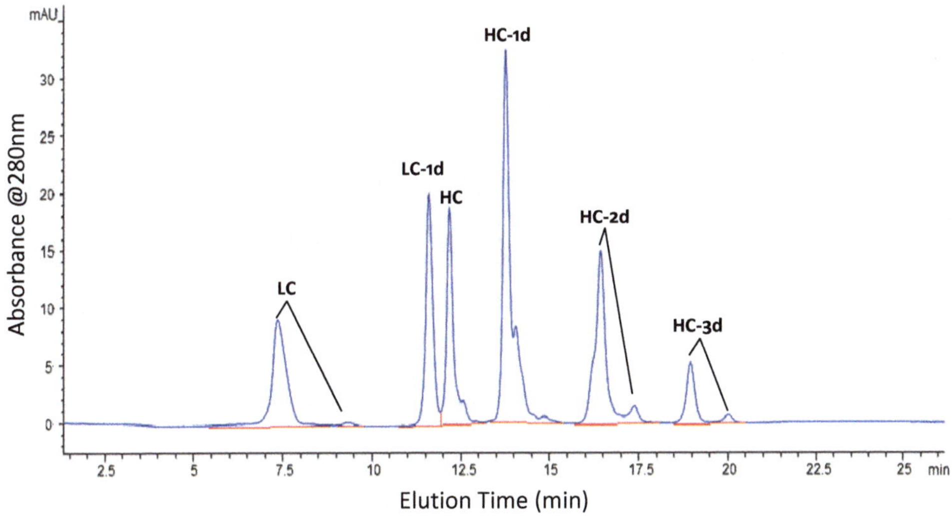

Fig. 4 A representative RP-HPLC chromatogram

Data analysis

1. Integrate peaks using either manual or automatic integration tools (Fig. 4).
2. Identify the light chain peaks and calculate the percentage peak area so that the total percentage sums to 100. Similarly, identify the heavy chain peaks and calculate the percentage peak area so that the total percentage sums to 100. As an example, Table 4 is shown: the information as described is transcribed in the 3rd column of Table 4.
3. Calculate weighted peak area of the light and heavy chains, separately, by multiplying the percentage peak area by the

Table 4
Example of DAR calculation from RP-HPLC analysis

Peak name	Drug load	Percentage peak area (%)[a]	Weighted peak area (drug load × peak area%)
LC	0	44.8	0.0
LC-1d	1	55.2	55.2
HC	0	20.6	0.0
HC-1d	1	48.3	48.3
HC-2d	2	22.3	44.6
HC-3d	3	8.8	26.4
Weighted average DAR			3.5

[a]Percentage peak area (%) represents the distribution of drug-loaded LC or HC, for example, LC-1d (light chain with 1 drug) accounts for 55.2 % of the entire LC forms and HC-2d (heavy chain with 2 drugs) accounts for 22.3 % of the entire HC forms

corresponding drug load and transcribe the information in the table (as an example in Table 4, the information is in the 4th column.).

4. Calculate the weighted average DAR using the equation below:

$$\mathrm{DAR} = 2 \times \left(\sum(\text{Weighted Peak Area of light chain}) + \sum(\text{Weighted Peak Area of heavy chain})\right)/100$$

4 Notes

1. For a new HIC column, it is recommended to run a few (3–5) injections of a standard sample for the best performance of subsequent analyses. A blank sample (e.g., formulation buffer without the ADC) injection is also recommended at the beginning and/or end of the sample analysis.
2. Minor peaks in Fig. 2 are Peaks (a) and (b) for 1-drug and 3-drug species, respectively. The assignments for the minor peaks can vary from one ADC to another. Using the identification method described in **step 5** in Data Analysis under Section 3.1 can aid the assignment. For some ADC molecules, Peak (a) may look more similar to species with 2-drug load and Peak (b) to 4-drug load. However, as the peak areas for these minor peaks only account for a small percent of the total percentage peak area (less than 2 % in this example, *see* Table 2), the final DAR value will not be affected regardless of their drug load assignments.

3. Figure 2 used manual integration in which a baseline was drawn from the beginning to the end points of the peak region. Vertical lines were dropped at the inflection points for each of the major peaks.

4. It has been our experience that DTT is the more effective reductant that primarily reduces the interchain disulfide bonds. It can, however, to a minimal extent, reduce the intra-chain disulfides (*see* Fig. 4 and **Note 7**). TCEP (tris(2-carboxyethyl)phosphine) hydrochloride may substitute DTT, but, in our experience, it is more likely to generate more peaks due to the intra-chain disulfide reduction that can potentially confound the data analysis.

5. Like HIC, for a new RP column, it is recommended to run a few (3–5) injections of a standard sample for the best performance of subsequent analyses. A blank sample (e.g., formulation buffer without the ADC) injection is also recommended at the beginning and/or end of the sample analysis.

6. The gradient conditions must be optimized thus can be different for each ADC molecule.

7. As shown in Fig. 4, minor peaks (or shoulders) immediately after the main peaks are observed. These peaks are due to small extent of intra-chain disulfide reduction (as confirmed by mass spectrometry analysis). Online liquid chromatography-mass spectrometry (LC-MS) can be conducted using the RP-HPLC conditions described in this article, as we chose to use formic acid which is amenable to MS. The small amount of TFA (0.025 %) is necessary to improve the peak shape without suppressing the MS signal. If MS data is not desired, replacing formic acid with 0.1 % TFA will provide similar results for the RP-HPLC analysis using the described running conditions.

8. For some ADCs, heavy chain may elute earlier than LC-1d. LC-MS is recommended to initially identify the peaks.

References

1. Senter PD (2009) Potent antibody drug conjugates for cancer therapy. Curr Op Chem Biol 13:1–10
2. Hamblett KJ, Senter PD, Chace DF, Sun MM, Lenox J, Cerveny CG, Kissler KM, Bernhardt SX, Kopcha AK, Zabinski RF, Meyer DL, Francisco JA (2004) Effects of drug loading on the antitumor activity of a monoclonal antibody drug conjugate. Clin Cancer Res 10:7063–7070
3. Sun MM, Beam KS, Cerveny CG, Hamblett KJ, Blackmore RS, Torgov MY, Handley FGM, Ihle NC, Senter PD, Alley SC (2005) Reduction-alkylation strategies for the modification of specific monoclonal antibody disulfides. Bioconj Chem 16:1282–1290
4. Wakankar A, Chen Y, Gokarn Y, Jacobson FS (2011) Analytical methods for physicochemical characterization of antibody drug conjugates. MAbs 3:161–172

Chapter 18

Drug-to-Antibody Ratio (DAR) and Drug Load Distribution by LC-ESI-MS

Louisette Basa

Abstract

This chapter describes an LC-ESI-MS method for the DAR and drug load distribution analysis that is suitable for lysine-linked ADCs. The ADC sample is desalted using a reversed-phase LC column with an acetonitrile gradient prior to online MS analysis. The MS spectrum is processed (deconvoluted) and converted to a series of zero charge state masses that corresponds to the increasing number of drugs in the ADC. Integration of the mass peak area allows the calculation of the DAR and drug load distribution of ADCs.

Key words Drug-to-antibody ratio (DAR), Drug load distribution, Electrospray ionization mass spectrometry (ESI-MS), Integration of mass spectra

1 Introduction

Liquid chromatography coupled to electrospray ionization mass spectrometry (LC-ESI-MS) is an orthogonal technique to UV/Vis spectroscopy, hydrophobic interaction chromatography (HIC), and reversed-phase-HPLC (RP-HPLC) in the analysis of drug-to-antibody ratio (DAR) and drug load distribution of antibody-drug conjugates (ADCs). DAR and drug load distribution are essential characteristics of ADCs as they determine the drug quantity to which the patient is exposed. They are also important to monitor as the various drug-loaded forms may differ in their PK/PD characteristics. The simplest analytical method to measure DAR is by UV/Vis spectroscopy [1–10]. Orthogonal methods to this technique depend on the linker-drug and the type of conjugation (e.g., lysine-linked or cysteine-linked). HIC [9, 22], RP-HPLC [11], LC-ESI-MS [12–15], and MALDI-TOF-MS [16–18] have all been used in addition to the UV/Vis method for determining DAR and drug load distribution of ADCs. HIC and RP-HPLC methods are used for ADCs with a limited number of

Laurent Ducry (ed.), *Antibody-Drug Conjugates*, Methods in Molecular Biology, vol. 1045,
DOI 10.1007/978-1-62703-541-5_18, © Springer Science+Business Media, LLC 2013

conjugation sites (e.g., at interchain cysteines or engineered cysteines), whereas the MS-based approach has been particularly useful in the analysis of the more heterogeneous lysine-linked ADCs [10, 19].

LC-ESI-MS of intact ADCs is essential in providing identification of the various drug-loaded forms of ADCs [10, 14, 15] (*see* **Note 1**). Lysine-linked ADCs are suitable for use with the denaturing RP-HPLC mobile phases typically used in LC-ESI-MS analysis. Unlike cysteine-linked ADCs that are held intact by both non-covalent and covalent interactions and tend to dissociate under typical LC-ESI-MS conditions [19], lysine-linked ADCs are stable and remain intact under these denaturing conditions. Consequently, the different drug-loaded forms of the intact lysine-linked ADC can be identified by their accurate masses.

Lysine-linked ADCs tend to be more heterogeneous than ADCs with limited site-specific conjugation and consequently, interpretation of the mass spectrum can be challenging. Additional sample preparation methods such as deglycosylation of the ADC [20] and removal of C-terminal lysine heterogeneity [21] are often needed to reduce the spectral complexity.

The mass spectra of lysine-linked ADCs typically include a series of ions with charge states from +45 to +60. Spectral processing or deconvolution of the mass spectra converts it to a series of zero charge state masses that shows a pattern of increasing number of linker-drugs. The spectral peak area can be integrated, thus, allowing a straightforward method for DAR and drug load distribution calculation. This approach, however, assumes that the MS ionization efficiency and MS response between the various intact drug forms are similar. The hydrophobic nature of the linker-drug and any changes in the overall net charge of the protein due to modifications to the lysine residues can affect the MS response and, consequently, the DAR and drug load distribution determination. Therefore, a comparison to the UV/Vis method is also performed. Studies have shown an acceptable correlation between the UV/Vis and LC-ESI-MS methods if the MS method utilizes the entire charge envelope for each drug-loaded species [13].

2 Materials

2.1 Equipment

1. Liquid chromatograph: Agilent 1100 Binary Gradient Pump with thermostated autosampler and column compartment (Agilent Technologies, Santa Clara, CA) or equivalent.
2. Mass spectrometer: Q-TOF Hybrid LC-MS/MS System (QSTAR, AB SCIEX, Framingham, MA) or equivalent.
3. HPLC column: PLRP-S (polystyrene-divinylbenzene reversed-phase column) 2.1 × 150 mm, 8 μm particle, 1,000 Å pore size (Agilent Technologies, Santa Clara, CA).

2.2 Reagents

Reagents for LC-ESI-MS must be of superior quality. Use >99 % or redistilled formic acid and trifluoroacetic acid (TFA). MS grade water and acetonitrile (p/n AH365-4 and 015-4, respectively, Burdick & Jackson, Muskegon, WI) are recommended.

1. Mobile phase A: 0.1 % formic acid, 0.025 % TFA in water. Prepare by adding 1 mL of formic acid and 0.25 mL of TFA (*see* **Note 2**) to 1,000 mL of water.
2. Mobile phase B: 0.1 % formic acid, 0.025 % TFA in acetonitrile. Prepare by adding 1 mL of formic acid and 0.25 mL of TFA (*see* **Note 2**) to 1,000 mL of acetonitrile.
3. PNGase F: Glycerol-free 500,000 u/mL (p/n P0705S, New England Biolabs, Ipswich, MA).
4. Carboxypeptidase-B (CpB): 5 mg/mL (p/n 10103233001, Roche Applied Science, Indianapolis, IN).
5. Digestion buffer stock solution: 1 M HEPES or 1 M Tris buffer pH 8.
6. Antibody-drug conjugate: Dilute to 1 mg/mL with water.

3 Methods

Deglycosylation of lysine-linked ADCs may be necessary prior to LC-ESI-MS analysis to reduce the carbohydrate contribution to the mass spectrum heterogeneity. N-linked deglycosylation is achieved with PNGaseF treatment of the ADC prior to analysis (*see* **Note 3**).

Removal of the C-terminal lysine heterogeneity in the heavy chain of the antibody prior to LC-ESI-MS analysis may also be necessary to reduce mass spectrum heterogeneity. This can be achieved with CpB treatment of the antibody (*see* **Note 3**).

3.1 Sample Preparation

1. *N-linked deglycosylation of ADCs prior to LC-ESI-MS*: Take 100 μg (100 μL of 1 mg/mL) of ADC and add 2 μL of 1 M HEPES or Tris buffer pH 8. Add 1 μL of PNGaseF (500,000 u/mL) and incubate at 45 °C for 1 h. Quench the deglycosylation reaction with TFA to a final concentration of 0.2 % TFA. Do not quench the reaction if the sample is to be followed with CpB treatment.
2. *CpB treatment of ADC prior to LC-ESI-MS*: Add 2 μL of 1 M HEPES or Tris buffer pH 8 to 100 μg (100 μL of 1 mg/mL) of ADC solution. Add 1.3 μL of CpB (1 mg/mL in water) and incubate at 37 °C for 20 min. Quench the reaction with TFA to a final concentration of 0.2 % TFA in the mixture.

3.2 LC-ESI-MS Analysis

1. Equilibrate the PLRP-S column at a flow rate of 250 μL/min at 75 °C (*see* **Note 4**).

2. Ensure that the LC column is well conditioned with several protein injections, if the column is new (*see* **Note 5**). Verify with at least two blank runs that a consistent back pressure plot or a stable baseline is achieved.
3. The Q-TOF MS source parameters must be optimized for intact antibody analysis. For the QSTAR (AB SCIEX), the declustering potential (DP) is set between 120 and 140 V, spray voltage is 4,500–5,000 V, source temperature is at 350 °C, and curtain and nebulizer gas are each set at 40 (*see* **Note 6**).
4. The MS should be calibrated to include the high mass range m/z (1,000–4,000). The expected spectral envelope for a typical antibody is between 2,000 and 3,500 m/z (~ +45 to +60 charge states).
5. For better mass accuracy, the MS should be calibrated prior to and kept in the scanning mode up until the sample analysis. The Q-TOF mass accuracy for intact antibodies is typically < 100 ppm.
6. Inject 15–20 μg of ADC solution onto the PLRP-S column. A typical LC gradient is shown in Table 1.
7. Figure 1 shows the total ion chromatogram (TIC) of the LC-ESI-MS analysis (*see* **Note** 7). Figure 2 shows the mass spectra of the entire TIC peak profile that is used for the MS software deconvolution. Charge states between +44 and +62 are often observed and, in most cases, included in the deconvolution.
8. Figure 3 shows the deconvoluted (zero charge state) mass spectra of an intact lysine-linked ADC. Using the ADC protein sequence and conjugate mass information, assign each of the mass peaks in the deconvoluted spectra with the appropriate number of drug load *n* (*see* **Note 8**).

Table 1
Typical LC gradient used for a PLRP-S column

Time	% mobile phase A	% mobile phase B
0	10	90
10	10	90
30	90	10
35	90	10
36	10	90
45	10	90

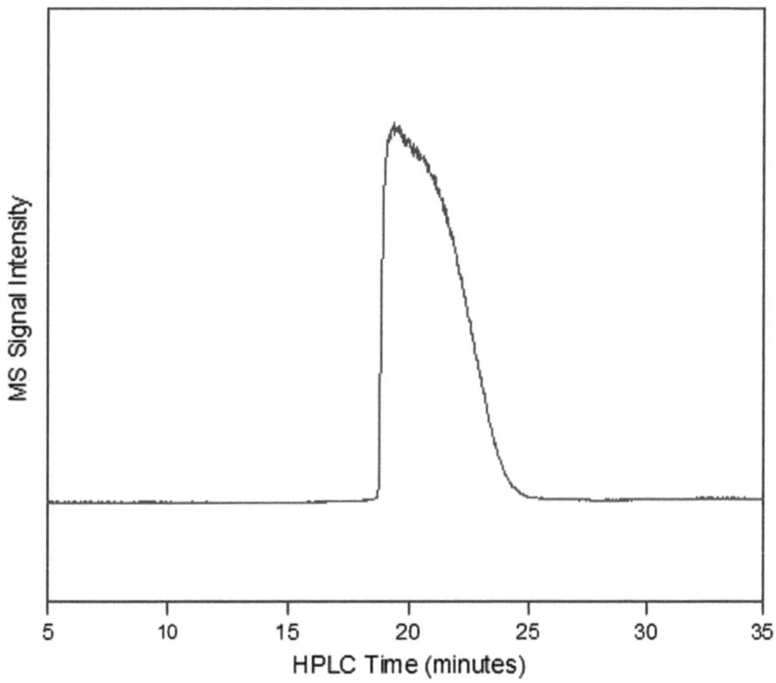

Fig. 1 LC-ESI-MS total ion chromatogram of a lysine-linked ADC

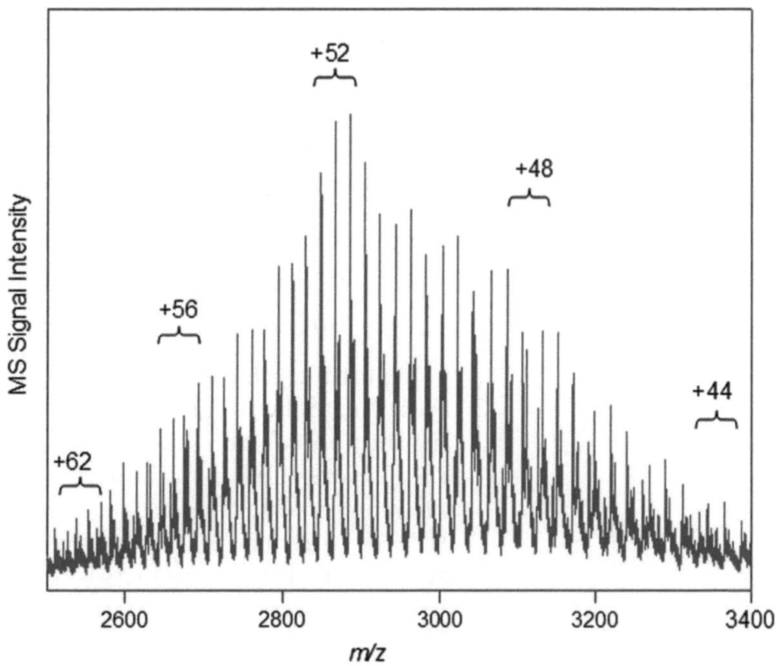

Fig. 2 Mass spectrum example of a lysine-linked ADC (Ab with drug load of 0–7 drugs) with a charge state envelope from +44 to +62

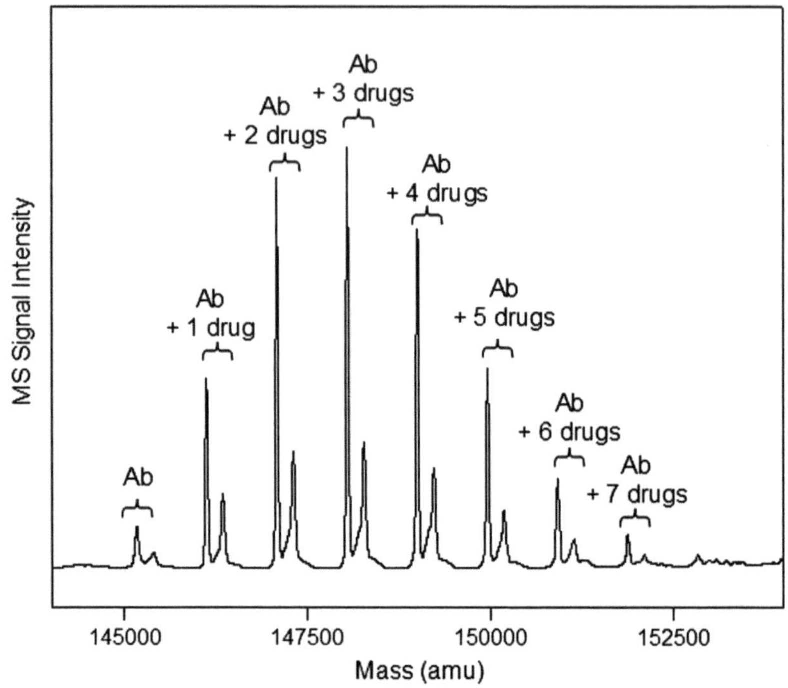

Fig. 3 Deconvoluted mass spectra of a lysine-linked ADC. The observed masses correspond to the antibody (Ab) with drug load (*n*) of 0–7

3.3 DAR and Drug Load Distribution Calculation

1. To determine the drug load distribution (%) for each antibody (Ab) with drug load *n*, integrate the mass peaks in the deconvoluted spectra (Fig. 3) to obtain the individual peak areas, then take the peak area of each Ab with drug load *n* and divide by the sum of all the peak areas, and finally multiply by 100 %:

$$\text{Drug load distribution}(\%) = (\text{peak area of Ab with drug load } n/\text{sum of all peak areas}) \times 100\ (\%) \text{ where n is number of drug load.}$$

   Repeat the calculation for each Ab with drug load *n*.

2. To calculate the weighted average DAR, first, the % drug load distribution of each Ab with drug load *n* (see Subheading 3.3.1) is multiplied by its corresponding drug load *n*. The resulting product represents the weighted contribution of each Ab with drug load *n* species to the ADC profile. Second, the sum of all these products is divided by 100. The resulting quotient represents the weighted average DAR of the ADC:

$$\text{DAR} = \sum(\text{drug load distribution } (\%) \text{ of each Ab with drug load } n)(n)/100$$

3. Whenever possible, correlate and validate the results against the values obtained by the UV/Vis method for DAR.

4 Notes

1. Aside from LC-ESI-MS of intact ADC, LC-ESI-MS of reduced ADC can also be used for determining the DAR. However, due to the difference in MS ionization efficiency between the drug-loaded light and heavy chains of the Ab, this approach may over- or underestimate the DAR. Both TCEP-HCl (tris(2-carboxyethyl)phosphine hydrochloride) and DTT (dithiothreitol) have been used successfully in our laboratory to reduce lysine-linked ADCs, when necessary. In general, 10 mM DTT in a 1 mg/mL ADC solution at pH 8 is sufficient to disrupt the interchain disulfide bonds when incubated at 37 °C for an hour, and 40 mM TCEP-HCl in a 1 mg/mL ADC solution is sufficient to disrupt both inter- and intra-chain disulfides when incubated at 60 °C for 10 min.
2. TFA is an excellent ion-pairing reagent for RP-HPLC of proteins and its use helps improve the chromatographic peak shape. However, under LC-ESI-MS conditions, TFA forms adducts and is associated with ion suppression. Use of formic acid as an ion-pairing agent improves the MS signal intensity but results in poorer chromatography. In general, a good compromise between sensitivity and chromatographic performance is to use a mixture of 0.1 % formic acid and 0.025 % TFA in the mobile phases [23]. For lysine-linked ADCs, since chromatographic separation is difficult to achieve, use of formic acid only for maximum sensitivity is a reasonable option.
3. Depending on the characteristics of the ADC, either deglycosylation, CpB treatment, or both may be necessary prior to the LC-ESI-MS analysis.
4. Poroshell 300SB-C8 1 × 75 mm and Pursuit 3 diphenyl 2 × 100 mm columns (both from Agilent Technologies) are excellent alternatives to the PLRP-S column. One advantage of the Poroshell column is that the analysis can be carried out using 1–5 μg of protein. Unlike the PLRP-S, which is a polystyrene-divinylbenzene macroporous column, the Poroshell is a C8 phase bonded to porous silica on a solid core column and the Pursuit diphenyl is a silica-based diphenyl matrix column. All three columns thus offer different protein selectivity and have been used in LC-ESI-MS of ADCs. In addition, all three columns are used at temperatures between 70 and 80 °C to minimize the chromatographic peak tailing and decrease the retention time elution of ADCs.
5. LC-ESI-MS is a very sensitive technique and typical HPLC grade reagents may not be clean enough for the system causing unnecessary adducts that complicate the spectra. Purchasing spectroscopy grade reagents diminish the likelihood of these contaminants.

6. MS source parameters must be optimized. Often, the source voltages that are needed to efficiently ionize and decluster the large antibody molecules are different from those needed for smaller than 30 kDa proteins or peptides. The MS is best optimized by infusing an antibody or ADC solution in an MS-compatible buffer such as 10–30 % acetonitrile with 0.1 % formic acid. The antibody or ADC should be desalted and free of nonvolatile salts such as phosphate, sulfate, and sodium.
7. The TIC trace of the LC-ESI-MS analysis often appears as a wide tailing peak due to the hydrophobic nature of the ADC.
8. The smaller of the doublet peak in each species corresponds to the antibody with unconjugated linker species (i.e., no drug(s) attached).

Acknowledgements

We thank Pat Rancatore, Richard Seipert, Boyan Zhang, and Andrea Ji for comments and help in preparing this review.

References

1. Laguzza BC, Nichols CL et al (1989) New antitumor monoclonal antibody-vinca conjugates LY203725 and related compounds: design, preparation and representative in vivo activity. J Med Chem 32:548–555
2. Greenfield RS, Kaneko T et al (1990) Evaluation in vitro of Adriamycin immunoconjugates synthesized using an acid-sensitive hydrazine linker. Cancer Res 50:6600–6607
3. Hudecz F, Garnett MC et al (1992) The influence of synthetic conditions on the stability of methotrexate-monoclonal antibody conjugates determined by reversed phase high performance liquid chromatography. Biomed Chromatogr 6:128–132
4. Chari RV, Martell BA et al (1992) Immunoconjugates containing novel maytansinoids: promising anticancer drugs. Cancer Res 52:127–131
5. Willner D, Trail PA et al (1993) (6-Maleimidocaproyl)hydrazine of doxorubicin—new derivative for the preparation of immunoconjugates of doxorubicin. Bioconjug Chem 4:521–527
6. Hinman LM, Hamann PR et al (1993) Preparation and characterization of monoclonal antibody conjugates of the calicheamicins; a novel and potent family of antitumor antibiotics. Cancer Res 53:3336–3342
7. Chari RV, Jackel KA et al (1995) Enhancement of the selectivity and antitumor efficacy of a CC-1065 analogue through immunoconjugate formation. Cancer Res 55:44079–44084
8. Moran J (2002) Presentation at the 224th American Chemical Society National Meeting, Boston, MA; 18–22 August 2002
9. Hamblett KJ, Senter PD et al (2004) Effects of drug loading on the antitumor activity of a monoclonal antibody drug conjugate. Clin Cancer Res 10:7063–7070
10. Wakankar A, Chen Y et al (2011) Analytical methods for physicochemical characterization of antibody drug conjugates. MAbs 3 (2):161–172
11. McDonagh CF, Turcott E et al (2006) Engineered antibody-drug conjugates with defined sites and stoichiometries of drug attachment. Protein Eng Des Sel 19:299–307
12. Wang L, Amphlett G et al (2005) Structural characterization of the maytansinoid-monoclonal antibody immunoconjugate, huN901-DM1, by mass spectrometry. Protein Sci 14:436–446
13. Lazar AC, Wang L et al (2005) Analysis of the composition of immunoconjugates using size-exclusion chromatography coupled to mass spectrometry. Rapid Commun Mass Spectrom 19:1806–1814
14. Junutula JR, Flagella KM et al (2010) Engineered thiotrastuzumab-DM1 conjugate with an improved therapeutic index to target human

epidermal growth factor receptor 2-positive breast cancer. Clin Cancer Res 16:4769–4778

15. Xu K, Liu L et al (2011) Characterization of intact antibody–drug conjugates from plasma/serum in vivo by affinity capture capillary liquid chromatography–mass spectrometry. Anal Biochem 412:56–66
16. Siegel MM, Hollander IJ et al (1991) Matrix-assisted UV-laser desorption/ionization mass spectrometric analysis of monoclonal antibodies for the determination of carbohydrate, conjugated chelator and conjugated drug content. Anal Chem 63:2470–2481
17. Quiles S, Raisch KP et al (2010) Synthesis and preliminary biological evaluation of high-drug-load paclitaxel-antibody conjugates for tumor-targeted chemotherapy. J Med Chem 53:586–594
18. Safavy A, Bonner JA et al (2003) Synthesis and biological evaluation of paclitaxel-C225 conjugate as a model for targeted drug delivery. Bionconjug Chem 14:302–310
19. Valliere-Douglass JF, McFee WA, Salas-Solano O (2012) Native intact mass determination of antibodies conjugated with monomethyl Auristatin E and F at interchain cysteine residues. Anal Chem 84:2843–2849
20. Jiang X, Song A et al (2011) Advances in the assessment and control of the effector functions of therapeutic antibodies. Nat Rev Drug Discov 10:101–111
21. Harris RJ (1995) Processing of C-terminal lysine and arginine residues of proteins isolated from mammalian cell culture. J Chromatogr A 705:129–134
22. Sun MM, Beam KS et al (2005) Reduction-alkylation strategies for the modification of specific monoclonal antibody disulfides. Bioconjug Chem 16:1282–1290
23. Duchateau ALL, Munsters BHM et al (1991) Selection of buffers and of an ion-pairing agent for thermospray liquid chromatographic–mass spectrometric analysis of ionic compounds. J Chromatogr A 552:605–612

Chapter 19

Determination of Charge Heterogeneity and Level of Unconjugated Antibody by Imaged cIEF

Joyce Lin and Alexandru C. Lazar

Abstract

Imaged capillary isoelectric focusing (icIEF) is capable of monitoring the charge heterogeneity profile of conjugated antibodies. The electropherogram from icIEF can be integrated to quantitate the amount of unconjugated antibody present in a conjugate sample. This chapter describes an icIEF method where a conjugate sample was first prepared by mixing with appropriate ampholytes, pI markers, and additives. Then, the sample was focused in a fluorocarbon-coated fused silica capillary, where absorbance images were taken. Quantitation of the unconjugated antibody was achieved by using a calibration curve.

Key words Imaged cIEF, Antibody–maytansinoid conjugates, Charge heterogeneity, Unconjugated antibody

1 Introduction

Immunoconjugates manufactured using ImmunoGen's Targeted Antibody Payload (TAP) technology contain antibodies to which cytotoxic maytansinoid molecules are attached through amino groups present in the protein (e.g., ε-amino groups of lysine residues and N-terminal amino groups) [1, 2]. Due to the inherent nature of the chemical process through which the antibody molecules are conjugated, the immunoconjugates are heterogeneous, containing antibody molecules that carry different numbers of the cytotoxic agent. Mass spectrometry has been successfully used to monitor the mass distribution profiles of the conjugated products [3]. Figure 1 shows a mass distribution profile of a typical immunoconjugate with an average of about 3.6 maytansinoid molecules (DM4 in this example) linked per antibody molecule. The profile shows that at this maytansinoid load, the immunoconjugate preparation contains low level of unconjugated antibody (D0) and that a small proportion of the antibody molecules can carry up to eight of the DM4 maytansinoids per antibody.

Laurent Ducry (ed.), *Antibody-Drug Conjugates*, Methods in Molecular Biology, vol. 1045, DOI 10.1007/978-1-62703-541-5_19, © Springer Science+Business Media, LLC 2013

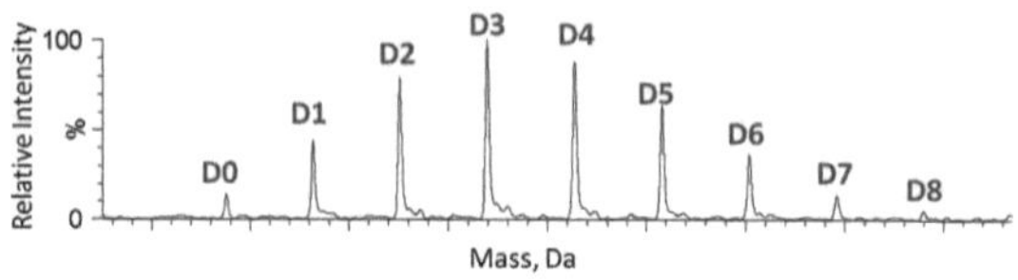

Fig. 1 Mass spectrum of deglycosylated MAb-DM4 conjugate. The *peak labels* indicate the number of DM4 molecules attached to the antibody: *D0* is the unconjugated antibody, while *Dn* corresponds to antibody molecules carrying *n* DM4 molecules (for $n = 1, 2, \ldots, 8$)

Conjugation of the amino groups to form amide bonds with a linker moiety eliminates basic sites in the proteins and changes the pI of the conjugated antibodies. Traditionally, analytical methods such as ion-exchange (IEX) chromatography and isoelectric focusing (IEF) in slab gel and capillary formats are routinely used to monitor charge heterogeneity in proteins and to measure their isoelectric point (pI) [4–6]. These methods have shown great success in characterizing antibodies. However, preliminary experiments have shown that neither IEX chromatography nor conventional IEF provides sufficient resolution to separate the charge variants in TAP products, due to the small differences in pI values between conjugated antibodies carrying different numbers of payload molecules.

In the past decade, the imaged capillary IEF (icIEF) instrument, iCE280 Analyzer (or more recently, iCE3), has been developed by ProteinSimple (Santa Clara, CA, USA). During isoelectric focusing, absorbance images of the full capillary are taken by a charged-couple device (CCD) camera at 280 nm, eliminating the need of mobilization of the focused samples before passing them in front of a detection window [7–9]. Compared to conventional cIEF, better peak separation can be achieved with this instrument because the mobilization step during conventional cIEF analysis often leads to peak broadening, poor reproducibility, and reduced resolution. Furthermore, with icIEF, the total run time for each sample is greatly reduced, since there is no mobilization step, providing more efficient sample analysis.

A typical icIEF run starts with rinsing the fluorocarbon-coated capillary with 1 % methyl cellulose (MC) solution. Then, the capillary is filled with the sample mixed with carrier ampholytes, pI marker, MC, and optional additives. After filling the capillary, focusing takes place in the length of the capillary between the electrodes, and absorbance images at 280 nm are taken by the instrument every 30 s during the course of focusing. The pI gradient in the final image can be calibrated by identifying the pI markers in the image, after which the peaks in the electropherogram can be integrated.

2 Materials

The reagents listed below can be purchased from ProteinSimple (Santa Clara, CA, USA). Please observe the manufacturer-recommended storage conditions and expiry dates. For preparation of solutions from chemicals obtained from other vendors, use electrophoresis grade reagents. Waste should be disposed in compliance with regulations.

1. Catholyte solution: 0.08 M phosphoric acid in 0.1 % (w/v) methyl cellulose (part of the Electrolyte Kit).
2. Anolyte solution: 0.1 M sodium hydroxide in 0.1 % (w/v) methyl cellulose (part of the Electrolyte Kit).
3. Transfer time measure solution: 8 % pH 3–10 Pharmalytes in 0.35 % (w/v) methyl cellulose (Transfer Time Measurement Solution Kit).
4. System suitability solution: hemoglobin stock solution, 8 % pH 3–10 Pharmalytes, 0.35 % (w/v) methyl cellulose, 4.22 pI marker, 9.46 pI marker (System Suitability Kit).
5. Capillary rinse buffer: 0.5 % (w/v) methyl cellulose (available as 1 % Methyl Cellulose Solution or 0.5 % Methyl Cellulose Solution Kit).
6. pI markers: lower marker 7.65 and upper marker 9.77 (*see* **Note 1**).
7. Carrier ampholyte: pH 8–10.5 Pharmalyte is the only carrier ampholyte used in this method (*see* **Note 2**).
8. cIEF cartridge: 50 mm, 100 μm I.D. fluorocarbon-coated capillary with built-in electrolyte tanks.
9. iCE280 Analyzer: the imaged cIEF instrument that is capable of taking 280 nm absorbance images using a CCD camera (*see* **Note 3**). The instrument control software (iCE280 CFR software) is also used to calibrate the pI scale in the electropherograms.
10. Autosampler: PrinCE autosampler was used in this experiment (*see* **Note 4**).
11. Empower software: used for integration of pI-calibrated electropherograms (Waters, Milford, MA, USA).

3 Methods

1. Initiate and set up the instrument following the step-by-step instructions on the software. It will walk through the steps of installing the capillary cartridge and setting up the rinse buffer, electrolytes, etc.

2. Prepare the immunoconjugate sample by combining the following components in a 0.5 mL centrifuge tube: 87.5 μL of 1 % methyl cellulose solution, 5.0 μL of pH 8.0–10.5 Pharmalyte, 1.0 μL of 7.65 pI marker, 1.0 μL of 9.77 pI marker, 10.0 μL of test analyte, and 145.5 μL of deionized water. The total volume of sample will be 250.0 μL. Mix the sample thoroughly by pipetting up and down gently for at least 15 times, or until the mixture is homogeneous. The concentration of the test analyte in the prepared sample is 200 μg/mL (*see* **Note 5**).
3. Prepare several concentrations of the monoclonal antibody standard solutions for the calibration curve by diluting the antibody using formulation buffer, to concentrations ranging from 0.05 to 5 mg/mL.
4. Prepare the diluted antibody samples from the previous step for calibration curve by combining the following components in a 0.5 mL centrifuge tube: 87.5 μL of 1 % methyl cellulose solution, 10.0 μL of pH 8–10.5 Pharmalyte, 1.0 μL of 7.65 pI marker, 1.0 μL of 9.77 pI marker, 5.0 μL of diluted antibody standard, and 145.5 μL of deionized water (*see* **Note 6**). The total volume of sample will be 250.0 μL. Mix the sample thoroughly by pipetting up and down gently for at least 15 times, or until the mixture is homogeneous. The antibody concentrations in the prepared standard solutions will range from 1 to 100 μg/mL.
5. Negative controls were prepared by using blank formulation buffers according to **step 3** for the conjugate and **step 4** for the antibody.
6. Transfer the prepared test analytes, standards, and controls to sample vials (*see* **Note 7**). Cap the vials and place them into the autosampler.
7. Set up a run sequence on the iCE software by entering the required sample information.
8. Isoelectric focusing method parameters: prefocus at 500 V for 1 min, and focus at 3,000 V for 10 min for antibody standards and 12 min for conjugate samples (*see* **Note 6**).
9. When the run is completed, process the images in the iCE software by identifying the lower and upper pI markers and calibrate the pI scale in all electropherograms (follow the User's Manual of the instrument) (Fig. 2).
10. Export all the processed electropherograms to *.cdf format from the iCE280 CFR software, and import them into Empower (*see* **Note 8**).
11. Integrate all the electropherograms, making sure that pI markers and peaks that are also present in the negative controls are not integrated.

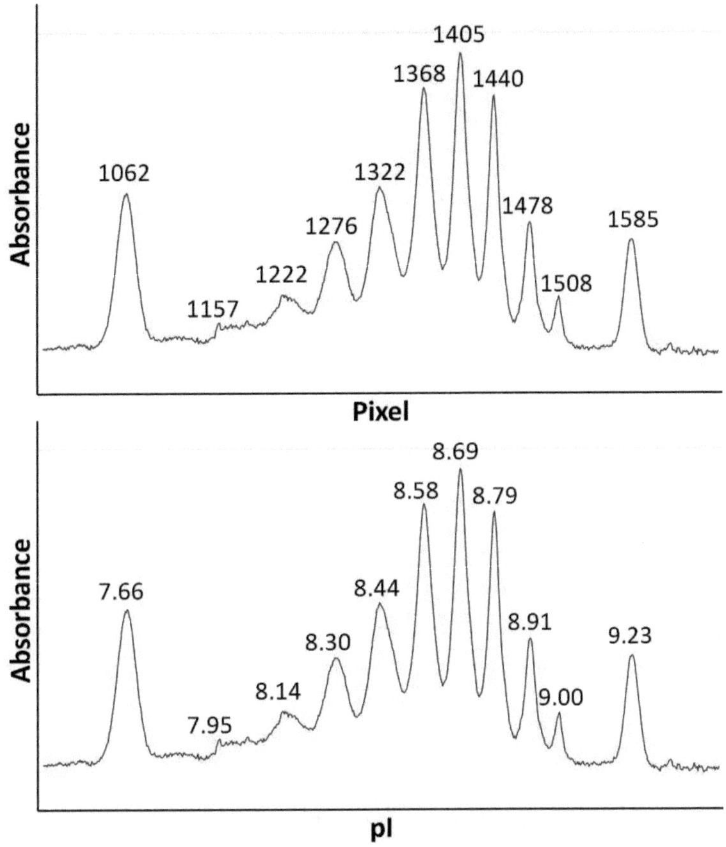

Fig. 2 Images of the electropherograms before (*top panel*) and after (*bottom panel*) calibration. After calibration, the horizontal axis is changed from "Pixel" to "pI"

12. Plot the peak areas of the main peak in all the antibody standard injections against the antibody concentration in the prepared standards to generate a calibration curve (*see* **Note 9**). Figure 3 shows the calibrated electropherograms of the antibody standards and the corresponding calibration curve.
13. Based on its pI value, identify the unconjugated antibody peak in the electropherogram of each conjugate sample (Fig. 4) and use the unconjugated antibody peak areas to calculate the concentrations of unconjugated antibody in each conjugate sample using the antibody calibration curve.
14. Divide the concentration of the unconjugated antibody in the conjugate sample (quantitated using the calibration curve) by the conjugate concentration in the prepared sample, which is 200 μg/mL. Multiply by 100 to obtain the percentage of unconjugated antibody in the conjugate sample.

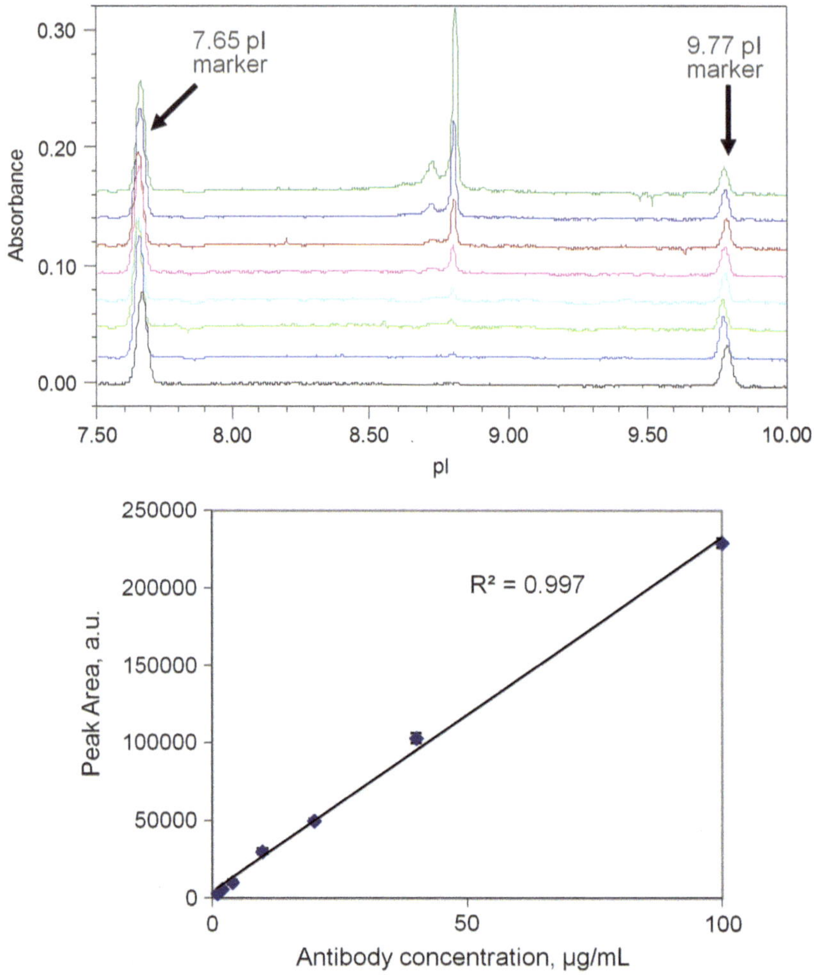

Fig. 3 Electropherograms of the antibody standards (*top panel*) and the corresponding calibration curve (*bottom panel*)

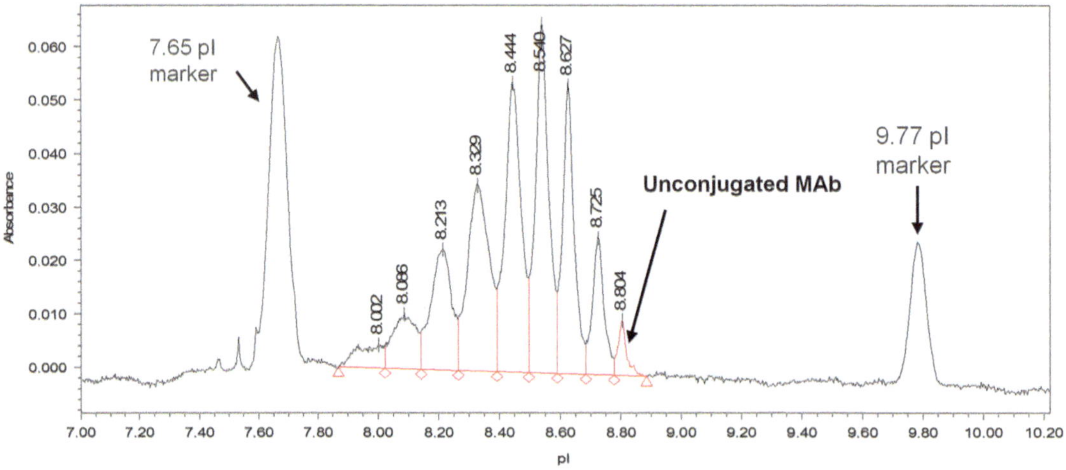

Fig. 4 Electropherogram of conjugate sample. The level of the unconjugated antibody was 3.2 %

4 Notes

1. Actual pI markers chosen for the sample depend on its theoretical pI. Two pI markers are needed for calibration of the pI scale of the electropherogram. The pI values of the markers should bracket the pI range of the sample.
2. The pI range of the carrier ampholytes can be varied to accommodate proteins with different pI values. Wide-range and narrow-range carrier ampholytes can also be used in the same sample to improve the resolution within a smaller range of pI.
3. Our work was performed with the iCE280 instrument. The method can be run also as described in this paper on the iCE3 instrument.
4. Other types of autosamplers are also available (e.g., Alcott autosampler).
5. Parameters such as carrier ampholyte concentration, sample concentration, and the use of additives can be optimized for each compound in order to improve resolution and sensitivity. Additives such as urea, Tween, or Pluronic are suggested additives by ProteinSimple to prevent precipitation of proteins during focusing.
6. The ampholyte concentrations and focusing times for the conjugate and antibody samples are slightly different, because the methods were optimized separately for the conjugate and antibody.
7. During transfer of solutions, avoid bubble formation. Bubbles injected into the capillary can interfere with focusing.
8. The default unit for the horizontal axis is "retention time" or "migration time." For the purpose of reporting, the horizontal axis is renamed "pI."
9. The antibody, besides the main peak, can contain basic and acidic components. For the calibration curve, only the peak area of the main peak is considered. It is assumed that the charge heterogeneity profile of the unconjugated antibody present in the conjugate sample is similar to that of the antibody standard.

References

1. Lambert J (2010) Antibody-maytansinoid conjugates: a new strategy for the treatment of cancer. Drugs Fut 35:471–480
2. Lambert J (2005) Drug-conjugated monoclonal antibodies for the treatment of cancer. Curr Opin Pharmacol 5:543–549
3. Lazar AC, Wang L, Blattler WA et al (2005) Analysis of the composition of immunoconjugates using size-exclusion chromatography coupled to mass spectrometry. Rapid Commun Mass Spectrum 19:1806–1814

4. Lyubarskaya Y, Houde D, Woodward J et al (2006) Analysis of recombinant monoclonal antibody isoforms by electrospray ionization mass spectrometry as a strategy for streamlining characterization of recombinant monoclonal antibody charge heterogeneity. Anal Biochem 348:24–39
5. Righetti PG (2004) Determination of the isoelectric point of proteins by capillary isoelectric focusing. J Chromatogr A 1037:491–499
6. Weinberger R (2000) Capillary isoelectric focusing. In: Practical capillary electrophoresis, 2nd edn. Academic Press, San Diego, p 209–243
7. Wu X, Huang T, Liu Z et al (2005) Whole-column imaging-detection techniques and their analytical applications. Trends Anal Chem 24(5):369–382
8. Li N, Kessler K, Bass L et al (2007) Evaluation of the iCE280 Analyzer as a potential high-throughput tool for formulation development. J Pharm Biomed Anal 43:963–972
9. Bo T, Pawliszyn J (2006) Characterization of bovine serum albumin-tryptophan interaction by capillary isoelectric focusing with whole column imaging detection. J Chromatogr A 1105:25–32

Chapter 20

Risk-Based Scientific Approach for Determination of Extractables/Leachables from Biomanufacturing of Antibody–Drug Conjugates (ADCs)

Weibing Ding

Abstract

Recent developments in biopharmaceutical processes twined with a desire to remove cleaning and cross-contamination issues from drug production have led to the widespread introduction of single-use technologies and systems within operations. One key area that end users need to address with the advent of these single-use solutions is the potential for increased levels of extractables and leachables within a process, which need to be evaluated and understood as part of any regulatory submission. A science-based and practical method for characterization of extractables and leachables from single-use systems used in manufacturing antibody–drug conjugates has been developed and described in detail. This risk-based approach minimizes the amount of test work while meeting the regulatory requirements to ensure the drug safety and quality. The test design is optimized and the analytical methods (gas chromatography/mass spectrometry, liquid chromatography/mass spectrometry, and inductively coupled plasma/mass spectrometry) are shown to be suitable for quantifying and identifying the extracted chemical compounds. Application of this characterization method speeds up the filing process for qualification and validation of single-use systems used in bioprocesses.

Key words Extractables, Leachables, Antibody–drug conjugates, Risk-based scientific approach, Analytical methods, Product safety, Single-use systems, Risk assessment

1 Introduction

Antibody–drug conjugates (ADC), an emerging type of biotherapeutic, bring an anticipated hope for a new class of drugs especially in the oncology category. An ADC consists of three parts: the antibody, the cytotoxic small molecule, and the linker. The manufacturing of all three parts as well as the final conjugation step involves both small molecule and biologic-based processes, which must all take place under cGMP [1]. Recently, single-use systems have been increasingly implemented in drug manufacturing processes because of a multitude of advantages, of which the elimination of cross

Laurent Ducry (ed.), *Antibody-Drug Conjugates*, Methods in Molecular Biology, vol. 1045,
DOI 10.1007/978-1-62703-541-5_20, © Springer Science+Business Media, LLC 2013

contamination between batches, the avoidance of large amount of toxic waste from cleaning process, and the minimization of the exposure of operators to the toxic drugs are particularly appealing to the manufacturing of ADCs. For these very reasons, single-use systems have been and will be more widely used in producing ADC.

The Food and Drug Administration (FDA) regulation on current Good Manufacturing Practice (cGMP) of Finished Pharmaceuticals (21 CFR Part 211) applies to process equipment including single-use systems. The section on Process Equipment 211.65(a) states: "Equipment shall be constructed so that surfaces that contact components, in-process materials, or drug products shall not be reactive, additive, or absorptive so as to alter the safety, identity, strength, quality, or purity of the drug product beyond the official or other established requirement" [2]. The European Medicines Agency (EMA) [3] has a similar statement: "Production equipment should not present any hazards to the product. The parts of the production equipment that come into contact with the product must not be reactive, additive or absorptive to such an extent that it will affect the quality of the product and thus present any hazard." Therefore, the chemical compounds leached from the process equipment including single-use system, which can be considered as additive, should be proved not altering the safety and quality of the ADC.

Specific to process equipment, BPSA (Bio-Process Systems Alliance) has defined extractables and leachables as follows [4]. Extractables are chemical compounds that migrate from any product contact material, including elastomeric, plastic, glass, and stainless steel or coating components, when exposed to an appropriate solvent under exaggerated conditions of time and temperature. Leachables, typically a subset of extractables, are chemical compounds that migrate into the drug formulation from any product contact material, including elastomeric, plastic, glass, and stainless steel or coating components, as a result of direct contact with the drug formulation under normal process conditions or accelerated storage conditions and are found in the final drug product.

A biological drug substance is typically manufactured through the following steps: upstream preparation, fermentation, harvest, downstream purification including clarification by filtration, concentration/diafiltration by tangential flow ultrafiltration, purification by chromatography, virus removal by nanofiltration, and formulation, frozen storage in biocontainer, and then filling. ADC manufacturing, unlike other biologicals, consists of a chemical conjugation reaction followed by a more standard downstream process. Single-use components or systems are increasingly used in these processes. Almost all these steps involve the contact of process stream with organic-based polymers, including both plastics and elastomers which are used to make filters, tubing, connectors, disconnectors, biocontainers, mixers, bioreactors, sensors, and filling needles. To evaluate extractables and leachables from the process equipment or single-use systems remains a challenging and daunting task due to the complexity of the process fluid, the process equipment, and the extractable compounds. This is of particular importance in the ADC area since an organic cosolvent is typically used in the conjugation process.

2 Risk-Based Scientific Approach

To minimize the cost and to shorten the time to get the drug to the market, risk assessment is essential for implementation and qualification/validation of single-use systems in ADC manufacturing. The main risk factors include the following:

1. Chemical Compatibility Between the Process Fluid and Single-Use Systems
   Because plastics and elastomers are typically formed by polymerizing monomers in the presence of suitable catalysts, these polymers may not be chemically compatible with certain solvents, some of which could even dissolve the polymers. In ADC manufacturing processes, solvents such as DMSO (dimethyl sulfoxide) and DMAC (*N*,*N*-dimethylacetamide) are often used. Both solvents, when present in high concentration, are not compatible with polyethersulfone (PES) and polyvinylidenefluoride (PVDF), which are the materials of construction of single-use components such as filters and sensors. In fact, pure DMSO and pure DMAC are solvents for PES and PVDF polymers. However, since the solvent strength is proportional to the volume fraction, solutions with lower concentrations of DMSO and DMAC may not attack these polymers. In any events, a prequalification of the single-use systems, which may consist of tubing, filter, sensors, connectors, and biocontainers, should be performed to confirm the systems will function as they are designed to. The single-use system is deemed as compatible only if all the components are compatible.
2. Product Composition
   The nature of the product has profound effect on the type and amount of extractables/leachables from single-use systems. According to the fundamental, "like dissolves like." While low-molecular-weight hydrocarbons will extract relatively significant amount of oligomers and additives from polyolefins such as polypropylene and polyethylene, water, as a polar solvent, extracts little from polyolefins.

3. Material Contact Area
   More contact areas typically lead to higher amount of extractables/leachables. Connectors have very low surface areas, while filters have relatively higher contact areas. Therefore, it is not surprising that filters normally generate more extractables/leachables than connectors.
4. Contact Time
   Longer contact time would typically result in more extractables/leachables. The kinetics of dissolution of a solute into a solvent will also depend on the location of the solute besides the solubility. If the solute is on the surface of the equipment, the extraction of the solute can happen very quickly. However, if the solute is inside of the polymer network, the solute needs to migrate to the surface and then be dissolved in the solvent. The latter, obviously, takes longer time.
5. Process Temperature
   In general, higher temperature will generate more extractables/leachables. At lower temperatures, for example, below the freezing point, although extractables/leachables concern is alleviated, it is recommended to evaluate the glass transition temperature to ensure the plastics will not become brittle and affect the functionality of the component. Some commercially available biocontainers were validated as suitable for applications at temperatures down to −80 °C [5].
6. Pre-sterilization Method
   Single-use systems are usually pre-sterilized by gamma irradiation, shipped, and ready to be used by the end user. During gamma irradiation, a high-energy electromagnetic radiation is imposed to the materials of construction of the single-use system. Some chemical bonds in larger molecules can be broken and eventually smaller molecules can form. These small molecules, as degradation products, are more likely to be extracted.
7. Proximity to the Final Container Closure System
   For the process equipment, the closer to the final container closure system, the higher risk in terms of generating leachables that could end up in the final container closure system. Process steps such as diafiltration can remove low-molecular-weight compounds. However, relevant test data should accompany such a claim.

After the risk assessment is completed, the detailed evaluation of extractables and leachables can be started. As defined, leachables are obtained when the actual process fluid is used for extraction. ADC formulation may contain proteins and salts, which are nonvolatile compounds. They will interfere with the quantitative gravimetric analysis of extractable compounds. In addition, proteins may present interference with analytical methods, especially LC/UV/MS (liquid chromatography/ultraviolet/mass spectrometry). As a result, leachable compounds, usually in trace amount, would be masked by these compounds and remain undetected, even though they are actually present in the process fluid. Therefore, extractables test employing a clean model solvent is essential to generate a complete list of probable leachables.

Single-use systems suppliers have published validation guides and technical articles for their single-use components [5–10]. Extractables study in model solvents such as water and ethanol is usually part of the product validation guides. The end user will need to perform a gap analysis looking at the conditions under which the generic extractables data has been generated. If these extractables study results are high quality data, meaning reasonable study design was used and analytical methods were qualified/validated (limit of detection, limit of quantitation, system suitability, linearity, and specificity), then the results can be used for initial qualification of the single-use component. If the test results are applicable to the ADC process (e.g., extractables test temperature is higher than the process temperature, test time is longer than the process time, and model solvent is relevant to the process fluid), then the results can be used for the specific process validation purpose. If not, to fill the gap, a process-specific extractables study should be initiated. After the relevant extractables data is obtained, the toxicity evaluation on these extractable compounds as a worst case is carried out. The detailed procedure is discussed in section 3. If there is a safety concern, then a leachables study should be carried out. If there is no safety concern, then an evaluation on whether there is a potential interaction between the extractables and process fluid should be performed. If the process fluid would not react with extractables to form a new leachable compound, then the extractables data will be the worst case for leachables, and no further leachables test is needed. For example, if the process fluid is a buffer solution consisting only of salts and water, then extractables data using water may be sufficient and the leachables testing using buffer solution will not be needed. Otherwise, if there is a potential chemical reaction between extractables and process fluid, then a leachables study should be performed.

3 Protocol for Running an Extractables and Leachables Study

The study protocol is relatively complex due to the nature of the system and a series of analytical techniques required.

1. The drawings of the single-use system should be studied. The actual system should be used for extraction unless the system consists of components too large to be tested in the laboratory. For example, if there is a 500 L biocontainer, then a smaller

biocontainer with the same materials of construction will be used as a scale-down version. Caution needs to be made to ensure that the surface area to volume ratio used in the test system is higher than that in the process system to represent a worst case.

2. The process fluid composition should be evaluated and a suitable model solvent chosen based on Pall's Model Solvent Approach^{sm} [11]. The volatile components will remain in the model solvent system, while nonvolatile components will be simulated by a volatile solvent that has the same functional group and with equal or higher extracting capability. For aqueous process fluids, pH should be evaluated since extreme pH (e.g., less than 3 or higher than 9) usually has significant effect on extraction. In these extreme cases, ammonium hydroxide, a volatile basic compound, and acetic acid or hydrochloric acid, a volatile acidic compound, can be used to simulate the pH effect for alkaline and acid solutions, respectively.
3. Inert materials such as glass reservoir, PTFE (polytetrafluoroethylene) tubing, and PTFE pump should be used to form the test setup as the fluid supply system to minimize background interference. Silicone tubing should be avoided in the test setup since the single-use system as the test article usually contains silicone tubing.
4. The test conditions should be chosen as reasonable worst case based on the process conditions. For example, if the process temperature is 15–20 °C, then the test temperature can be 20–25 °C. If the process time is 6 h, then the test time can be 8 h. The test assembly should be gamma irradiated at 50 kGy, which is typically the maximum expected dose for any commercially available single-use systems.
5. When performing the extraction, the test solvent should be recirculated through the system (including filter, tubing, connectors, and disconnectors) excluding the biocontainer, which can be extracted separately by static soak with appropriate agitation. Care must be taken to avoid any potential cross contamination since this test involves trace analysis.
6. For extractables test, flush step is not incorporated to represent a worst case.
7. For leachables test, if there is a flush step to remove potential leachables during the actual process, then this flush step is incorporated in the test procedure.
8. The extracts from the system (combining the extracts from the biocontainer and the rest of the system) will be subjected to detailed analyses. The analytical methods for extractables are listed in Table 1. If the solvent is water, then TOC (total organic carbon), pH, conductivity, and ion chromatography

Table 1
Analytical methods used to assess extractables or leachables

Analytical method	Target compounds or property
Nonvolatile residue (NVR) measurement	Total mass of extractables after evaporation of the test solvent. Not applicable to leachables analysis when nonvolatile components are present in the process fluid, such as proteins and salts
Fourier transform infrared spectroscopy (FTIR)	Qualitative analysis of unknowns, including oligomers of polymers. Not applicable to leachables analysis when nonvolatile components are present in the process fluid, such as proteins and salts
Ultraviolet spectroscopy (UV)	Compounds with chromophores
Direct injection gas chromatography/mass spectrometry (direct injection GC/MS)	Semi-volatile organic compounds
Headspace gas chromatography/mass spectrometry (GC/MS)	Volatile organic compounds
Derivatization gas chromatography/mass spectrometry (derivatization GC/MS)	Organic acids, especially long-chain fatty acids
Liquid chromatography/ultraviolet/mass spectrometry (LC/UV/MS)	Part of semi-volatile and nonvolatile organic compounds, usually additives from polymers, oligomers, and degradation products
Inductively coupled plasma/mass spectrometry (ICP/MS)	Metal ions

(IC) will also be conducted [12]. For leachables analysis, the methods listed in Table 1 will be used except for NVR and FTIR. This is because the components present in the process fluid typically have interference with these analytical methods. Some most likely extractables/leachables from the most common single-use filter, tubing, and biocontainer are listed in Table 2.

9. The results should be presented as total amount of each compound from the whole system. For example, under the conditions, the system will not leach more than 0.05 mg of isopropyl alcohol into the process fluid.
10. Toxicity and safety assessment of leachables (or extractables if leachables test is justified as not needed) should be performed by the end user (this is not generally provided by the system supplier as they do not normally have specific details regarding the route of administration, dosage level, or toxicity of the proposed drug compound). The ICH approach of using "No-Observable-Effect Level" (NOEL) or "Lowest-Observed-Effect Level" (LOEL) of each leachable compound

Table 2
Some extractables/leachables from common single-use components

Components	Extractables/leachables
Filter with polypropylene support/drainage layers [8]	2-Ethylhexanoic acid; 1,3-di-tert-butyl-benzene; 2,4-di-tert-butyl-phenol; lauryl acetate; lauryl acrylate; oxalic acid; malonic acid; lauric acid; succinic acid; myristic acid; palmitic acid; stearic acid
Thermoplastic tubing [9]	2,3,4-Trimethylpentane; 1,3-di-tert-butyl-benzene; 2,4-di-tert-butyl-phenol; low-molecular-weight aliphatic hydrocarbons; 1-tridecanol; lauryl acrylate; Irgafos[a] antioxidant; myristic acid; palmitic acid; stearic acid
Biocontainer with polyethylene contact layer [9]	2-Methylpentane; hexane; trimethylpentane; 3-methylheptane; 1-octene; n-octane; 1,3-di-tert-butyl-benzene; 2,4-di-tert-butyl-phenol; 2-octanone; 1-heptadecanol; 1-octadecanol; succinic acid; palmitic acid; stearic acid

[a]Irgafos is a proprietary stabilizer and trademark of Ciba Holding AG in Basel, Switzerland

to calculate the permissible daily exposure (PDE) can be used [12]. By comparing the PDE with the patient's maximum daily intake of leachable compound, a safety factor for each leachable compound can be obtained [13]. Another approach developed by PQRI (Product Quality Research Institute) can also be used (2006) as a reference although it was specifically developed for orally inhaled and nasal drug products [13]. The recommendation for injectables and ophthalmics is currently being developed by PQRI.

4 Conclusion

A risk-based scientific approach for determination of extractables/leachables from biomanufacturing of ADC has been developed. This method, which has been successfully applied to validate many drug manufacturing processes, can help end users to minimize the cost and shorten the time to deliver drugs to the market.

Acknowledgment

The author appreciated the direction and guidance from Dr. Helene Pora, the constructive review from Bruce Rawlings, and the support from Sharon Klugewicz.

References

1. Ritter A (2012) Antibody–drug conjugates. Pharma Technol 36(1):42–47
2. FDA (2006) Code of federal regulations food and drugs title 21, Part 211.65. US Government Printing Office, Washington, DC. http://www.accessdata.fda.gov/scripts/cdrh/cfdocs/cfCFR/CFRSearch.cfm?fr=211.65&utm_campaign=Google2&utm_source=fdaSearch&utm_medium=website&utm_term=211.65&utm_content=1. Accessed 26 April 2012
3. EMA (1998) EUDRALEX Volume 4, Chap 3–Premise and Equipment, Section 3.39–Revised Directive 2003/94/EC: Good Manufacturing Practices, Medicinal Products for Human and Veterinary Use. European Commission: Brussels, Belgium. http://ec.europa.eu/health/files/eudralex/vol-4/pdfs-en/cap3_en.pdf. Accessed 26 April 2012
4. BPSA (2010) BPSA Extractables Guide 2010. Recommendations for testing and evaluation of extractables from single-use process equipment. http://www.bpsalliance.org/. Accessed 26 April 2012
5. Pall Life Sciences (2009) Validation guide. Allegro^{TM} 2D Biocontainers. USTR 2475a.
6. Pall Life Sciences (2009) Validation guide. Kleenpak™ Connector for Use with 13 mm (12 inch) Nominal Tubing. USTR 2232a
7. Ding W, Nash R (2009) Extractables from integrated single-use systems in biopharmaceutical manufacturing Part I. Study on components (Pall KleenpakTM Connector and Kleenpak Filter Capsule). PDA J Pharm Sci Technol 63(4):322–338
8. Ding W, Martin J (2008) Implementing single-use technology in biopharmaceutical manufacturing: an approach to extractables/leachables studies, part one—connectors and filters. Bioprocess Int 6(9):34–42
9. Ding W, Martin J (2009) Implementation of single-use technology in biopharmaceutical manufacturing: an approach to extractables/leachables studies, Part two—tubing and biocontainers. Bioprocess Int 7(5):46–55
10. Ding W, Martin J (2010) Implementation of single-use technology in biopharmaceutical manufacturing an approach to extractables and leachables studies, Part three—single-use systems. Bioprocess Int 8(10):52–61
11. Pall Life Sciences (2012) Scientific and technical report. Extractables and Leachables from Single-Use Systems
12. ICH Q3C(R5) (2011) Impurities: guideline for residual solvents. http://www.ich.org/fileadmin/Public_Web_Site/ICH_Products/Guidelines/Quality/Q3C/Step4/Q3C_R5_Step4.pdf. Accessed 26 April 2012
13. Product Quality Research Institute Leachables and Extractables Working Group (2006) Safety thresholds and best practices for extractables and leachables in orally inhaled and nasal drug products. http://www.pqri.org/pdfs/LE_Recommendations_to_FDA_09-29-06.pdf. Accessed 26 April 2012

INDEX

Laurent Ducry (ed.), *Antibody-Drug Conjugates*, Methods in Molecular Biology, vol. 1045,
DOI 10.1007/978-1-62703-541-5, © Springer Science+Business Media, LLC 2013

O

P

Q

R

S

T

U

V

MIX
Papier aus verantwortungsvollen Quellen
Paper from responsible sources
FSC® C105338

If you have any concerns about our products,
you can contact us on
ProductSafety@springernature.com

In case Publisher is established outside the EU,
the EU authorized representative is:
Springer Nature Customer Service Center GmbH
Europaplatz 3, 69115 Heidelberg, Germany

Printed by Libri Plureos GmbH
in Hamburg, Germany